# Emerging Trends in Global Cancer Epidemiology

# Emerging Trends in Global Cancer Epidemiology

Guest Editor

**Syed Ahsan Raza**

MDPI

Basel • Beijing • Wuhan • Barcelona • Belgrade • Novi Sad • Cluj • Manchester

*Guest Editor*
Syed Ahsan Raza
Department of Medicine
Baylor College of Medicine
Houston
United States

*Editorial Office*
MDPI AG
Grosspeteranlage 5
4052 Basel, Switzerland

This is a reprint of the Special Issue, published open access by the journal *Cancers* (ISSN 2072-6694), freely accessible at: https://www.mdpi.com/journal/cancers/special_issues/N946HDMKIS.

For citation purposes, cite each article independently as indicated on the article page online and as indicated below:

| Lastname, A.A.; Lastname, B.B. Article Title. *Journal Name* **Year**, *Volume Number*, Page Range. |
|---|

**ISBN 978-3-7258-4387-9 (Hbk)**
**ISBN 978-3-7258-4388-6 (PDF)**
**https://doi.org/10.3390/books978-3-7258-4388-6**

Cover image courtesy of Syed Ahsan Raza

# Contents

# About the Editor

**Syed Ahsan Raza**

Syed Ahsan Raza is a physician scientist, epidemiologist, and educator with over two decades of global experience in clinical research, cancer epidemiology, and population health. Dr. Raza holds an MD from the University of Karachi, a PhD in Epidemiology from the University of Montreal, and a Diploma in Tropical Medicine & Hygiene from Baylor College of Medicine. He is a Fellow of American College of Epidemiology (FACE) and serves on their Board of Directors.

Dr. Raza's research spans clinical trials, cancer outcomes, infectious disease epidemiology, and geospatial analytics. His global work includes projects funded by the Bill and Melinda Gates Foundation, International Agency for Research on Cancer (IARC), WHO, and the Quebec Health Research Fund. He has served as faculty, staff scientist and fellow at institutions such as the University of Pittsburgh Medical Center, International Agency for Research on Cancer, Union for International Cancer Control, University of Montreal, and Aga Khan University.

He has authored more than 50 peer-reviewed publications and book chapters in high-impact journals and has been invited to speak at leading international conferences. Dr. Raza is also an ad hoc reviewer for several journals, including *The Lancet Regional Health, International Journal of Surgery, Pediatric Infectious Diseases, Medical Education and Annals of Epidemiology*. He currently chairs the Publications Committee of the American College of Epidemiology and has taught at the London School of Hygiene and Tropical Medicine.

As the editor of this Special Issue, *Emerging Trends in Global Cancer Epidemiology*, Dr. Raza brings together diverse voices and novel insights from across the world, fostering interdisciplinary collaboration to inform evidence-based cancer control strategies.

# Preface

The increasing cancer incidence and mortality rates worldwide underscore the urgent need to better understand the complex interplay of biological, environmental, social, and behavioral determinants of cancer. This Reprint, *Emerging Trends in Global Cancer Epidemiology*, brings together a collection of diverse and thought-provoking studies that reflect the evolving landscape of cancer research across different regions and populations. It includes analyses of incidence, mortality, and survival trends, as well as investigations into the influence of lifestyle, environmental exposures, and social determinants of health.

The primary aim of this volume is to provide an up-to-date and comprehensive overview of the key developments in global cancer epidemiology. It is intended to serve not only as a scholarly reference but also as a practical guide for public health professionals, oncologists, cancer researchers, and students who are seeking to understand the broader trends and emerging challenges in the field.

This compilation was motivated by the growing recognition that cancer control must be informed by sound epidemiological evidence and must be contextualized within the diverse social and geographic settings in which cancer occurs. It is my hope that the findings and perspectives presented in this volume will stimulate further research, guide effective policies, and ultimately contribute to reducing the global burden of cancer.

I am deeply grateful to the contributing authors and peer reviewers for their dedication and insights, and to the editorial team at *Cancers* for their support in bringing this Reprint into fruition.

**Syed Ahsan Raza**
*Guest Editor*

*cancers*

MDPI

*Editorial*

# Emerging Trends in Global Cancer Epidemiology

**Syed Ahsan Raza**

Section of Epidemiology and Population Sciences, Department of Medicine, Baylor College of Medicine, Houston, TX 77546, USA; s.ahsanraza@gmail.com

Cancer continues to be one of the most pressing global public health challenges, with an increasing number of new cases and deaths each year. As the global burden of cancer grows, so too does the need for robust epidemiological research that illuminates patterns in incidence, mortality, prevalence, and survival across diverse populations and regions (Contribution 1). This Special Issue, entitled 'Emerging Trends in Global Cancer Epidemiology', brings together insightful research that collectively reflects the dynamic landscape of cancer epidemiology worldwide. These contributions offer novel perspectives on cancer trends, highlight innovative methods—including the use of big data, genomics, and machine learning—and explore the influence of environmental, lifestyle, and social determinants on cancer outcomes. From analyses of population-level disparities to evaluations of prevention strategies, each study in this issue adds a unique piece to the global cancer puzzle. The full collection of articles featured in this Special Issue can be accessed at the following link: https://www.mdpi.com/journal/cancers/special_issues/N946HDMKIS.

In one study in this Special Issue, Aldhaleei et al. explore the rising burden of early-onset colorectal cancer (EO-CRC) among individuals aged 20 to 44 in the United States over a three-decade period (Contribution 2). Using data from the Global Burden of Disease Study 2021 and an age–period–cohort (APC) modeling approach, the authors revealed a 49% increase in EO-CRC cases from 1990 to 2021, with age-standardized incidence rates rising by 34%. These findings emphasize the complex interplay of age, generational cohort, and period in shaping EO-CRC trends and highlighting the urgency of developing targeted prevention strategies to address this growing incidence in younger populations.

Beltran-Ontiveros et al. present a comprehensive analysis of cancer trends in Mexico over a 30-year period, also drawing on data from the Global Burden of Disease Study 2019 (Contribution 3). From an epidemiological standpoint, this study is a critical reminder of how national-level data can offer valuable insights into shifting cancer dynamics. It also reflects the growing complexity of cancer epidemiology in middle-income countries like Mexico, where demographic transitions, urbanization, and health system challenges may be driving these divergent trends. This research underscores the importance of cancer control strategies that are sensitive to both sex-specific trends and the heterogeneous nature of cancer burden across different cancer types. As countries like Mexico move toward universal health coverage, this kind of granular evidence will be instrumental in shaping equitable cancer prevention and control policies.

Abboud et al. carried out analyses to investigate an emerging and somewhat under-recognized trend in the U.S.—the rising incidence of rectal neuroendocrine tumors (RNETs) in younger adults under the age of 55 (Contribution 4). Using data from the United States Cancer Statistics (USCS) database from 2001 to 2020, the authors conducted a detailed analysis stratified by age, sex, race, and tumor stage. This paper raises important questions about what might be fueling the rise of RNETs in younger demographics. The age-specific divergence in incidence trends is compelling, especially given the growing body of literature pointing to earlier onset patterns across several gastrointestinal malignancies. The fact that the increase is largely driven by early-stage diagnoses suggests that enhanced detection may play a role—but it also hints at possible shifts in risk exposures, lifestyle factors, or even gut microbiome changes in younger generations. This study underscores the need for more targeted research into the etiology and risk profile of RNETs in young adults, and it serves as a call to action for clinicians to revisit current screening thresholds and symptom awareness strategies for this tumor type.

Interesting research carried out by Hussan et al. explores the relationship between obesity, bariatric surgery (BRS), and the development of colorectal polyps—a precursor to colorectal cancer using a large, propensity-matched U.S. nationwide cohort from the 2012–2020 MarketScan Insurance Claims Research Database (Contribution 5). From a clinical epidemiological perspective, this study offers important insights into the preventive potential of bariatric surgery beyond metabolic improvements. It challenges us to think of obesity not just as a risk factor for colorectal cancer, but as a modifiable exposure with early pathological consequences that may be mitigated with timely intervention. The finding of the absence of a significant change in polyp rates pre- vs. post-BRS is particularly thought-provoking—it may suggest that while bariatric surgery halts further risk accumulation, it does not necessarily reverse established polyp pathology. This highlights the need for continued colorectal surveillance, even after weight loss interventions and calls for more research into the biological mechanisms linking obesity, metabolic dysfunction, and early neoplastic changes in the colon.

A population-based study in Eastern Sicily, was carried out to explore cancer burden among migrant populations in a group often underrepresented in epidemiological research (Contribution 6). Using data from the regional cancer registry spanning 2004 to 2019, the study assessed proportionate morbidity ratios (PMRs) and odds ratios (ORs) for various cancers in migrants compared to non-migrants. This study provides an important lens into the intersection of migration and cancer epidemiology. The analysis speaks to the need for culturally appropriate cancer prevention strategies. The markedly higher odds of cervical cancer highlight gaps in HPV vaccination and screening among migrant women, while the elevated lung cancer risk suggests environmental or occupational exposures that warrant closer scrutiny.

Marino et al. delve into the critical yet often overlooked dimension of patient-centered communication (PCC) in intercultural cancer care settings in Italy (Contribution 7). Using the ONCode coding system, the researchers analyzed 42 video-recorded oncology consultations involving both Italian and foreign patients to assess how communication dynamics vary by patient background, type of visit (first vs. follow-up), and presence of companions. Interestingly, quantitative analyses revealed no significant differences in PCC quality between Italian and foreign patients. However, qualitative findings uncovered meaningful distinctions, particularly in the nature of interruptions during encounters with foreign patients, which tended to be more frequent and potentially disruptive. The study emphasizes that while language competence is essential, it should not be the sole indicator of communication effectiveness in multicultural medical settings. This research can be seen as a compelling argument for deeper structural sensitivity in care delivery. In a world of increasingly diverse patient populations, achieving true patient-centricity demands more than protocols; it requires active, empathetic listening and a commitment to minimizing avoidable power imbalances in clinical encounters.

In England, Smith et al. address a critical issue in cancer health disparities by examining how diagnostic pathways mediate the impact of comorbidity on survival among patients with diffuse large B-cell lymphoma (DLBCL) and follicular lymphoma (FL)

(Contribution 8). This paper unpacks a subtle but powerful mechanism through which structural inequities manifest in clinical outcomes. From an epidemiological standpoint, this is impactful because it highlights a modifiable point in the cancer care continuum, i.e., diagnostic timeliness, that could yield substantial survival gains if addressed effectively. The mediation analysis strengthens the case for interventions that prioritize early, elective cancer detection in patients with complex health profiles. This evidence should inform not just public health programs, but also clinical training and system-level reforms that aim to anticipate diagnostic risk in vulnerable populations.

The fact that rural residents in developed nations face barriers akin to those in low- and middle-income countries such as delayed diagnosis, limited specialist care, and lower health literacy speaks volumes about the persistent structural gaps in healthcare systems. The study by Ramamurthy et al. from Australia is both insightful and concerning (Contribution 9). They conducted a scoping review to examine how rurality influences oral cancer trends across OECD member countries. Drawing from 18 studies selected from an initial pool of over 1100, the review highlights a troubling pattern: despite residing in high-income countries, individuals in rural and remote areas experience disproportionately higher incidence and poorer outcomes for oral and oropharyngeal cancers. The review points to rising rates of tobacco and alcohol use, low awareness of HPV-related cancer risks, and limited access to advanced cancer care as key drivers of this disparity. The burden is especially high among older adults in rural regions of the United States, Australia, Canada, and several European nations emphasizing that geography remains a powerful determinant of cancer inequity, even in well-resourced settings.

Drăgan and Drăgan from Romania provide a comprehensive narrative review on the assessment of venous thromboembolism (VTE) risk in ambulatory cancer patients, an area often under-addressed in clinical practice (Contribution 10). While VTE is a well-recognized complication in hospitalized and perioperative cancer settings with clear guidelines supporting thromboprophylaxis, the same clarity does not extend to ambulatory patients. The review examines existing tools like the Khorana score, highlighting its limitations, and explores emerging risk stratification models, including those incorporating biomarkers, genetic profiles, clinical parameters, and even machine learning approaches. The authors also discuss the potential role of imaging and biomolecular screening in improving risk prediction and guiding individualized patient care.

Finally, Gupta et al. present a novel population-based study exploring the relationship between environmental temperature and survival outcomes in gastroesophageal cancers (GECs) across the United States (Contribution 11). Using data from over 17,000 esophageal and more than 20,000 gastric cancer patients in the SEER database (1996–2015), combined with county-level temperature data from the National Centers for Environmental Information, their study found that warmer average annual temperatures (AAT) were significantly associated with improved overall survival (OS) and disease-specific survival (DSS). Specifically, patients living in regions with an AAT above 53.5 °F experienced an 11–13% improvement in survival outcomes for esophageal cancer and 13–14% for gastric cancer. Moreover, survival improved incrementally by 3–4% with every 5 °F increase in temperature. These associations held true across histological subtypes and were robust to adjustments for key demographic and clinical variables. While the biological plausibility draws on preclinical evidence that cold stress impairs antitumor immunity, this is one of the first large-scale studies to demonstrate a temperature–survival relationship in human cancer populations (Contribution 11). It introduces an environmental and potentially modifiable factor into the complex equation of cancer prognosis. While the retrospective design and potential for confounding must be acknowledged, the implications are far-reaching. These findings encourage us to consider the broader ecological context in which patients live and receive care. They also spark intriguing questions: Could thermal interventions, such as maintaining thermoneutrality or avoiding cold exposure, complement existing treatment strategies? How might these results influence cancer survivorship planning, especially for vulnerable populations in colder regions? This study opens the door for a new interdisciplinary dialogue between oncology, climate science, and environmental health, one that we are only just beginning to understand.

Collectively, the studies featured in this Special Issue weave a rich and diverse tapestry of emerging trends in global cancer epidemiology. They underscore how cancer risk, burden and outcomes are shaped not only by biological and clinical factors, but also by geography, social determinants, lifestyle, environment, and access to care. From rising early-onset cancers in younger populations to disparities rooted in migration, rurality, comorbidity, and even environmental temperature, these studies challenge us to think beyond traditional risk factors and to adopt a more holistic approach in cancer research and control. As cancer epidemiologists, clinicians, and public health practitioners, we must remain agile and innovative in our methods, while grounded in the realities of patients' lived experiences. Ultimately, advancing the science of cancer in a truly global context requires embracing complexity, fostering collaboration across disciplines, and translating evidence into cancer prevention and care strategies for all populations.

**Conflicts of Interest:** The author declare no conflict of interest at the time manuscript was written.

**List of Contributions:**

1. Raza, S.A.; da Costa, W.L.; Thrift, A.P. Editorial: Sex differences in cancer incidence, mortality, and survival: Methodological perspectives. *Front. Oncol.* **2024**, *14*, 1441965. https://doi.org/10.3389/fonc.2024.1441965.
2. Aldhaleei, W.A.; Wallace, M.B.; Bhagavathula, A.S. Trends and Age-Period-Cohort Effect on the Incidence of Early-Onset Colorectal Cancer (20-44 Years) from 1990 to 2021 in the United States. *Cancers* **2024**, *16*, 2883. https://doi.org/10.3390/cancers16162883.
3. Beltran-Ontiveros, S.A.; Contreras-Gutierrez, J.A.; Lizarraga-Verdugo, E.; Gutierrez-Grijalva, E.P.; Lopez-Lopez, K.; Lora-Fierro, E.H.; Trujillo-Rojas, M.A.; Moreno-Ortiz, J.M.; Cardoso-Angulo, D.L.; Leal-Leon, E.; et al. National Burden and Trends for 29 Groups of Cancer in Mexico from 1990 to 2019: A Secondary Analysis of the Global Burden of Disease Study 2019. *Cancers* **2023**, *16*, 149. https://doi.org/10.3390/cancers16010149.
4. Abboud, Y.; Pendyala, N.; Le, A.; Mittal, A.; Alsakarneh, S.; Jaber, F.; Hajifathalian, K. The Incidence of Rectal Neuroendocrine Tumors Is Increasing in Younger Adults in the US, 2001–2020. *Cancers* **2023**, *15*, 5286. https://doi.org/10.3390/cancers15215286.
5. Hussan, H.; McLaughlin, E.; Chiang, C.; Marsano, J.G.; Lieberman, D. The Risk of Colorectal Polyps after Weight Loss Therapy Versus Obesity: A Propensity-Matched Nationwide Cohort Study. *Cancers* **2023**, *15*, 4820. https://doi.org/10.3390/cancers15194820.
6. Collatuzzo, G.; Ferrante, M.; Ippolito, A.; Di Prima, A.; Colarossi, C.; Scarpulla, S.; Boffetta, P.; Sciacca, S. Cancer in Migrants: A Population-Based Study in Italy. *Cancers* **2023**, *15*, 3103. https://doi.org/10.3390/cancers15123103.
7. Marino, F.; Alby, F.; Zucchermaglio, C.; Scalisi, T.G.; Lauriola, M. Navigating Intercultural Medical Encounters: An Examination of Patient-Centered Communication Practices with Italian and Foreign Cancer Patients Living in Italy. *Cancers* **2023**, *15*, 3008. https://doi.org/10.3390/cancers15113008.
8. Smith, M.J.; Rachet, B.; Luque-Fernandez, M.A. Mediating Effects of Diagnostic Route on the Comorbidity Gap in Survival of Patients with Diffuse Large B-Cell or Follicular Lymphoma in England. *Cancers* **2022**, *14*, 5082. https://doi.org/10.3390/cancers14205082.
9. Ramamurthy, P.; Sharma, D.; Clough, A.; Thomson, P. Influence of Rurality on Oral Cancer Trends among Organisation for Economic Co-Operation and Development (OECD) Member Countries-A Scoping Review. *Cancers* **2024**, *16*, 2957. https://doi.org/10.3390/cancers16172957.

10. Dragan, A.; Dragan, A.S. Novel Insights in Venous Thromboembolism Risk Assessment Methods in Ambulatory Cancer Patients: From the Guidelines to Clinical Practice. *Cancers* **2024**, *16*, 458. https://doi.org/10.3390/cancers16020458.
11. Gupta, K.; George, A.; Attwood, K.; Gupta, A.; Roy, A.M.; Gandhi, S.; Siromoni, B.; Singh, A.; Repasky, E.; Mukherjee, S. Association between Environmental Temperature and Survival in Gastroesophageal Cancers: A Population Based Study. *Cancers* **2023**, *16*, 74. https://doi.org/10.3390/cancers16010074.

cancers

MDPI

Article

# Mediating Effects of Diagnostic Route on the Comorbidity Gap in Survival of Patients with Diffuse Large B-Cell or Follicular Lymphoma in England

Matthew J. Smith [1,*], Bernard Rachet [1] and Miguel Angel Luque-Fernandez [1,2]

1 Inequalities in Cancer Outcomes Network, Department of Non-Communicable Disease Epidemiology, London School of Hygiene and Tropical Medicine, Keppel Street, London WC1E 7HT, UK
2 Department of Statistics and Operations Research, University of Granada, 18071 Granada, Spain
* Correspondence: matt.smith@lshtm.ac.uk

**Simple Summary:** There are inequalities in cancer survival between patients with or without comorbidities. The healthcare pathway (i.e., diagnostic route) of a patient is thought to explain some of these inequalities. We explore how much of the effect of comorbidity on survival of patients with diffuse large B-cell lymphoma (DLBCL) or follicular lymphoma (FL) is explained by the diagnostic route (i.e., emergency diagnosis). We used mediation analysis to separate the effect of comorbidity on survival from its effect through diagnostic route. We found that, for DLBCL and FL, emergency diagnosis accounted for 24% and 16% of the inequalities in survival between comorbidity groups within 12 months since cancer diagnosis. This proportion reduced over time and was small after 5 years of follow up. Comorbidities can complicate the diagnosis and management of patients with DLBCL or FL. Our results show that greater research is needed to ensure patients with comorbidities have a timely diagnosis and will help to reduce the inequalities in cancer survival.

**Abstract: Background:** Socioeconomic inequalities in survival from non-Hodgkin lymphoma persist. Comorbidities are more prevalent amongst those in more deprived areas and are associated with diagnostic delay (emergency diagnostic route), which is also associated with poorer survival probability. We aimed to describe the effect of comorbidity on the probability of death mediated by diagnostic route (emergency vs. elective route) amongst patients with diffuse large B-cell (DLBCL) or follicular lymphoma (FL). **Methods:** We linked the English population-based cancer registry and hospital admission records (2005–2013) of patients aged 45–99 years. We decomposed the effect of comorbidity on survival into an indirect effect acting through diagnostic route and a direct effect not mediated by diagnostic route. Furthermore, we estimated the proportion of the comorbidity effect on survival mediated by diagnostic route. **Results:** For both DLBCL ($n$ = 27,379) and FL ($n$ = 14,043), those with any comorbidity, or living in more deprived areas, were more likely to experience diagnostic delay and poorer survival. The indirect effect of comorbidity on mortality through diagnostic route was highest at 12 months since diagnosis (DLBCL: Odds Ratio 1.10 [95% CI 1.07–1.13], FL: OR 1.09 [95% CI 1.04–1.14]). Within the first 12 months since diagnosis, emergency diagnostic route accounted for 24% (95% CI 17.5–29.5) and 16% (95% CI 6.0–25.6) of the comorbidity effect on mortality, for DLBCL and FL, respectively. **Conclusion:** Efforts to reduce diagnostic delay (emergency diagnosis) amongst patients with comorbidity would reduce inequalities in DLBCL and FL survival by 24% and 16%, respectively. Further public health programs and interventions are needed to reduce diagnostic delay amongst lymphoma patients with comorbidities.

**Keywords:** diffuse large B-cell lymphoma; follicular lymphoma; mediation analysis; epidemiology; comorbidity; survival

## 1. Introduction

Non-Hodgkin lymphoma (NHL) is a heterogeneous group of malignancies, two of the most common types are diffuse large B-cell lymphoma (DLBCL) and follicular lymphoma (FL). For both DLBCL and FL, survival has steadily increased and, at 5 years since diagnosis, is substantially higher amongst those with FL compared to DLBCL [1–3]. However, there has been a differential increase in better health outcomes between patient characteristics, which has exacerbated deprivation and comorbidity inequalities in survival [1]. For other cancers, differences in comorbidity status partly explain the deprivation gap in survival yet inequalities remain [4]. Research has suggested that inequalities are partly due to the interaction between the patient, with certain characteristics, and the healthcare pathway (for example, accessing a GP appointment) [5].

The presence of a comorbidity impacts on a timely diagnosis, which then impacts on survival length [6]. For example, having a comorbidity that exacerbates the symptoms of lymphoma could hasten an appointment with a healthcare professional, potentially leading to an earlier diagnosis and a longer survival time. On the other hand, a comorbidity that obscures symptoms of lymphoma could delay an appointment with a healthcare professional, eventually leading to a shorter survival time. In other words, the effect of patient characteristics (e.g., comorbidity status) on survival is mediated by the access to the healthcare system (e.g., route to diagnosis).

Understanding the interaction between patients with certain characteristics and the healthcare pathway is crucial for enhancing public health policies. Quantifying the effect of comorbidity status on survival that is attributable to route to diagnosis is important for the healthcare system to investigate sources of inequity, contrast, and target routes to diagnosis, and allocate essential resources.

Applying conventional methodological approaches is limited to analyses that do not account for factors on the causal pathway. Mediation analysis has been developed to disentangle the effect of an exposure on an outcome that is mediated by another factor [7–9]. We aimed to mechanistically describe whether the impact of comorbidity on the probability of death is attributed to its direct effect on the chances of survival or rather its indirect effect that is mediated through the route of cancer diagnosis (i.e., emergency vs. elective).

## 2. Methods

### 2.1. Study Design, Participants, Data, and Setting

We used data from a retrospective population-based cohort study of patients diagnosed with DLBCL or FL between 1 January 2005 and 31 December 2013, followed up to 31 December 2015. DLBCL and FL diagnoses were made according to the International Classification of Diseases for Oncology (ICD-O), 3rd edition, based on codes C82.0–C85.9 (Supplementary Table S1) [10]. Patients entered the study on the date of their diagnosis and were followed up until death or administratively right censored at the 31st of December 2015 whichever occurred first.

Data was obtained from population-based cancer registries within the English National Cancer Registry and Analysis Service (CAS) [11] and linked to patient's electronic health records from Hospital Episode Statistics (HES) [12]. CAS contains patient and tumour information (i.e., birth, diagnosis, and vital status dates) and sex, age at diagnosis, and ethnicity. HES data (for the period 2003 to 2015) was used for the assessment of comorbid conditions according to ICD codes (Supplementary Table S2) and contained clinical and administrative information. Using HES data, we assessed, retrospectively, the presence of any record of a comorbidity diagnosis for all patients with DLBCL and FL: certain comorbidities must be recorded even if they are not related to the reason for the hospital admission. In HES, the diagnostic fields are completed from admission and throughout the patient's episode during secondary care. HES can include up to 20 different diagnostic codes within one episode: 1 main clinical code (indicating the reason for the admission), 19 secondary clinical codes, and up to 24 operation/procedural codes. Episodes are coded at admission and then each time a patient moves between different hospital units. We restricted the inclusion of comorbidity records to those diagnosed prior to 6 months, and up to 2 years, before the date of cancer diagnosis; this restriction aims to capture non-cancer related comorbidities and to minimise the introduction of selection bias [13].

### 2.2. Outcome, Exposure, and Other Variables

The outcome of this study was time since diagnosis up to death observed within (i) 1 year, (ii) 3 years given survival at 1 year, and (iii) 5 years given survival at 3 years. The main exposure was comorbidity status, and the mediator was route to diagnosis (i.e., emergency diagnostic route versus other). Based on data availability and clinical reasoning, we included age at diagnosis, sex, deprivation level and ethnicity as confounders.

*Comorbidity status* was classified according to the Royal College of Surgeons (RCS) Charlson score (Supplementary Table S1): an adapted score that reduces the number of relevant comorbidities (in comparison to the Charlson comorbidity score [14]) by removing a category (peptic ulcer disease) and groups diseases together (e.g., diabetes mellitus codes with or without complications are grouped into a single category). The score represents the count of comorbidities of a patient. Unlike the Charlson comorbidity score, the RCS Charlson score does not weigh the comorbidities: making the assumption that any comorbidity has the same impact on short-term mortality [15]. For the interest of the analytical approach, we dichotomised the score (no comorbidities vs. one or more comorbidities).

*Route to diagnosis* (NCRAS dataset), or *diagnostic route*, was originally recorded as one of eight routes to diagnosis [16]. Patients diagnosed on a 'death certificate only' were excluded to remove bias. There is no nationally recognised screening programme for NHL, thus no patients were diagnosed via a 'screen-detected' route. The remaining routes were dichotomised into a binary variable indicating whether the patient was diagnosed following an emergency or elective presentation: elective presentation consisted of patients diagnosed through two-week-wait, general practitioner referral, inpatient, or outpatient.

*Deprivation level* is based on the Lower Super Output Area [17] (*LSOA*) of residence of the patient at the date of cancer diagnosis. This is information is publicly available from the Office for National Statistics. An LSOA is a geographical location with a median of 1500 inhabitants. From the Index of Multiple Deprivation [18] (IMD), the income domain was classified into one of five quintiles based on the national distribution of ranked deprivation scores in the 32,844 LSOAs. Each patient was linked with one of the 209 Clinical Commissioning Groups (CCG) where their LSOA resides [19].

*Ethnicity* (HES dataset), due to data sparsity amongst ethnic minorities, was recorded as white or other.

### 2.3. Causal Diagram

The assumed causal relationships between the variables are shown in Figure 1. The main exposure, comorbidity status, causally influences the diagnostic route and death at a certain follow-up time. For simplicity in the graph only (i.e., not in the analysis), we group the baseline confounders (age at diagnosis, gender, ethnicity, and deprivation level) but note that they will not have the same level of effect on other variables, specifically diagnostic route, treatment, and mortality. The number of GP appointments represents the number of interactions between the patient and the primary care system. For other cancers, the number of GP appointments up to 4 months prior to diagnosis is associated with emergency presentation [20]. We structured the causal diagram from left to right in accordance with the assumed time frame in which these events are expected to occur. The omission of confounders that are unobserved, such as previous GP appointments, and unmeasured mediators, such as stage at diagnosis and treatment, represent our causal assumptions. For example, we assume that the number of GP appointments prior to diagnosis does not affect survival except through its effect on diagnostic route. For graphical illustration we include the unmeasured confounders of the mediator-outcome relationship, U. The omission of an arrow from comorbidity status to U represents our assumption that the effect of comorbidity status on survival acts solely direct, or indirect, through diagnostic route.

We assume that there are no unmeasured confounders (U) for the (i) comorbidity-survival, (ii) route-survival, and (iii) comorbidity-route relationships. Additionally, we assume that (iv) the effect of comorbidity on survival is either direct or indirect through diagnostic route only. For example, this assumption states there is no unmeasured confounder for the route-survival relationship that is itself effected by comorbidity. Lastly, we assume that (v) there is consistency of a patient's record of survival, such that survival is not altered if we set the comorbidity and route to the values they would naturally take.

To define the assumption of no unmeasured confounding, we define the potential outcome $Y_i(a)$ represent the value of $Y$ if $A$ were set to $a$ for patient $i = 1, 2, \ldots, n$. Firstly, we assume no interference (i.e., the potential outcome for patient $i$ does not depend on the comorbidity status, $A_i$, of patient $i$). Secondly, we assume consistency, such that for those who have comorbidity status $A = a$, their observed $Y$ is the same as what it would have been had they had comorbidity status $A = a$ via the hypothetical intervention. Furthermore, we assume conditional exchangeability, such that comorbidity status $A$ is independent of each of the potential outcomes, conditional on the baseline confounders. Finally, since we used conditional survival time (i.e., survival at 5 years conditional on surviving the first 3 years after diagnosis), we assumed that censoring was non-informative during this time interval [21].

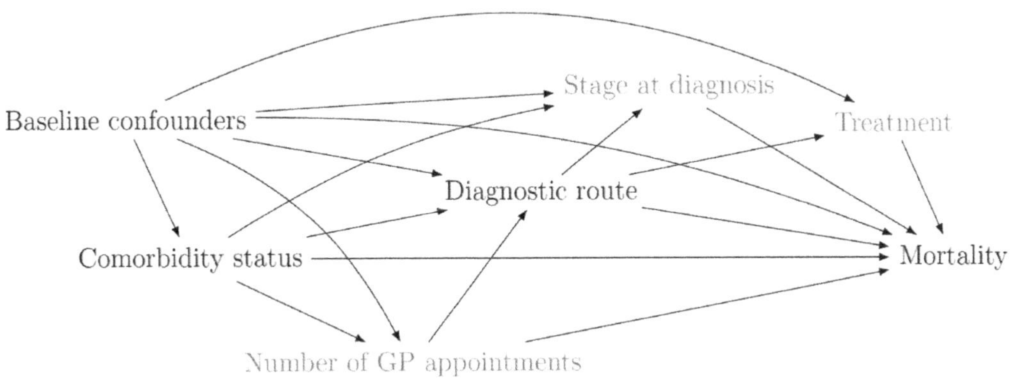


**Figure 1.** For patients diagnosed with DLBCL or FL in England between 2005 and 2013, this causal diagram represents the total effect of comorbidity on death mediated by diagnostic route, adjusted for baseline confounders (i.e., age at diagnosis, sex, deprivation, and ethnicity). Unmeasured confounders are stage at diagnosis, treatment, and number of general practitioner appointments.

## 3. Statistical Analysis

### 3.1. Descriptive Statistics

We described the characteristics of DLBCL and FL patients, separately, using counts and proportions, and calculated the odds ratios of having at least one comorbidity along with Wald test $p$-values. The proportion of patients diagnosed with DLBCL, or FL, was graphed by diagnostic route, over comorbidity status, and stratified by deprivation level (i.e., least compared to most deprived). We then estimated 5-year net survival (for least and most deprived) DLBCL or FL patients for each comorbidity status and diagnostic route using a cohort approach (administratively censored at 31 December 2015) and the Pohar Perme estimator [22] in the Stata [23] package *stns* [24].

### 3.2. Natural Effect Estimates and Proportion Mediated

We examined what proportion of the comorbidity gap in survival was explained by diagnostic route amongst patients diagnosed with DLBCL or FL. As the outcome, exposure, and mediator are binary variables, we focused on the decomposition of the *total causal effect* (TCE) into the *natural direct*, and *indirect*, *effects* (i.e., NDE and NIE, respectively) [25].

The natural effects are calculated using the *gformula* Stata command [26]. To illustrate the decomposition, we first define the natural direct and indirect effects in terms of nested counterfactuals, $Y(a, M(a^*))$, which indicates the outcome $Y$ if $A$ took the value of $a$ and $M$ took the value it would have taken if $A$ took the value of $a^*$. Here, A relates to the presence of comorbidities (i.e., A = 1 for one or more comorbidities, A = 0 for no comorbidities) and M related to the diagnostic route (i.e., M = 1 for emergency vs. M = 0 for other diagnostic route). The direct effect is then the comparison of $Y(a, M(a^*))$ to $Y(a^*, M(a^*))$, which measures the direct effect of changing the comorbidity status. The indirect effect is the comparison of $Y(a^*, M(a))$ to $Y(a^*, M(a^*))$, which measures the indirect effect of changing the diagnostic route. The total effect is the summation of the direct and indirect effects.

We first define the logistic regression model for the outcome Y with mediator covariables C

$$logit[E\{Y(a, M(a^*))|C\}] = \beta_0 + \beta_1 a + \beta_2 a^* + \beta_3 C + \beta_4 a \cdot a^* + \beta_5 a \cdot C + \beta_6 a^* \cdot C$$

this gives the NDE odds ratio

$$\frac{odds\{Y(a, M(a^*)) = 1 \mid C\}}{odds\{Y(a^*, M(a^*)) = 1 \mid C\}} = exp\{(\beta_1 + \beta_4 a^* + \beta_5 C)(a - a^*)\}$$

and the NIE odds ratio

$$\frac{odds\{Y(a, M(a)) = 1 \mid C\}}{odds\{Y(a, M(a^*)) = 1 \mid C\}} = exp\{(\beta_2 + \beta_4 a + \beta_6 C)(a - a^*)\}.$$

Their product measures the total effect: $odds\{Y(a) = 1 \mid C\}/odds\{Y(a^*) = 1 \mid C\}$.

The proportion mediated (PM) captures what would happen to the effect of comorbidity status on mortality (i.e., by how much it would be reduced) if we were to disable the pathway between comorbidity status and diagnostic route (i.e., setting it to its natural value in the absence of comorbidity). The PM captures how much of the effect of comorbidity status on mortality is because of the effect of comorbidity on diagnostic route. On the risk difference scale, the PM is the ratio of the NIE to the TCE (i.e., $PM = \frac{NIE}{TCE}$). As the outcome is binary and the measure is the odds ratio, the ratio scale is used, but the PM is calculated using a transformation, such that

$$PM = \frac{OR_{NDE}(OR_{NIE} - 1)}{(OR_{NDE} \times OR_{NIE}) - 1}.$$

As the comorbidity gap in survival changes over time since diagnosis, the binary outcome (mortality) was stratified into death within (i) 12 months, (ii) 36 months given 12 months survival, and (iii) 60 months given 36 months survival. Analyses were performed on each of the three binary conditional survival outcomes. Since cause of death records are often unreliable or unavailable in population-based cancer registry data, the estimation of net survival in the relative survival setting reduces bias arising from background population mortality. However, the interpretation of net survival estimates within mediation analysis is not yet well understood; thus, we used a binary indicator of all-cause mortality within specific time periods. No patients were lost to follow up (i.e., there was no right censoring). The outcome (all-cause mortality) and the mediator (diagnostic route) were modelled using logistic regression. Missing records of diagnostic route (5.8%) were imputed using single stochastic imputation within the g-computation procedure, and all variables were included in the imputation model.

We used Stata v.17 (StataCorp, College Station, TX, USA) for statistical analysis. The code used for this analysis is provided for reproducibility at https://github.com/mattyjsmith/Proportion-mediated-NHL (accessed on 23 August 2022).

# 4. Results

## 4.1. Summary Statistics

Overall, 41,422 patients in England, aged from 45 to 99 years, were diagnosed with Diffuse Large B-cell lymphoma ($n$ = 27,379) or Follicular lymphoma ($n$ = 14,043), between 1 January 2005 and 31 December 2013 (Table 1). The prevalence of at least one comorbidity was 11.4% and 8.2% for DLBCL and FL, respectively. For both DLBCL and FL, those with comorbidities were those diagnosed at an older age and living in more deprived areas. For DLBCL, the probability of the presence of a comorbidity was lower amongst females. Emergency diagnostic route was more likely amongst those with comorbidity (both DLBCL and FL).

Amongst FL patients with any comorbidity, the more deprived the area, the more likely the patients were to have an emergency presentation (Figure 2), Amongst DLBCL patients with any comorbidity, there was no apparent trend in diagnostic route by deprivation level. For both DLBCL and FL patients without any comorbidity, the proportion of patients in each deprivation level were similar when comparing emergency and elective diagnostic routes.

Net survival differed between the least and most deprived for DLBCL and FL (Figure 3). Of those without comorbidity, the difference in survival at 1 year since diagnosis amongst the most deprived patients was 6.4% (71.3% vs. 64.9%) and 2.4% (94.1% vs. 91.7%) lower than least deprived for DLBCL and FL, respectively (Table 2). For both DLBCL and FL, the deprivation gap in survival was apparent from 1 year and remained similar through to 5 years since diagnosis, except for those with at least one comorbidity where there was no apparent deprivation gap through 5 years (Table 2 and Figure 3).

**Table 1.** Age at diagnosis, sex, deprivation level and ethnicity according to the comorbidity status amongst patients with Diffuse Large B-cell ($n$ = 27,379) or Follicular lymphomas ($n$ =14,043) in England between 2005 and 2013.

| | No Comorbidity N (%) | Comorbidity N (%) | Total N (%) | OR † (95% CI) | p-Value * |
|---|---|---|---|---|---|
| **Diffuse large B-cell lymphoma** | | | | | |
| **Age** *** | | | | | |
| Mean (SD) | 70.3 (11.3) | 74.1 (10.6) | 70.7 (11.0) | 1.35 (1.31–1.41) ** | <0.001 |
| **Sex** | | | | | |
| Male | 12,904 (53.2) | 1748 (56.2) | 14,652 (53.5) | Ref | - |
| Female | 11,365 (46.8) | 1362 (43.8) | 12,727 (46.5) | 0.88 (0.82–0.95) | 0.001 |
| **Deprivation** | | | | | |
| Least deprived | 5348 (22.0) | 547 (17.6) | 5895 (21.5) | Ref | - |
| 2 | 5586 (23.0) | 652 (21.0) | 6238 (22.8) | 1.14 (1.01–1.29) | 0.031 |
| 3 | 5115 (21.1) | 641 (20.6) | 5756 (21.0) | 1.23 (1.09–1.38) | 0.001 |
| 4 | 4665 (19.2) | 676 (21.7) | 5341 (19.5) | 1.42 (1.26–1.60) | <0.001 |
| Most deprived | 3555 (14.7) | 594 (19.1) | 4149 (15.2) | 1.63 (1.44–1.85) | <0.001 |
| **Route** | | | | | |
| Elective | 15,495 (67.3) | 1785 (58.8) | 17,280 (66.3) | Ref | - |
| Emergency | 7547 (32.8) | 1252 (41.2) | 8799 (33.7) | 1.44 (1.33–1.56) | <0.001 |
| Missing | 1227 (5.1) | 73 (2.4) | 1300 (4.7) | - | - |

**Table 1.** *Cont.*

| | No Comorbidity N (%) | Comorbidity N (%) | Total N (%) | OR † (95% CI) | *p*-Value * |
|---|---|---|---|---|---|
| **Follicular lymphoma** | | | | | |
| **Age** *** | | | | | |
| Mean (SD) | 66.2 (11.0) | 72.0 (10.3) | 66.7 (10.7) | 1.62 (1.53–1.71) ** | <0.001 |
| **Sex** | | | | | |
| Male | 5980 (46.4) | 532 (46.5) | 6512 (46.4) | Ref | - |
| Female | 6918 (53.6) | 613 (53.5) | 7531 (53.6) | 1.00 (0.88–1.12) | 0.949 |
| **Deprivation** | | | | | |
| Least deprived | 3091 (24.0) | 193 (16.9) | 3284 (23.4) | Ref | - |
| 2 | 3025 (23.5) | 203 (17.7) | 3228 (23.0) | 1.07 (0.88–1.32) | 0.487 |
| 3 | 2759 (21.4) | 254 (22.2) | 3013 (21.5) | 1.47 (1.21–1.79) | <0.001 |
| 4 | 2356 (18.3) | 253 (22.1) | 2609 (18.6) | 1.71 (1.42–2.09) | <0.001 |
| Most deprived | 1667 (12.9) | 242 (21.1) | 1909 (13.6) | 2.32 (1.91–2.83) | <0.001 |
| **Route** | | | | | |
| Elective | 10,332 (87.2) | 889 (81.0) | 11,221 (86.7) | Ref | - |
| Emergency | 1518 (12.8) | 209 (19.0) | 2407 (18.6) | 1.60 (1.36–1.88) | <0.001 |
| *Missing* | 1058 (8.2) | 47 (4.1) | 1105 (7.9) | - | - |

* Chi-squared test of association; ** Odds ratio for each 10-year increase in age; *** Range of 45 to 99 years; † Odds ratio of one or more comorbidities compared to none.

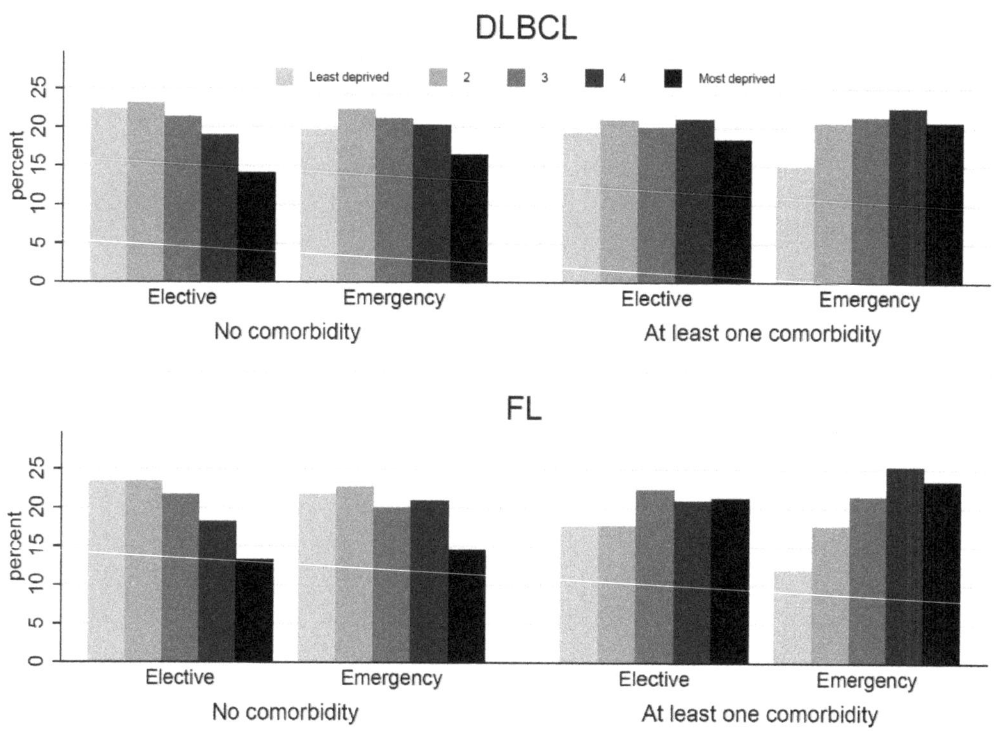


**Figure 2.** Distribution of deprivation levels by diagnostic route stratified over comorbidity status amongst patients diagnosed with DLBCL ($n$ = 27,379) or FL ($n$ = 14,043) in England between 2005 and 2013.

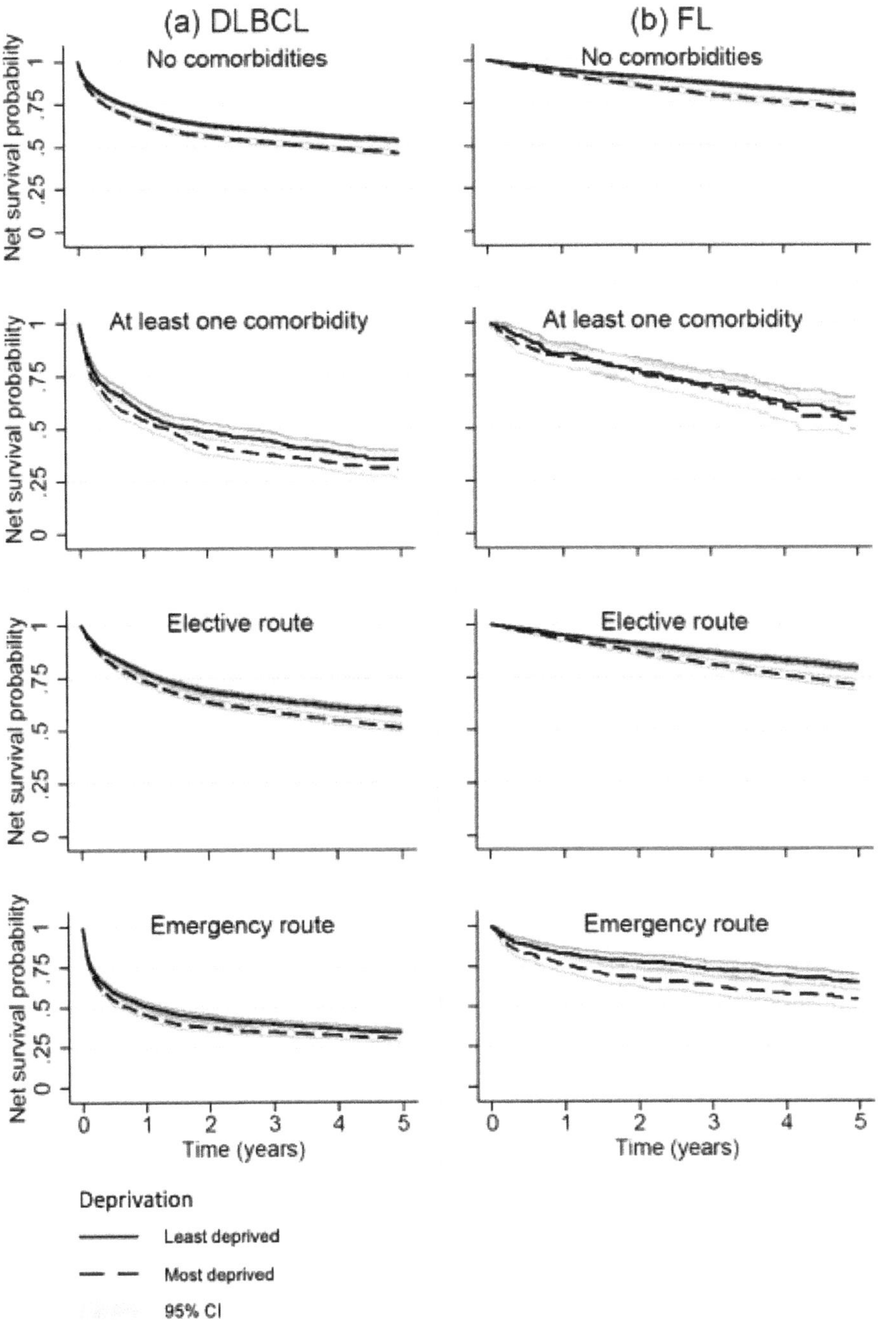


**Figure 3.** Net survival probabilities by comorbidity status and diagnostic route, stratified by deprivation level, amongst patients diagnosed with DLBCL ($n$ = 27,379) or FL ($n$ = 14,043) in England between 2005 and 2013.

**Table 2.** Net survival estimates by comorbidity status and diagnostic route amongst patients diagnosed with DLBCL ($n$ = 27,379) or FL ($n$ = 14,043) in England between 2005 and 2013.

| | 1 Year NS (95% CI) | | 3 Years NS (95% CI) | | 5 Years NS (95% CI) | |
|---|---|---|---|---|---|---|
| | Least Deprived | Most Deprived | Least Deprived | Most Deprived | Least Deprived | Most Deprived |
| DLBCL | | | | | | |
| Comorbidity | | | | | | |
| None | 71.3 (70.1–72.5) | 64.9 (63.4–66.5) | 58.9 (57.6–60.4) | 52.5 (50.9–54.2) | 53.3 (51.9–54.7) | 45.7 (44.0–47.4) |
| At least one | 58.0 (53.8–62.1) | 54.2 (50.2–58.2) | 44.1 (39.9–48.3) | 37.4 (33.5–41.3) | 35.4 (31.0–39.7) | 30.4 (26.4–34.4) |
| Route | | | | | | |
| Elective | 77.8 (76.5–79.1) | 73.6 (71.9–75.3) | 64.8 (63.3–66.3) | 59.2 (57.3–61.1) | 58.8 (57.2–60.4) | 51.1 (49.1–53.2) |
| Emergency | 51.0 (48.6–53.4) | 45.3 (42.8–47.8) | 39.4 (37.1–41.8) | 34.6 (32.2–37.0) | 34.3 (32.0–36.7) | 30.2 (27.8–32.6) |
| Follicular | | | | | | |
| Comorbidity | | | | | | |
| None | 94.1 (93.3–95.0) | 91.7 (90.3–93.0) | 86.3 (85.0–87.5) | 79.6 (77.7–81.6) | 79.0 (77.5–80.5) | 70.5 (68.2–72.9) |
| At least one | 85.0 (80.0–90.0) | 83.5 (78.8–88.2) | 70.5 (64.0–77.0) | 68.4 (62.5–74.3) | 56.6 (48.9–64.3) | 53.7 (46.8–60.7) |
| Route | | | | | | |
| Elective | 94.7 (93.9–95.6) | 93.1 (91.9–94.4) | 86.6 (85.3–88.0) | 81.0 (79.0–82.9) | 78.8 (77.1–80.5) | 70.9 (68.4–73.3) |
| Emergency | 82.8 (78.9–86.7) | 75.9 (70.9–81.0) | 72.9 (68.2–77.5) | 62.7 (56.9–68.5) | 64.2 (58.9–69.5) | 53.5 (47.2–59.7) |

DLBCL: diffuse large B-cell lymphoma; FL: follicular lymphoma; NS: net survival; 95% CI: confidence interval.

### 4.2. Natural Effect Estimates

**Total causal effect (TCE).** The total effect of comorbidity on survival is the summation of the effects shown in Figure 1. Amongst those with comorbidity, for DLBCL, the odds of death within 12 months were 1.50 (95% CI: 1.39–1.61) times that of those without comorbidity; for FL, it was 1.71 times (95% CI: 1.45–2.02) (Table 3 and Figure 4). Over time, the comorbidity effect slightly increased for patients with DLBCL, however, for FL, the comorbidity effect was lowest at 3 years conditional on 1 year survival. At 5 years conditional on 3-year survival, the comorbidity effect remained strong at 1.57 (95% CI 1.39–1.79) and 1.62 (95% CI 1.38–1.90) for DLBCL and FL, respectively.

**Natural indirect effect (NIE).** The indirect effect of comorbidity status through diagnostic route decreased as time since diagnosis increased for both DLBCL and FL (Table 3 and Figure 4). For both DLBCL and FL, the indirect effect was highest within 12 months since diagnosis (DLBCL: OR 1.10 [95% CI 1.07–1.13], FL: OR 1.09 [95% CI 1.04–1.14]) and gradually reduced through to 5 years since diagnosis (DLBCL: OR 1.01 [95% CI 1.00–1.02], FL: OR 1.00 [95% CI 0.99–1.01]).

**Proportion mediated (PM).** For DLBCL and FL, the proportion mediated was highest within the first 12 months since diagnosis and decreased over time since diagnosis (Figure 5). Within the first 12 months since diagnosis, about a quarter (95% CI 17.5–29.5) and a sixth (95% CI 6.0–25.6) of the effect of comorbidity on survival was mediated by diagnostic route, for DLBCL and FL, respectively. With increasing time since diagnosis, the proportion of the comorbidity effect mediated by diagnostic route decreased to 1.3% (95% CI 0.0–2.8) and 0.3% (95% CI −1.0–1.5) after 5 years since diagnosis of DLBCL and FL, respectively.

**Table 3.** Natural effect estimates for the odds ratio of conditional mortality since diagnosis, comparing comorbidity to no comorbidity mediated by diagnostic route, amongst patients diagnosed between 2005 to 2013 in England with DLBCL patients ($n$ = 27,379) or FL patients ($n$ = 14,043).

| | 1 Year OR (CI) | 3 Years OR (CI) | 5 Years OR (CI) |
|---|---|---|---|
| **DLBCL** | | | |
| TCE | 1.50 (1.39–1.61) | 1.41 (1.28–1.57) | 1.57 (1.39–1.79) |
| NDE | 1.36 (1.27–1.46) | 1.39 (1.26–1.54) | 1.56 (1.38–1.78) |
| NIE | 1.10 (1.07–1.13) | 1.02 (1.01–1.03) | 1.01 (1.00–1.02) |
| PM | 23.5% (17.5–29.5) | 4.8% (2.3 –7.2) | 1.3% (0.0–2.8) |
| **FL** | | | |
| TCE | 1.71 (1.45–2.02) | 1.41 (1.23–1.62) | 1.62 (1.38–1.90) |
| NDE | 1.57 (1.34–1.85) | 1.40 (1.22–1.61) | 1.62 (1.38–1.90) |
| NIE | 1.09 (1.04–1.14) | 1.01 (1.00–1.02) | 1.00 (0.99–1.01) |
| PM | 15.8% (6.0–25.6) | 3.0% (0.0–6.0) | 0.3% (−1.0–1.5) |

NDE: natural direct effect; NIE: natural indirect effect; TCE: Total causal effect; PM: Proportion mediated; OR: odds ratio; CI: 95% confidence interval; DLBCL: diffuse large B-cell lymphoma; FL: follicular lymphoma.

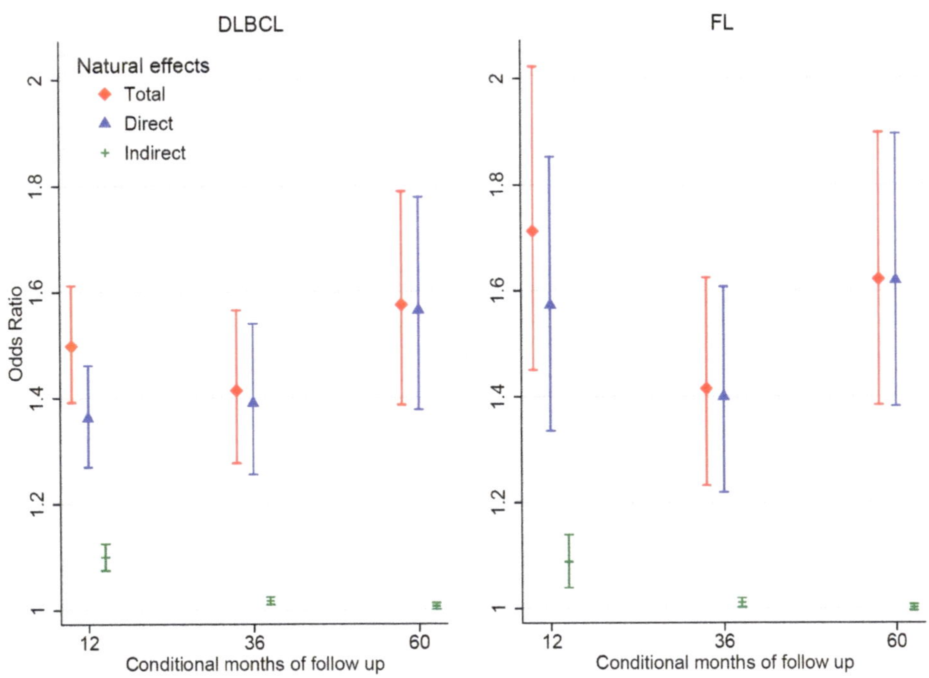


**Figure 4.** Effect of comorbidity status on odds of death at different conditional months of follow up since diagnosis amongst DLBCL ($n$ = 27,379) or FL ($n$ = 14,043) patients in England between 2005 and 2013.

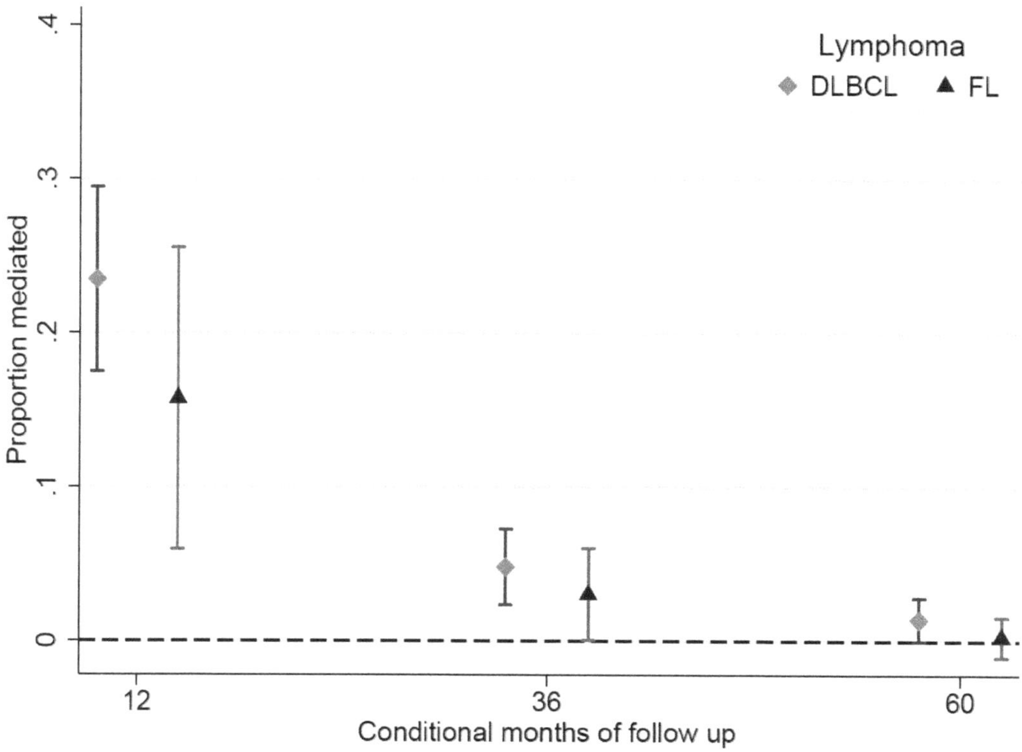


**Figure 5.** Proportion of the effect of comorbidity status on survival mediated by diagnostic route amongst patients diagnosed with DLBCL ($n$ = 27,379) or FL ($n$ = 14,043) in England between 2005 and 2013.

## 5. Discussion

We aimed to estimate the proportion of the effect of comorbidity on survival that is mediated by diagnostic route amongst patients diagnosed with diffuse large B-cell (DLBCL) or follicular lymphoma (FL) in England.

Our results suggest that an elective (compared to an emergency) diagnostic route would reduce the odds of mortality within the first 12 months since diagnosis by 24% and 16%, for DLBCL and FL, respectively. This effect reduced over a longer follow-up time but was still apparent at 3 years since diagnosis, given these patients had survived 1 year. Patients with FL are often, at least initially, managed via watch-and-wait, whereas DLBCL is commonly treated with intensive immunochemotherapy, which may depend on the presence of comorbidities. The difference in the comorbidity effect between the two lymphoma subtypes (i.e., 24% vs. 16%) might be explained by the lack of information on treatment allocation.

The proportion mediated estimates how much of the total effect of comorbidity on survival operates through diagnostic route. If the proportion were large in our study, then the effect of comorbidity on survival would primarily be through the diagnostic route. However, in our study, since the proportion was small there may be other pathways through which comorbidity is acting on survival. Since diagnostic route is thought to be a process that identifies, and separates, comorbidity from cancer-related symptoms, a small value for the proportion mediated shows that comorbidity does not have a large effect on diagnostic route. Implying that, during the healthcare interaction (e.g., a general practitioner consultation), comorbidity symptoms are being identified as separate from cancer related symptoms for most patients. On the other hand, since there is still an ostensive value for the proportion mediated, this implies that comorbidity does influence diagnostic route for some patients, possibly for those with milder or obscure cancer symptoms.

Other pathways for the effect of comorbidity on survival could be through its effect on treatment allocation, quality and number of general practitioner examinations, or stage at cancer diagnosis. Firstly, information within the data was not available for the prevalence of treatment allocation (e.g., immunotherapies such as rituximab). Treatment allocation may explain little of the comorbidity gap in survival for patients with FL because these patients are managed via a watch and wait approach, unless they have a high-grade lymphoma. For DLBCL, the first line recommended treatment is immunochemotherapy (i.e., R-CHOP); however, a patient's history of cardiac conditions might explain the comorbidity gap in survival because these patients are more likely to be allocated less intensive (i.e., less cardiotoxic) treatments (e.g., R-CVP). For example, patients at risk of cardiotoxicity (i.e., patients with underlying cardiac conditions) are likely to receive less intensive immunochemotherapies (e.g., combination chemotherapy without doxorubicin). Secondly, the quality of general practitioner examinations prior to cancer diagnosis is associated with the possibility of missed opportunities for early diagnoses, leading to a higher proportion of emergency diagnoses [27]. Information on the quality of the examination may explain the effect of comorbidity on diagnostic route thereby reducing the proportion mediated that was found in this study. Thirdly, it is possible that similar results would be obtained with stage at diagnosis as a mediator. Stage at diagnosis is closely associated with route to diagnosis; for example, patients diagnosed via emergency presentation are likely to have severe symptoms and an advanced cancer presenting with a late stage [28]. Lastly, completion of a treatment plan is crucial for optimal chances of survival. Performance status is known to be associated with the failure to complete the planned treatment of R-CHOP, and treatments are often made less intensive due to the toxicity [29]. In this study, information on performance status was not available; since this was not accounted for, performance status might explain the comorbidity gap in survival through treatment allocation and completion.

Our aim was to study the causal effect of comorbidity on survival whilst studying intermediate pathways, this made the application of causal mediation analysis a natural choice. Another strength of this study was the large population-based data incorporating all patients diagnosed with DLBCL or FL between 2005 and 2013. To our knowledge, this study is the first to disentangle the effects of comorbidity on survival of patients with NHL. The effect of diagnostic route on survival of patients with NHL is well known; emergency presentation is strongly associated with poorer health outcomes and worse survival probability [16,30]. Moreover, the effects of comorbidity on a patient's diagnostic route are becoming clearer: the presence of comorbidities can either hasten the cancer diagnosis (due to the patient having more numerous interactions with the healthcare system) or delay the cancer diagnosis (due to comorbidities with similar symptoms) [31–33]. The multi-faceted interactions along a lymphoma patient's pathway is not well known but this study highlights the need for further research into this. For other cancers, and in England, a study found that when using stage at diagnosis as a mediator for the deprivation gap in survival, stage explained little of the survival inequalities.[4] This could suggest that including stage as a mediator in this study would not add further information beyond that of diagnostic route.

Comorbidities, though more prevalent in patients who are elderly or live in more deprived areas, have been shown to explain little in age- and deprivation-related inequalities in DLBCL or FL outcomes [34–36]. For policy purposes, further research could investigate how our findings from mediation analysis varies by deprivation (and age). More complex mediation analyses would however require more detailed information on individual clinical factors and system-level factors. Such factors may act as barriers to help-seeking behaviour, particularly among more deprived and elderly populations [33].

This study has its limitations. Firstly, we used an ecological measure of a patient's deprivation level, which was geographically defined using the patient's LSOA at the time of cancer diagnosis. Ecological bias could be present in this study because area-based income deprivation is possibly a poor predictor of individual income status [37]. However, since deprivation level was a confounder, misclassification is expected to have only a small influence on our conclusions in this study. Secondly, we did not include patients diagnosed through death certificates. It is possible that these patients could have had a short disease course and a more severe ill health, leading to an emergency presentation. For these patients, the length of time that they lived with the disease before death (i.e., their survival) is unknown, and including these patients would give an underestimate of the true survival probability. Moreover, there was a small proportion of patients diagnosed through DCO (DLBCL 0.8%, FL: 0.3%): including these patients would have a negligible effect on our results.

We used hospital episode records (i.e., Hospital Episode Statistics data) to determine a patient's comorbidity history. These records have universal coverage, allow for longitudinal linkage (ideal for cohort studies), and adheres to standardised coding practices [38]. These records are primarily collated for reimbursement purposes within the National Health Service rather than for research purposes and it is possible that some comorbidities are poorly recorded. However, administrative data (such as HES) has been suggested as the best available option, in comparison to clinical records, to ascertain comorbidity status for the Charlson comorbidity index [39,40].

Although diagnostic routes are well-defined, the process to identify the route is often complex [16]. A 'route to diagnosis' is a sequence of interactions between the patient and the healthcare system, but for analytical purposes are grouped into eight broad categories. This study focused on the comparison of emergency diagnostic route compared to other routes. There are close similarities in the qualitative definition between two-week-wait (TWW) referrals by a general practitioner and emergency route to diagnosis. For example, if HES records indicate an emergency route but a TWW record exists, then the TWW record takes priority if the emergency record date is more than 28 days prior to the decision to treat date. Given than comorbidity and deprivation can contribute to a delay in treatment, it is possible that some of these patients (who were recorded as TWW) should have been recorded as emergency diagnosis. Further studies could investigate this hypothesis by assuming different proportions of those patients diagnosed through TWW were emergency diagnosis, and measuring the proportion mediated accordingly.

In conclusion, our results show the effect of comorbidity status on survival of patients with lymphoma in England are partly explained by diagnostic route. Efforts to reduce diagnostic delay amongst patients with comorbidity would reduce DLBCL and FL survival inequalities by roughly 24% and 16% within the first 12 months since diagnosis, for DLBCL and FL, respectively. The proportion of the mediated effect reduces over time but is still apparent at 36 months since diagnosis. Public health programs could be redefined and implemented to reduce diagnostic delay amongst lymphoma patients with comorbidities. Further research should examine whether our findings differed in underserved areas.

**Supplementary Materials:** The following supporting information can be downloaded at: https://www.mdpi.com/article/10.3390/cancers14205082/s1, Table S1. Comorbidities and their diagnostic ICD-10 codes; Table S2. Distribution of non-Hodgkin lymphoma subtypes for patients diagnosed from 2005–2013, with respective morphology and topography ICD-O-3 codes.

**Author Contributions:** Conceptualization, M.J.S., B.R. and M.A.L.-F.; methodology, M.J.S. and M.A.L.-F.; software, M.J.S.; validation, M.J.S., B.R. and M.A.L.-F.; formal analysis, M.J.S.; investigation, M.J.S.; resources, M.J.S.; data curation, M.J.S.; writing—original draft preparation, M.J.S.; writing—review and editing, M.J.S.; visualization, M.J.S.; supervision, M.A.L.-F.; project administration, M.J.S.; funding acquisition, B.R. All authors have read and agreed to the published version of the manuscript.

**Funding:** This research was funded by Cancer Research UK (Reference C7923/A18525). Funders had no role in the study design, data collection, data analysis, data interpretation, or writing of the report.

**Institutional Review Board Statement:** We obtained the statutory approvals required for this research from the Confidentiality Advisory Group (CAG) of the Health Research Authority (HRA): PIAG 1–05(c) 2007. Ethical approval was obtained from the Research Ethics Committee (REC) of the Health Research Authority (HRA): 07/MRE01/52.

**Informed Consent Statement:** Informed consent from participants was waived by the ethics committee. This work uses the data provided by patients and collected by the National Health Service as part of their care and support. We used anonymized National Cancer Registry and Hospital Episode Statistics data. No consent to participate was sought from patients. All methods were carried out in accordance with relevant guidelines and regulations.

**Data Availability Statement:** The data that support the findings of this study are available via application to the Public Health England Office for Data Release, but restrictions apply to the availability of these data.

**Conflicts of Interest:** The authors declare no conflict of interest.

## References

1. Rachet, B.; Mitry, E.; Shah, A.; Cooper, N.; Coleman, M.P. Survival from non-Hodgkin lymphoma in England and Wales up to 2001. *Br. J. Cancer* **2008**, *99*, S104–S106. [CrossRef] [PubMed]
2. Rachet, B.; Ellis, L.; Maringe, C.; Chu, T.; Nur, U.; Quaresma, M.; Shah, A.; Walters, S.; Woods, L.; Forman, D.; et al. Socioeconomic inequalities in cancer survival in England after the NHS cancer plan. *Br. J. Cancer* **2010**, *103*, 446–453. [CrossRef] [PubMed]
3. Smith, A.; Crouch, S.; Lax, S.; Li, J.; Painter, D.; Howell, D.; Patmore, R.; Jack, A.; Roman, E. Lymphoma incidence, survival and prevalence 2004–2014: Sub-type analyses from the UK's Haematological Malignancy Research Network. *Br. J. Cancer* **2015**, *112*, 1575–1584. [CrossRef] [PubMed]
4. Li, R.; Daniel, R.; Rachet, B. How much do tumor stage and treatment explain socioeconomic inequalities in breast cancer survival? Applying causal mediation analysis to population-based data. *Eur. J. Epidemiol.* **2016**, *31*, 603–611. [CrossRef]
5. Renzi, C.; Lyratzopoulos, G.; Hamilton, W.; Maringe, C.; Rachet, B. Contrasting effects of comorbidities on emergency colon cancer diagnosis: A longitudinal data-linkage study in England. *BMC Health Serv. Res.* **2019**, *19*, 311. [CrossRef]
6. Renzi, C.; Kaushal, A.; Emery, J.; Hamilton, W.; Neal, R.D.; Rachet, B.; Rubin, G.; Singh, H.; Walter, F.M.; de Wit, N.J.; et al. Comorbid chronic diseases and cancer diagnosis: Disease-specific effects and underlying mechanisms. *Nat. Rev. Clin. Oncol.* **2019**, *16*, 746–761. [CrossRef]
7. Robins, J.M.; Greenland, S. Identifiability and Exchangeability for Direct and Indirect Effects. *Epidemiology* **1992**, *3*, 143–155. [CrossRef]
8. VanderWeele, T.J. Mediation Analysis: A Practitioner's Guide. *Annu. Rev. Public Health* **2016**, *37*, 17–32. [CrossRef]
9. Richiardi, L.; Bellocco, R.; Zugna, D. Mediation analysis in epidemiology: Methods, interpretation and bias. *Int. J. Epidemiol.* **2013**, *42*, 1511–1519. [CrossRef]
10. International Agency for Research on Cancer International Classification of Diseases for Oncology. 2013. Available online: http://codes.iarc.fr/ (accessed on 4 October 2019).
11. Public Health England National Cancer Registration and Analysis Service. 2019. Available online: https://www.gov.uk/guidance/national-cancer-registration-and-analysis-service-ncras#cancer-registration (accessed on 30 March 2020).
12. NHS Digital Hospital Episode Statistics. 2015. Available online: https://digital.nhs.uk/data-and-information/data-tools-and-services/data-services/hospital-episode-statistics (accessed on 4 October 2019).
13. Maringe, C.; Fowler, H.; Rachet, B.; Luque-Fernandez, M.A. Reproducibility, reliability and validity of population-based administrative health data for the assessment of cancer non-related comorbidities. *PLoS ONE* **2017**, *12*, e0172814. [CrossRef]
14. Charlson, M.E.; Pompei, P.; Ales, K.L.; MacKenzie, C.R. A new method of classifying prognostic comorbidity in longitudinal studies: Development and validation. *J. Chronic Dis.* **1987**, *40*, 373–383. [CrossRef]
15. Armitage, J.N.; van der Meulen, J.H. Identifying co-morbidity in surgical patients using administrative data with the Royal College of Surgeons Charlson Score. *Br. J. Surg.* **2010**, *97*, 772–781. [CrossRef] [PubMed]
16. Elliss-Brookes, L.; McPhail, S.; Ives, A.; Greenslade, M.; Shelton, J.; Hiom, S.; Richards, M. Routes to diagnosis for cancer—Determining the patient journey using multiple routine data sets. *Br. J. Cancer* **2012**, *107*, 1220–1226. [CrossRef] [PubMed]
17. National Health Service: Data dictionary Lower Super Output Area. 2018. Available online: https://www.datadictionary.nhs.uk/data_dictionary (accessed on 4 October 2019).
18. English Indices of Multiple Deprivation. 2015. Available online: https://www.gov.uk/government/statistics/english-indices-of-deprivation-2015 (accessed on 4 October 2019).
19. Office for National Statistics Clinical Commissioning Group Population Estimates. 2020. Available online: https://www.ons.gov.uk/peoplepopulationandcommunity/populationandmigration/populationestimates/datasets/clinicalcommissioninggroupmidyearpopulationestimates (accessed on 30 March 2020).

20. Sheringham, J.R.; Georghiou, T.; Chitnis, X.A.; Bardsley, M. Comparing primary and secondary health-care use between diagnostic routes before a colorectal cancer diagnosis: Cohort study using linked data. *Br. J. Cancer* **2014**, *111*, 1490–1499. [CrossRef] [PubMed]
21. Hernán, M.A. The hazards of hazard ratios. *Epidemiology* **2010**, *21*, 13–15. [CrossRef] [PubMed]
22. Pohar-Perme, M.; Janez, S.; Jacques, E. On Estimation in Relative Survival. *Biometrics* **2012**, *68*, 113–120. [CrossRef]
23. StataCorp. *Stata Statistical Software*, Version 17; StataCorp LLC.: College Station, TX, USA, 2021.
24. Clerc-Urmès, I.; Grzebyk, M.; Hédelin, G. Net survival estimation with stns. *Stata J.* **2014**, *14*, 87–102. [CrossRef]
25. Robins, J. A new approach to causal inference in mortality studies with a sustained exposure period—Application to control of the healthy worker survivor effect. *Math. Model* **1986**, *7*, 1393–1512. [CrossRef]
26. Daniel, R.M.; de Stavola, B.L.; Cousens, S.N. gformula: Estimating causal effects in the presence of time-varying confounding or mediation using the g-computation formula. *Stata J.* **2011**, *11*, 479–517. [CrossRef]
27. Renzi, C.; Lyratzopoulos, G.; Card, T.; Chu, T.P.C.; Macleod, U.; Rachet, B. Do colorectal cancer patients diagnosed as an emergency differ from non-emergency patients in their consultation patterns and symptoms? A longitudinal data-linkage study in England. *Br. J. Cancer* **2016**, *115*, 866. [CrossRef]
28. Kane, E.; Howell, D.; Smith, A.; Crouch, S.; Burton, C.; Roman, E.; Patmore, R. Emergency admission and survival from aggressive non—Hodgkin lymphoma: A report from the UK's population-based Haematological Malignancy Research Network. *Eur. J. Cancer* **2017**, *78*, 53–60. [CrossRef] [PubMed]
29. Wästerlid, T.; Harrysson, S.; Andersson, T.M.L.; Ekberg, S.; Enblad, G.; Andersson, P.O.; Jerkeman, M.; Eloranta, S.; Smedby, K.E. Outcome and determinants of failure to complete primary R-CHOP treatment for reasons other than non-response among patients with diffuse large B-cell lymphoma. *Am. J. Hematol.* **2020**, *95*, 740–748. [CrossRef] [PubMed]
30. Hamilton, W. Emergency admissions of cancer as a marker of diagnostic delay. *Br. J. Cancer* **2012**, *107*, 1205–1206. [CrossRef] [PubMed]
31. Gurney, J.; Sarfati, D.; Stanley, J. The impact of patient comorbidity on cancer stage at diagnosis. *Br. J. Cancer* **2015**, *113*, 1375–1380. [CrossRef]
32. Sarfati, D.; Koczwara, B.; Jackson, C. The impact of comorbidity on cancer and its treatment. *CA Cancer J. Clin.* **2016**, *66*, 337–350. [CrossRef]
33. Salika, T.; Lyratzopoulos, G.; Whitaker, K.L.; Waller, J.; Renzi, C. Do comorbidities influence help-seeking for cancer alarm symptoms? A population-based survey in England. *J. Public Health* **2017**, *40*, 340–349. [CrossRef]
34. Smith, M.J.; Fernandez, M.A.L.; Belot, A.; Quartagno, M.; Bonaventure, A.; Majano, S.B.; Rachet, B.; Njagi, E.N. Investigating the inequalities in route to diagnosis amongst patients with diffuse large B-cell or follicular lymphoma in England. *Br. J. Cancer* **2021**, *125*, 1299–1307. [CrossRef]
35. Smith, A.; Crouch, S.; Howell, D.; Burton, C.; Patmore, R.; Roman, E. Impact of age and socioeconomic status on treatment and survival from aggressive lymphoma: A UK population-based study of diffuse large B-cell lymphoma. *Cancer Epidemiol.* **2015**, *39*, 1103–1112. [CrossRef]
36. Smith, M.J.; Belot, A.; Quartagno, M.; Fernandez, M.A.L.; Bonaventure, A.; Gachau, S.; Majano, S.B.; Rachet, B.; Njagi, E.N. Excess Mortality by Multimorbidity, Socioeconomic, and Healthcare Factors, amongst Patients Diagnosed with Diffuse Large B-Cell or Follicular Lymphoma in England. *Cancers* **2021**, *13*, 5805. [CrossRef]
37. Ingleby, F.C.; Belot, A.; Atherton, I.; Baker, M.; Elliss-Brookes, L.; Woods, L.M. Assessment of the concordance between individual-level and area-level measures of socio-economic deprivation in a cancer patient cohort in England and Wales. *BMJ Open* **2020**, *10*, e041714. [CrossRef]
38. Herbert, A.; Wijlaars, L.; Zylbersztejn, A.; Cromwell, D.; Hardelid, P. Data Resource Profile: Hospital Episode Statistics Admitted Patient Care (HES APC). *Int. J. Epidemiol.* **2017**, *46*, 1093–1093i. [CrossRef] [PubMed]
39. Sarfati, D. Review of methods used to measure comorbidity in cancer populations: No gold standard exists. *J. Clin. Epidemiol.* **2012**, *65*, 924–933. [CrossRef] [PubMed]
40. Bannay, A.; Chaignot, C.; Blotiere, P.O.; Basson, M.; Weill, A.; Ricordeau, P.; Alla, F. The Best Use of the Charlson Comorbidity Index with Electronic Health Care Database to Predict Mortality. *Med. Care* **2016**, *54*, 188–194. [CrossRef] [PubMed]

cancers

MDPI

*Article*

# Navigating Intercultural Medical Encounters: An Examination of Patient-Centered Communication Practices with Italian and Foreign Cancer Patients Living in Italy

**Filomena Marino, Francesca Alby, Cristina Zucchermaglio, Teresa Gloria Scalisi and Marco Lauriola ***

Department of Social and Developmental Psychology, Sapienza Università di Roma, 00185 Roma, Italy; filomena.marino@uniroma1.it (F.M.); francesca.alby@uniroma1.it (F.A.); cristina.zucchermaglio@uniroma1.it (C.Z.); gloria.scalisi@uniroma1.it (T.G.S.)

* Correspondence: marco.lauriola@uniroma1.it

**Simple Summary:** Good communication is key in cancer care, especially when doctors and patients come from different cultures or speak different languages. We studied 42 videos of doctors talking to Italian and foreign cancer patients during their visits. We looked at how they talked to each other, whether they misunderstood anything, whether there were interruptions, and how much trust and emotion were shown. The type of appointment and the doctor's personal style mattered more than whether the patient was Italian or foreign. This tells us that even when foreign patients can speak the language well, doctors cannot only rely on this to communicate effectively. Doctors should pay attention to interruptions and focus on taking care of the patient as a whole person. The methods we used in this study could help doctors improve their communication skills, which will lead to better care for all patients.

**Abstract:** Effective communication is crucial in cancer care due to the sensitive nature of the information and the psychosocial impact on patients and their families. Patient-centered communication (PCC) is the gold standard for providing quality cancer care, as it improves patient satisfaction, treatment adherence, clinical outcomes, and overall quality of life. However, doctor–patient communication can be complicated by ethnic, linguistic, and cultural differences. This study employed the ONCode coding system to investigate PCC practices in oncological visits (doctor's communicative behavior, patient's initiatives, misalignments, interruptions, accountability, and expressions of trust in participants' talk, Markers of uncertainty in doctor's talk, markers of emotions in doctor's talk). Forty-two video-recorded patient–oncologist encounters (with 22 Italian and 20 foreign patients), including both first and follow-up visits, were analyzed. Three discriminant analyses were conducted to assess differences in PCC between patient groups (Italian or foreign patients) according to the type of encounter (first visit or follow-up) and the presence or absence of companions during the encounters. Multiple regression analyses were performed to evaluate the PCC differences by oncologist age, patient age, and patient sex, controlling for the type of encounter, the presence of a companion during the visit, and patient group on ONCode dimensions. No differences were found in PCC by patient group in discriminant analyses and regressions. Doctor communication behavior, interruptions, accountability, and expressions of trust were higher in first visits than in follow-ups. The disparities in PCC were primarily linked to the type of visit and the age of the oncologist. However, a qualitative analysis showed notable differences in the types of interruptions during visits with foreign patients compared to Italian patients. It is essential to minimize interruptions during intercultural encounters to foster a more respectful and conducive environment for patients. Furthermore, even when foreign patients demonstrate sufficient linguistic competence, healthcare providers should not solely rely on this factor to ensure effective communication and quality care.

**Keywords:** patient-centered communication; oncology encounters; intercultural communication; ONCode coding system; video-recorded visits; communication barriers; cancer care quality

## 1. Introduction

Oncology visits offer a unique ecology for studying communication and its effects. The unique characteristics of cancer care influence the communication process between doctors and patients. Neoplasms are serious and potentially life-threatening diseases, but they also hold the possibility of cure. Therapies involve numerous treatment modalities and different professionals (oncologists, surgeons, radiotherapists, nurses, etc.). Furthermore, during these encounters, high stress levels, uncertainty, complex information, and life-changing medical decisions are involved. During oncology visits, physicians and patients engage in an intense communication activity that involves providing, understanding, and remembering information about the disease and treatments. Effective communication can alleviate suffering by improving the emotional well-being of patients. It can also indirectly improve treatment adherence [1].

Recognizing the importance of effective communication in oncology, ASCO [2] published guidelines for physicians on Patient-Centered Communication practices (PCC). PCC is a multidimensional construct that involves the co-construction and integration of instrumental, affective, and participation behaviors [1,3–5]. PCC aims to improve the effective exchange of information between participants, respond to the emotions expressed by the patient, and manage the uncertainty of the encounter. Moreover, PCC contributes to building a lasting relationship between the parties and involves the patient in the care process and therapeutic decisions through discussion and shared understanding of the disease and available treatments [1,6–10].

The importance of PCC practices is reflected in studies that demonstrate its positive impact on patient well-being. It is well established that PCC can have a positive influence on post-visit health outcomes, including satisfaction, reduced emotional distress, anxiety, and improved physical and psychological quality of life [6,11–13]. In addition, patients who are more involved in the decision-making process tend to be more satisfied with the encounter. They are more knowledgeable about their disease, exhibit higher treatment compliance, are better able to control their condition, and experience an improved quality of life after diagnosis and treatment [14,15]. Finally, empathic listening, addressing patients' concerns and fears, and providing reassurance all contribute to the establishment of a trusting relationship. This, in turn, leads to greater compliance with medical treatment, better psychological health, reduced emotional distress, and decreased anxiety [16–19].

Providing a diagnosis and clear, written information about treatment, giving space for the patient to ask questions, seek clarification and express doubts, as well as accepting the patient's concerns and emotional states are communicative activities that, along with other actions such as: explaining and discussing the severity of the disease, providing comprehensive information about the available options and the treatment pathway, would define lower levels of cancer-related anxiety and depression, higher levels of satisfaction following the encounter, and greater competence, compliance, adherence, and self-management of the proposed therapy [4,20,21]. In turn, adherence to treatment increases the chances of survival, enables better management and quality of therapeutic outcomes and, from a broader perspective, leads to a reduction in healthcare costs and unnecessary treatments [1,7,19,22–31].

In this sense, there is a "virtuous circle of PCC" [32] in which the more the oncologist integrates and co-constructs a PCC with patients and caregivers during visits characterized by affective, instrumental, and participative behaviors, the greater the chances of establishing a solid relationship of trust between the parties; that the patient will have a better understanding of the illness and the therapies that the patient will comply with the proposed medical treatments, and that there will be positive results on his or her health and psychological well-being over time.

The virtuous circle of PCC tends to be challenged when communication takes place between doctors and foreign patients. Studies conducted in an intercultural context illustrated the complexity of doctor–patient communication when the latter is a foreigner and there are linguistic, communicative, interpretative, and relational barriers [33]. Studies of migrant patients have shown that they face multiple sources of stress when engaging with healthcare, including difficulties in understanding or navigating the local healthcare system, communication challenges, and language barriers. Other factors that contributed to inequalities in health outcomes among foreign patients included an inaccurate understanding of diagnosis and treatment and an increased incidence of communicative misunderstandings regarding the causes of cancer. These barriers, in turn, affect the comprehension of diagnosis and treatment, resulting in poor long-term health outcomes [34–40]. Such barriers are also associated with more significant psychological distress and lower quality of life among foreign cancer patients [41–43]. Furthermore, the different linguistic, ethnic, and cultural identities of patients and physicians influenced the expectation of mutual understanding [39,44,45]. On the one hand, foreign patients exhibit less assertiveness and verbal expressiveness and experience difficulties in using effective conversation strategies. On the other hand, physicians showed greater emotional detachment, adopted more directive behavior, and spent less time explaining the disease and treatment to foreign patients.

The few studies investigating PCC in the intercultural context underline physicians' difficulties in building patient-centered interactions and the communication needs of foreign patients during medical visits. Research with migrant women highlighted barriers to the implementation of PCC due to language, the poor training of doctors, and organizational difficulties within hospitals and the health care system. Research also highlighted the need for doctors to have more knowledge about how to establish a PCC with migrant patients and the lack of attention given by health professionals to their concerns and questions. These patients also emphasized the need for more information and time to discuss their condition with professionals [46]. Studies conducted in the US on PPC in ethnic minorities showed that compared to white men, black and Hispanic/Latino patients reported fewer experiences of patient-centered medical visits, greater unmet needs, more significant experiences of discrimination, and dissatisfaction with treatment discussions [47]. Similarly, studies conducted in the US and Canada with Asian-American and Asian-Canadian cancer patients (male and female) reported that they were less likely to be involved in treatment decisions compared to white patients, and language was the main factor contributing to perceived disparities [47–51]. On the other hand, studies investigating the positive effects of PCC on the experiences of migrant patients showed that satisfaction with the care received increased, regardless of the racial concordance between the doctor and the patient. This increase was observed when the specialist spent time with the patient, informed and explained the patient's health condition, showed support, and involved the patient in treatment decisions [52,53].

Drawing on a corpus of video recording of oncology visits, the present study aims to contribute to the literature by exploring PCC practices in the Italian medical context. Italian medical context is understudied in relation to PCC practices with ethnically diverse groups. Our first objective is to explore potential differences in PCC practices in two kinds of medical encounters: oncology visits between Italian doctors and Italian patients and oncology visits between Italian doctors and foreign patients. Our second objective is to verify if the differences in PCC depend on the type of visit and the presence/absence of companions. Finally, we analyzed the effects on the PCC of six non-interacting variables, including the type of encounter, age of the oncologist, age of the patient, patient's gender, the presence of a companion, and the nationality of the patient.

## 2. Materials and Methods

### 2.1. Participants

The video-recorded medical visits analyzed in this study were collected in the oncology unit of a medium-sized Italian hospital operated by a Religious Order during ethnographic research in 2019. The research received approval from the Ethics Committee of the hospital (Prot. No. 1886/CE Lazio) and the Ethics Committee of the Department of Social and Developmental Psychology, Sapienza University of Rome (Prot. No. 0000944). These videos included interactions between eight different oncologists (equally distributed by gender) and 42 patients, of which 22 were Italian (17 women, age M = 57 years; 5 men, M age = 71) and 20 foreigners (15 women, M age = 52 years; 5 men, M age = 61). The foreign patients' countries of birth were Romania, Peru, Albania, USA, Moldova, Cameroon, Bulgaria, Ecuador, Kosovo, Egypt, Poland, the Philippines, Ukraine, Mexico, and Paraguay. The heterogeneity of the ethnic background of these patients reflects the inhomogeneity of the Italian context. According to census data [54], foreigners residing in Italy as of 1 January 2022, number 5,030,716 and account for 8.5 percent of the total population. Except for Romanians, who account for about 20% of all foreign residents, there are four groups each representing 5–10%, and 12 groups each representing between 1 and 5%. Friends or relatives accompanied eleven Italian and nine foreign patients in the examination room. The most common neoplasms among the participants were breast cancer (42.9%), followed by gastrointestinal stromal tumors (21.4%), gynecological cancers (11.9%), lung cancer (11.9%) and head and neck cancer, urological cancers, neuroendocrine tumors, liver cancer and lymphoma tumors (2.4% each). Italian language proficiency was assessed retrospectively to avoid selection bias. Specifically, video-recorded visits were coded using the indicators included in the Common European Reference Framework for Languages [55], and a language proficiency score (encompassing both comprehension and production) was assigned to each patient. Ninety percent of the patients demonstrated at least a sufficient knowledge of the Italian language, and 65% of them were highly proficient. Generally, patients with lower competence in the Italian language were those who were accompanied most frequently.

### 2.2. Materials and Procedure

This corpus consisted of 42 video recordings, selected to represent a diverse range of encounters, such as follows: (a) first-time, post-surgical encounters; (b) follow-up oncological visits; (c) intercultural oncological encounters with foreign patients; (d) oncological visits with Italian patients. By including diverse encounters, our goal was to provide comprehensive coverage of communication dynamics in different contexts within the oncology setting. We collected data during the first time post-surgical visits (20 in total, equally distributed by foreign and Italian patients) and follow-up visits (22 in total, ten with foreign patients and twelve with Italian patients). Oncologists, patients, and companions were invited to participate in the study while waiting for their appointment. Those who agreed to participate were asked to sign a written informed consent form to take part in the study and allow video recording of the visit. A video camera was placed in the examination room, focusing on the patients, companions, and physicians interacting.

We used the ONCode tool to assess PCC during over 13,000 interaction turns, amounting to a total of 18 h of oncological visits. ONCode is a new coding system specifically developed to capture doctor–patient communication practices in post-surgical oncological encounters [56]. It was developed based on video-recorded consultations in Italian hospitals from 2012 to 2020. ONCode is grounded in emic notions of PCC, together with evidence and definitions provided by the literature [57–59]. Moreover, previous studies provided the ground for a situated definition of the PCC dimensions used in ONCode. Prior work provided an empirical ground for understanding how patient-centered communication unfolds within the cultural, organizational, and medical constraints of oncological consultations in Italy [60–64] while also documenting the overall structural organization of these oncology consultations, which routinely include a sequence of stages and activities [65–68]. By examining the extent to which and how each participant (i.e., doctor, patient, and companion, if present) participated in various communicative actions, ONCode provides the following interactive dimension scores: physician's communicative behavior (DCB), patient's initiatives (PI), misalignments between doctor and patient (MIS), interruptions in visits (INT), accountability and expressions of trust in the talk (ACC), markers of uncertainty in doctor's talk (MOU), and markers of emotions in doctor's talk (MOE). In a previous study [56], ONCode scores displayed good reliability even when employed by a single observer and had incremental validity above other existing coding systems for analyzing

PCC. Table 1 reports a thorough description of each score, including operative definitions and examples. In the present study, we also considered the following non-interactional variables as potentially affecting PCC: the age of the oncologist, patient's age, patient's sex, type of encounter, presence of a companion during the visit, and patient's nationality.

**Table 1.** ONCode dimensions, operative definitions, and examples.

| ONCode Dimension | Operative Definition | Examples |
|---|---|---|
| Doctor's communicative behavior (DCB) | We observed how the doctor accomplished the activities at each stage of the consultation. It concerns affective, instrumental and participation verbal and non-verbal behaviors, which can be present about the activity in progress in each phase. | Some communicative actions included how the doctor recommended a treatment, prescribed the following examinations, or delivered the diagnosis. We relied on linguistic actions, such as questions, meta-pragmatic formulations, explanations, and recommendations. Additionally, we noted whether and how the doctor engaged in small talk, used humor, and allowed the patient to propose questions and initiatives of interest to her or him. |
| Patient's initiatives (and companion) (PI) | We observed whether and how the patient and companion co-constructed the encounter. | We examined each patient and companion communication action during each stage of the visit, including whether patients and their companion took initiatives, such as asking questions, expressing concerns, proposing a topic, or simply aligning with what the doctor said or asked. |
| Misalignments (MIS) | We observed whether a fracture in the co-orientation of participants toward the same activity or in the understanding of the topic had occurred. | What is evaluated is whether, and with what effort, the participants repaired the fracture and reached an agreement or, instead, remained in distant positions. |
| Interruptions (INT) | We observed interruptions in all the moments in which the consultation was suspended due to matters that did not concern the current consultation and the patient. We checked for interruptions at each stage of the consultation. | Interruptions included phone calls, the doctor leaving the room, exchanges with the nurse, or other doctors entering the room. Interruptions due to systematic organizational routines (e.g., the doctor goes out to photocopy the patient's exams) were not counted. |
| Accountability and expressions of trust in participants' talk (ACC) | We observed how the doctor made her/himself accountable to the patient by providing access to her/his medical knowledge and reasoning. We also assessed if the patient topicalized trust and confidence in the doctor discourse. | The accountability involves explaining the rationale used for recommending treatment, providing alternative options for treatment, and using metapragmatic markers that help the patient orient themselves within the consultation activities. Furthermore, we coded expressions of trust and confidence in patient discourse in the oncology, such as "If the doctor says so, I will do it" or "You are the doctor, and I trust what you say". |
| Markers of uncertainty in doctor's talk (MOU) | We observed mentions of uncertainty in the doctor's talk, that is, when the doctor showed uncertainty about the treatment outcomes, test results, or treatment possibilities | They refer to all those occasions when the doctor showed uncertainty in their speech by using modalized or evidential moods, reference to probability, emphasizing small benefits, expressing uncertainty of outcomes and test results (e.g., "The recommendation for treatment is not absolute in my opinion, but I tend to prescribe it"). |
| Markers of emotions in doctor's talk (MOE) | We observed whether there were occasions during the doctor's conversation when he/she expressed verbal and non-verbal socio-affective behaviors | We observed whether there were sequences of reassurance (e.g., the doctor highlights positive sides of the situation), jokes or humor, the doctor's response to emotional concerns expressed by the patient, and whether the doctor gestures of support such as touching hands. |

### 2.3. Statistical Analysis

The skewness and kurtosis statistics of the seven ONCode scores ranged between −2 and +2, suggesting that the assumption of normality has not been violated, and parametric statistics can be applied [69]. Furthermore, the presence of heteroscedasticity was checked, and it was found that all the residuals were homoscedastic. To determine whether there are differences in PCC between visits with Italian and foreign patients, a discriminant analysis was carried out on the seven ONCode scores, considered simultaneously. Similarly, to examine whether there were differences in the PCC within the corpus based on the type of visit and the presence of the companion, two additional discriminant analyses were carried out on the seven ONCode interactive dimensions, considering them simultaneously. Finally, to analyze the effect of the noninteractive variables (i.e., age of the oncologist, patient's age, patient's sex, type of encounter, presence of companion during the visit, and patient's nationality) on the ONCode interactive dimensions, seven separate multiple standard regressions were performed for each interactive dimension of the system, while ruling out multicollinearity issues. All of the analyses were performed using STATISTICA 13.

## 3. Results

### 3.1. Discriminant Function Analyses

In the first discriminant analysis, the investigation focused on examining the presence of differences in PCC between the Italian patient group and the foreign patient group using the patient's nationality as the group factor. However, Fisher's F value was found to be nonsignificant, $F (7, 34) = 0.446$, $p = 0.86$. The seven ONCode scores did not discriminate between the groups, nor did they make a unique significant contribution to the discrimination between the groups. Thus, no differences in PCC were found during visits depending on whether the patients belonged to the Italian or foreign group of patients.

In the second discriminant analysis, the presence or absence of the accompanying person considered during the visits was considered the grouping factor. The main results are reported in Table 2. The overall model was not statistically significant in discriminating between the groups based on the presence of a companion, $F (7, 34) = 1.62$, $p < 0.16$. A closer examination of the individual variables showed that none of them individually contributed significantly to the discrimination between the groups, except for interruptions (INT) with partial Lambda of 0.84, $p < 0.01$. The frequency of interruptions played a role in differentiating between the groups, and this variable's contribution to distinguishing unaccompanied patients from accompanied ones was independent of any contributions made by other variables.

As shown in Table 3, the number of interruptions during visits increased when the patient was accompanied.

The last discriminant analysis considered the type of encounter, comparing the group of first visits with the group of follow-up visits (Table 4). The significant omnibus test, $F (7, 34) = 3.17$, $p = 0.01$, indicated that the set of variables considered discriminated between the types of encounters. The analysis also revealed that interruptions (INT) had the highest F-remove value (3.18) and the lowest $p$-level (0.08), suggesting that they may be the most important ONCode variable to distinguish between first visits and follow-ups. Other variables, such as doctor's communicative behavior (DCB), accountability and expressions of trust in participants' talk (ACC), and markers of uncertainty in doctor's talk (MOU), also had relatively high F-remove values and low $p$-levels, indicating that they may contribute to the differences between the two groups as well.

Although no individual variable (partial Lambda) reached the conventional levels of statistical significance, the overall analysis of discriminant functions was significant, indicating a significant difference between the two groups when considering all variables collectively. This finding suggests that a multivariate effect may have obscured the univariate effects of the variables, making it challenging to determine the individual contributions of each variable to the differences between the two groups.

**Table 2.** Discriminant Function Analysis Summary for presence of accompanying person (Unaccompanied Patient vs. accompanied Patient).

| N = 42 | **Discriminant Function Analysis Summary<br>No. of Vars in Model: 7; Grouping: Companion (2 Groups)<br>Wilks' Lambda: 0.75 Approx. F (7, 34) = 1.62 *p* = 0.164** | | | | | |
|---|---|---|---|---|---|---|
| | **Wilks' Lambda** | **Partial Lambda** | **F-Remove (1, 34)** | ***p*-Level** | **Toler.** | **1-Toler (R-Sqr.)** |
| Doctor's communicative behavior (DCB) | 0.76 | 0.99 | 0.34 | 0.56 | 0.50 | 0.50 |
| Patient's initiatives (and companion) (PI) | 0.76 | 0.98 | 0.61 | 0.44 | 0.58 | 0.42 |
| Misalignments (MIS) | 0.78 | 0.96 | 1.44 | 0.24 | 0.89 | 0.11 |
| Interruptions (INT) | 0.90 | 0.84 | 6.69 | 0.01 | 0.80 | 0.20 |
| Accountability and expressions of trust in participants' talk (ACC) | 0.76 | 0.99 | 0.31 | 0.59 | 0.61 | 0.39 |
| Markers of uncertainty in doctor's talk (MOU) | 0.79 | 0.95 | 1.85 | 0.18 | 0.90 | 0.10 |
| Markers of emotions in doctor's talk (MOE) | 0.76 | 0.99 | 0.35 | 0.56 | 0.81 | 0.19 |

**Table 3.** Means for the presence of an accompanying person (Unaccompanied patient vs. accompanied patient).

| **Companion** | **Means** | | | | | | | |
|---|---|---|---|---|---|---|---|---|
| | **DCB** | **PI** | **MIS** | **INT** | **ACC** | **MOU** | **MOE** | **Valid N** |
| Unaccompanied | 8.63 | 4.58 | 3.63 | 0.54 | 1.33 | 0.33 | 1.63 | 24 |
| Accompanied | 9.17 | 4.78 | 3.00 | 1.11 | .22 | 0.50 | 1.78 | 18 |
| all Groups | 8.86 | 4.67 | 3.36 | 0.79 | 1.29 | 0.41 | 1.69 | 42 |

Legend: DCB = doctor's communicative behavior; PI = patient initiatives (and companion); MIS = misalignments; INT = interruptions; ACC = accountability and expressions of trust in participants' talk; MOU = markers of uncertainty in the doctor's talk; MOE = markers of emotions in doctor's talk (MOE).

**Table 4.** Discriminant Function Analysis Summary for type of encounter (Follow-up vs. First Visit).

| N = 42 | **Discriminant Function Analysis Summary<br>No. of Vars in Model: 7; Grouping: Type of Encounter (2 Groups)<br>Wilks' Lambda: 0.61 Approx. F (7, 34) = 3.12 *p* < 0.05** | | | | | |
|---|---|---|---|---|---|---|
| | **Wilks' Lambda** | **Partial Lambda** | **F-Remove (1, 34)** | ***p*-Level** | **Toler.** | **1-Toler (R-Sqr.)** |
| Doctor's communicative behavior (DCB) | 0.65 | 0.93 | 2.69 | 0.11 | 0.56 | 0.44 |
| Patient initiatives (and companion) (PI) | 0.63 | 0.97 | 1.08 | 0.31 | 0.58 | 0.42 |
| Misalignments (MIS) | 0.62 | 0.98 | 0.81 | 0.37 | 0.90 | 0.10 |
| Interruptions (INT) | 0.66 | 0.92 | 3.18 | 0.08 | 0.77 | 0.23 |
| Accountability and expressions of trust in participants' talk (ACC) | 0.65 | 0.93 | 2.66 | 0.11 | 0.71 | 0.29 |
| Markers of uncertainty in doctor's talk (MOU) | 0.65 | 0.93 | 2.63 | 0.11 | 0.93 | 0.71 |
| Markers of emotions in doctor's talk (MOE) | 0.63 | 0.96 | 1.48 | 0.23 | 0.79 | 0.21 |

Examining the standardized coefficients of the discriminant function reported in Table 5 can be an appropriate analytic approach to identify the variables that contributed the most to discrimination between first visits and follow-ups within the context of a significant multivariate effect. This approach allowed us to better understand the complexity of the multivariate effect and gain insights into the relative importance of each variable in differentiating PCC by type of encounter.

**Table 5.** Standardized Coefficients for Canonical Variables.

| ONCode Dimensions | Standardized Coefficients for Canonical Variables |
|---|---|
| | Root 1 |
| Doctor's communicative behavior (DCB) | 0.58 |
| Patient's initiatives (and companion) (PI) | −0.37 |
| Misalignments (MIS) | −0.26 |
| Interruptions (INT) | 0.53 |
| Accountability and expressions of trust in participants' talk (ACC) | 0.51 |
| Markers of uncertainty in doctor's talk (MOU) | 0.44 |
| Markers of emotions in doctor's talk (MOE) | −0.37 |

Using a cut-off point of 0.50 for interpretation, Table 5 revealed that doctor communicative behavior (DCB), interruptions (INT), and accountability and expressions of trust in participants' talk (ACC) had the strongest positive coefficients, indicating that these variables were more prominent in distinguishing the two groups. The markers of uncertainty in doctor's talk (MOU) had a moderate positive coefficient, indicating a moderate contribution to the differences between the groups. On the other hand, patient's initiatives (and companion) (PI), misalignments (MIS), and markers of emotions in doctor's talk (MOE) had negative coefficients, suggesting that these variables were less influential in differentiating between encounters.

As shown in Table 6, the ONCode dimensions that had the greatest influence on the discriminant function (i.e., doctor communication behavior, interruptions, accountability, and expressions of trust) were higher in first-visit encounters. Similarly, markers of uncertainty were higher during first-visit encounters, but this ONCode dimension had a lower weight on the discriminant function.

**Table 6.** Means for type of encounter (follow-up vs. first visit).

| Type of Encounter | Means | | | | | | | |
|---|---|---|---|---|---|---|---|---|
| | DCB | PI | MIS | INT | ACC | MOU | MOE | Valid N |
| Follow-up | 8.09 | 4.55 | 3.59 | 0.64 | 0.91 | 0.27 | 1.77 | 22 |
| First Visit | 9.70 | 4.80 | 3.10 | 0.95 | 1.70 | 0.55 | 1.60 | 20 |
| all Groups | 8.86 | 4.67 | 3.36 | 0.79 | 1.29 | 0.41 | 1.69 | 42 |

Legend: DCB = doctor's communicative behavior; PI = patient's initiatives (and companion); MIS = misalignments; INT = interruptions; ACC = accountability and expressions of trust in participants' talk; MOU = markers of uncertainty in doctor's talk; MOE = markers of emotions in doctor's talk (MOE).

Anticipating the discussion, more interruptions occurred during initial oncology visits than during follow-up visits, possibly due to the longer duration of first-time encounters or the increased participation of companions. Furthermore, oncologists used more PCC strategies during initial consultations than during follow-up visits. This was also related to the presence of trust and responsibility expressions in the conversations. In fact, during the initial appointments, doctors provided diagnostic explanations that supported the choice of medical treatments that patients would need to follow over time.

The ONCode scores were able to correctly classify 82% of the follow-up visits, while first visits were correctly classified in 75% of the cases. This result underscores the strong discriminatory ability of all dimensions of the ONCode in distinguishing between types of visits. Additionally, the square of the canonical correlation coefficient (Canonical $R^2 = 0.39$;

$Chi^2 = 18.32$, df = 7, $p < 0.05$) indicated that the set of variables explained approximately 40% of the variance in the PCC due to differences in the type of encounters.

*3.2. Regression Analyses*

We conducted seven multiple standard regression analyses, one for each dimension of the ONCode, using the non-interactive variables collected in the present study as predictors: oncologist age, patient age, patient sex, type of interaction, presence of a companion during the visit, and patient nationality. The only significant analysis was for interruptions (INT) as the dependent variable. As shown in Table 7, there was a significant relationship between interruptions and several variables, namely the age of the oncologist, the nationality of the participant, and the presence of the companion. These variables significantly contributed to the prediction of interruptions, $R^2 = 0.37$, $p < 0.01$, and F (6, 35) = 3.47. The beta coefficient for each variable was positive, indicating that higher values on these variables were associated with a higher frequency of interruptions. Specifically, older oncologists ($\beta = 0.44$), patients from foreign countries ($\beta = 0.31$), and the presence of a companion during the visit ($\beta = 0.49$) were associated with more interruptions during the medical encounters. The other variables, including the type of encounter, patient's age, and patient's sex, did not significantly contribute to the prediction of interruptions.

**Table 7.** Regression summary for dependent variable interruption.

| N = 42 | **Regression Summary for Dependent Variable: Interruption R = 0.61 $R^2$ = 0.37 Adjusted $R^2$ = 0.26 F (6, 35) = 3.47 *p* < 0.01 Std. Error of Estimate: 0.62** | | | | | |
|---|---|---|---|---|---|---|
| | **Beta** | **Std. Err. of Beta** | **B** | **Std. Err. of B** | **t(35)** | ***p*-Level** |
| Intercept | | | −1.21 | 0.83 | −1.47 | 0.15 |
| Type of Encounter | −0.05 | 0.15 | −0.07 | 0.22 | −0.34 | 0.73 |
| Oncologist's age | 0.44 | 0.15 | 0.03 | 0.01 | 2.94 | 0.01 |
| Patient's age | −0.01 | 0.16 | 0.00 | 0.01 | −0.04 | 0.97 |
| Patient's sex | 0.05 | 0.15 | 0.08 | 0.24 | 0.32 | 0.75 |
| Companion's presence | 0.49 | 0.15 | 0.70 | 0.21 | 3.30 | 0.00 |
| Patient's nationality | 0.31 | 0.15 | 0.44 | 0.21 | 2.13 | 0.04 |

All independent variables had relatively low levels of redundancy, as shown in Table 8, and each made a unique contribution to the prediction of interruptions.

**Table 8.** Redundancy of independent variables and DV interruption.

| **Variable** | **Redundancy of Independent Variables; DV: Interruption The R-Square Column Contains the R-Square of the Respective Variable with All Other Independent Variables** | | | |
|---|---|---|---|---|
| | **Toleran.** | **R-Square** | **Partial Cor.** | **Semipart Cor** |
| Type of Encounter | 0.77 | 0.23 | −0.06 | −0.05 |
| Oncologists' age | 0.82 | 0.19 | 0.45 | 0.39 |
| Patients' age | 0.72 | 0.28 | −0.01 | −0.01 |
| Patients' gender | 0.85 | 0.15 | 0.06 | 0.04 |
| Companions' presence | 0.81 | 0.19 | 0.49 | 0.44 |
| Patients' nationality | 0.85 | 0.15 | 0.34 | 0.29 |

Since the beta values of the three variables were significant, we can compare their unique contributions by squaring the semipartial correlations shown in Table 9. The results indicated that the presence of a companion had the highest semi-partial correlation (0.44), followed by oncologist age (0.39) and patient nationality (0.29). These variables were the most important predictors of oncological visits, and there were no collinearity issues in the analysis.

**Table 9.** Semi-partial correlations between the VIs and the DV interruption.

| Independent Variables | Semipartial Correlation | % Explained Variance |
|---|---|---|
| Type of Encounter | −0.05 | 0.21 |
| Oncologists' age | 0.39 | 15.46 |
| Patients' age | −0.01 | 0.00 |
| Patients' gender | 0.04 | 0.19 |
| Companions' presence | 0.44 | 19.44 |
| Patients' Nationality (groups) | 0.29 | 8.13 |

It should be noted that in the discriminant analyses, the ONCode variables (including interruptions) did not differentiate patients by nationality. However, in the regression, belonging to the Italian or foreign patient group appears to be a significant predictor of the "interruptions" variable. This discrepancy is likely due to the contribution of the other variables included in the regression, such as the patient's age and gender, which may have acted as "suppressors" [70] of the variance related to nationality that was not directly associated with the "interruptions" variable. As a result, there was an increase in the component of "unique" variance shared between nationality and interruptions.

### 3.3. *Qualitative Analyses*

Prompted by regression analysis, we conducted a qualitative analysis of the interruption occurrences to gain a deeper understanding of the interruptions that occurred throughout the encounters. Our analysis revealed that oncologists aged over 40 experienced interruptions more frequently than their younger counterparts. The interruptions experienced by older oncologists included requests for advice, comments, and comparisons from peers in the same specialty about other patients, consultations from other specialists (such as radiotherapists) regarding ongoing treatments for shared patients, the secretary entering the room to ask for information and/or resolve issues with patients and/or appointments, the secretary entering the room to collect or return medical records, a patient leaving the room. The head of the department, being one of the senior oncologists, experienced the most interruptions during visits. These interruptions were not only for the reasons mentioned above but also due to the need to address issues related to the management and organization of the oncology department. The "nature" of the interruptions, especially those involving requests from other coworkers (such as seeking advice on another patient's ongoing treatment or seeking information on a specific case) and/or consultations from other specialists (such as discussing the possibility of performing radiotherapy on a patient), was a practice that, in this corpus, was observed only in the visits of experienced oncologists with several years of clinical practice and who had been collaborating with other oncologists for an extended period. The consultations with younger oncologists (under 40 years old) were occasionally interrupted and typically for non-organizational reasons, such as the secretary entering the room or the doctor's mobile phone ringing.

To gain a better understanding of the reasons for interruptions during visits with foreign patients, we focused on distinguishing between different sources of interruptions. Specifically, we categorized interruptions into two groups: those originating from outside the examination room (e.g., the secretary knocking on the door or phone ringing) and those originating from inside the room (e.g., the doctor leaving the room or making unrelated phone calls during the consultation). Our findings indicated that interruptions during visits with Italian patients were primarily attributed to external events that involved only the oncologist or hospital staff. However, in four instances during intercultural visits, the interruption of the visit could be attributed to phone calls made to the private mobile phones of patients and caregivers. Additionally, visits with foreign patients experienced interruptions due to internal events that originated from the oncologists themselves. For instance, on six occasions, the oncologist made phone calls for professional or organizational activities that were unrelated to the ongoing visit. Thus, in contrast to visits with Italian patients, visits with foreign patients were more susceptible to interruptions caused by both external events affecting patients and their companions as well as internal events initiated by the oncologist.

## 4. Discussion

Using a corpus of video recordings of oncology visits and a recently developed observational coding system (ONCode), the present study aimed to explore PCC practices with cancer patients in an Italian religious-order-operated hospital. Our first objective was to investigate differences in PCC practices in medical encounters between Italian doctors and Italian patients and those involving Italian doctors and foreign patients. Previous research addressing this issue has reported differences in communication practices during intercultural encounters with foreign patients, highlighting the role of linguistic, cultural, and ethnic backgrounds [33–40]. Language has been identified as a primary contributing factor to difficulties in PCC [48–51]. However, doctor training and organizational challenges within hospitals and healthcare systems have also been reported as barriers to effective PCC [46,48–51]. For example, foreign patients have expressed the need for more information and time to discuss their condition with healthcare professionals rather than complaining about linguistic problems [46]. Furthermore, studies conducted internationally have shown that patients from ethnic minorities typically report fewer patient-centered medical visits and more experiences of discrimination compared to white men. For example, qualitative analyses in oncology indicated that black and Hispanic men had more unmet needs during interactions with physicians, received fewer inquiries about their preferences and priorities, and expressed greater dissatisfaction with long-term treatment discussions [47,71,72].

Our research found limited evidence of differences in PCC practices between medical encounters with Italian and foreign patients. In fact, we observed that factors such as nationality and ethnic background had less influence on PCC practices compared to other interactive and non-interactive variables. This contrasts with the findings of most international studies that have emphasized the impact of nationality and ethnic background on PCC practices [33–43]. However, it is important to note that implementing PCC has the potential to bridge the racial and cultural differences between doctors and patients, and it can have a positive impact not only on both native and foreign patients. In this vein, our results align with previous research that has highlighted the positive effects of PCC on patients with a migrant background in the US [46,52,53]. Paraphrasing Chu et al. [53], PCC "is key to reducing disparities and improving immigrant patients' satisfaction level with medical care".

In addition to that, it is critical to recognize that our study was conducted within a specific context with its own unique constraints, and further research is needed to gain a comprehensive understanding of PCC in intercultural contacts in Italy. First, the lack of discernible changes between visits by Italian and foreign patients could be attributed to specific features of organizational culture. This religious hospital claims and emphasizes in its mission the centrality of each person in the care process, with particular attention to minority and vulnerable groups, including migrant and foreign patients. This aligns with recent research suggesting that religious hospitals promote a more inclusive and respectful atmosphere, leading to a higher quality of care. This interpretation is consistent with a recent Italian study that examined the differences in the provision of support to cancer patients undergoing chemotherapy between oncologists in a religious hospital and those in a government-operated hospital [73]. Second, it is worth noting that research on PCC with foreign patients in Italy is still in its early stages, and there is a lack of studies specifically examining the impact of language difficulties. While it is possible that linguistic factors may have been less influential in our study, as almost all patients had sufficient knowledge of the Italian language and had good proficiency levels, it is crucial to recognize that patients with good proficiency may still struggle to understand medical terminology in a foreign language. These language barriers can lead to misunderstandings, difficulties in fully comprehending medical information, and a potential lack of trust in healthcare professionals. More research is needed to understand how language difficulties can affect PCC for foreign patients in Italy.

The second objective of the present study was to determine whether PCC was different between first visits and follow-ups or dependent on the presence or absence of an accompanying person. In fact, companions can both facilitate doctor–patient communication and provide support to cancer patients while sometimes being seen as obtrusive, particularly with elderly or vulnerable patients in advanced stages of illness [66,74–76]. Therefore, we speculated that the presence of an accompanying person could facilitate intercultural encounters, providing informational and affective support to foreign patients. In our study, however, the presence of an accompanying person and being a foreign patient were found to play a role only in relation to interruptions during the visit. Before discussing this finding, it is worth noting that the oncologist's age, and thus their role as an organizational senior, was also found to predict PCC categories, and in particular, the interruptions.

In the ONCode framework, interruptions included events such as phone calls, the doctor leaving the room because of matters that did not concern the current consultation and the patient, exchanges with the nurse, or other doctors entering the room. During first-time visits, interruptions occurred more frequently than during follow-up visits. This finding might be attributed to the longer duration of these encounters, which could make them more likely to be interrupted by external events. The fact that the doctor's age predicted the frequency of interruptions could be attributed to the recognized expertise within the medical team and their greater involvement in organizational matters, a finding that resonates with previous research that considered organizational challenges to be impeding effective PCC [46,48–51].

To gain further insight into interruptions in terms of PCC practices, we conducted a qualitative analysis to examine the specific nature of interruptions during the visits. Our analysis revealed that encounters with younger oncologists were characterized by sporadic interruptions, such as the secretary entering the room or the doctor's mobile phone ringing for consultations. In contrast, older oncologists experienced more frequent interruptions due to a variety of reasons, including requests for consultation, expert opinions, and discussions with colleagues in the same specialty, consultations from other specialists, secretaries entering the room for information, problem solving, or medical record collection, and occasionally personal mobile phone ringing. Among senior oncologists, the head of the department experienced the most frequent interruptions, which were often related to additional responsibilities associated with their organizational position and management of the oncology department. These types of interruptions were only observed in oncology visits involving doctors with extensive clinical experience and long-term collaboration with the oncology department.

The finding that older oncologists faced more interruptions could indicate their greater experience and the demand for their advice and consultations. However, it could also imply a lack of adequate organizational support to effectively manage their time and minimize interruptions. Additionally, the observation of interruptions from colleagues and specialists exclusively in visits of oncologists with several years of clinical practice and long-term collaboration with the oncology department raises interesting questions about the influence of professional networks and organizational culture on clinical practice. These insights highlight the need for further research to enhance our understanding of the factors contributing to interruptions in oncology encounters and their implications for patient care.

Understanding why the frequency of interruptions increased in the presence of foreign patients was more challenging. While visits with Italian patients were predominantly interrupted from outside and involved only the oncologist or hospital staff, visits with foreign patients were interrupted from outside but also involved the patient and the companion. In fact, on four occasions, the interruption of the visit can be traced to the telephone calls made to the private mobile phones of patients and companions. Furthermore, on six occasions, it was necessary to interrupt the interaction due to events occurring during the visit; that is, the oncologist interrupted the communicative action with the patient to devote themselves to activities not related to the event in progress. However, on one occasion, the researcher in the room interrupts the visit. Therefore, unlike what happens in visits with Italian patients, it is possible that in the presence of foreign patients, visits are more likely to be interrupted by: (a) external events that also affect patients and their companions, (b) internal events that concern interruptions made by the doctors and sometimes by other participants in the visit. In the first case, contrary to what happened in visits with Italian patients, foreign patients and their companions contributed to interrupting the visit in the same way as the oncologists did: by maintaining contact with the outside world during the interaction and by answering the telephone. In the second case, only in cross-cultural visits did we observe within-site interruptions that originated from the oncologist.

All these findings were unexpected and emerged only after a qualitative analysis. It is possible that in the encounter between an Italian doctor and foreign patients, there are implicit signals on both sides that prime interruptions. Previous research has often interpreted the suspensions of the visit as negative events for PCC [77–79]. However, interruptions should not necessarily be seen as negative events. For example, communication interruptions can lead to more patient (or companion) initiatives, such as asking questions or seeking clarification or explanation [80]. The qualitative analysis suggested notable differences in the types of interruptions that occur during visits with foreign patients compared to Italian patients. Interruptions during visits with Italian patients were primarily due to external events caused by hospital staff or the oncologist. On the contrary, visits with foreign patients were disrupted by both external events and internal events initiated by the oncologist. These findings may suggest that foreign patients require additional attention from healthcare professionals to maximize the quality of patient-centered care. If these differences are replicated, an avenue for future research could investigate the antecedents of interruptions in both same the culture and intercultural encounters.

*Limitations*

Although this work provided encouraging results on PCC in intercultural medical encounters, it is important to highlight the limitations of our research and the possibilities for future studies to address these problematic knots. The sensitivity of the collected data and the complexity of the context in which the oncological encounters were videotaped determined the first limitation of this study, represented by the limited number of participants. While the limited number of participants and the partial repetition of oncologists' communication characteristics and behaviors pose research limitations, this data set is valuable, despite the statistical constraint on the number of visits. Future research could leverage larger data sets and ensure enough visits per oncologist. However, it is worth noting that the study's novelty and importance lie in its analysis of over 13,000 interaction turns from 18 h of oncological visits, providing a rare view of the negotiation and co-construction of PCC in real intercultural interactions. Despite its complexity, such research into PCC as a multidimensional construct is scarce, underlining this study's value.

Another aspect to be considered is the use of oncologists in the analyses as partially repeated measures. Given that there were eight oncologists, it would be expected that each would show 'consistent' behaviors from one visit to the next, thus contributing to the results to some extent. With a larger corpus of available data, each oncologist would have had more visits. It would have been possible to evaluate the effects of the oncologists' characteristics as clusters, separately from those of the other variables, using multilevel analysis. With these considerations in mind, future research could look at larger datasets with enough visits per oncologist. Finally, the study highlighted the role of interruptions during encounters as opportunities especially exploited by foreign patients.

Future qualitative research could explore further which kind of use participants make of such breaks in the ongoing communication during the visits.

## 5. Conclusions

The use of ONCode provided statistically significant results that illustrated how PCC was negotiated and co-constructed between all participants in the visit. In fact, the doctor, the patient, and the companion contributed equally to the development of the oncological encounter. Our findings shed new light on oncology visits and the challenges oncologists must manage daily in clinical practice. These challenges result in concerns about interactional and local features of the unfolding communication event rather than individual patient characteristics (i.e., nationality). Managing the sequential unfolding of the activities of the different types of visits while handling organizational matters and maintaining a patient-centered focus in communication could be quite challenging for physicians.

Based on the findings of the present study, we can suggest some practical implications for healthcare providers to improve PCC in oncology. First, doctors should pay attention to the interruptions during visits, especially with foreign patients, and to the overall management of the unfolding interaction in intercultural encounters. Medical education interventions might target this topic by sustaining doctors' reflexive awareness of their interactional practices while helping them to create a more conducive and respectful environment for the patient. Second, although linguistic issues have been highlighted as a contributing factor to PCC difficulties, our study discovered that even when foreign patients have enough linguistic competence, healthcare providers should not rely only on this element to assume good communication and quality care. Instead, they should prioritize PCC, especially in international interactions, to maintain patient-centeredness. Third, the finding was that PCC was similar between Italian and foreign patients in the context of a religious-operated hospital. Future studies are needed to verify and further explore this finding that, if confirmed, might contribute to support and promote the humanization of health care.

**Author Contributions:** F.M.: Conceptualization, Methodology, Validation, Formal Analysis, Investigation, Data Curation, Writing—original draft, Writing—Review and editing; F.A.: Conceptualization, Methodology, Validation, Investigation, Data Curation, Writing—Review and editing; C.Z.: Conceptualization, Methodology, Validation, Investigation, Data Curation, Writing—Review and editing, Supervision; T.G.S.: Methodology, Software, Formal Analysis, Writing—Review and editing; M.L.: Writing—Review and editing, Project Administration, Funding Acquisition. All authors have read and agreed to the published version of the manuscript.

**Funding:** The research leading to these results received funding from Sapienza University of Rome under Grant Agreement No. RM11916B7E07E816.

**Institutional Review Board Statement:** The study protocol was approved by the Ethics Committee of Lazio Region (1886/CE Lazio) and the Ethics Committee of the Social and Developmental Psychology, Sapienza University of Rome (Prot. No.0000944).

**Informed Consent Statement:** Informed consent was obtained from all oncologists, patients, and accompanying persons.

**Data Availability Statement:** The entire data corpus used in this study is not publicly available for privacy reasons. The collected video recordings of oncology encounters contain sensitive information that cannot be shared because it could compromise the privacy of the research participants. The data that support the findings of this study are available from the corresponding author, F.M., upon request.

**Acknowledgments:** The authors wish to thank all medical professionals and healthcare teams involved in the study. The authors also express sincere gratitude to all patients and their accompanying persons for participating in this study.

**Conflicts of Interest:** The authors declare no conflict of interest.

## References


1. Epstein, R.M.; Street, R.L. *Patient-Centered Communication in Cancer Care: Promoting Healing and Reducing Suffering*; National Cancer Institute, NIH Publication: Bethesda, MA, USA, 2007.
2. American Society of Clinical Oncology. *Patient-Clinician Communication: American Society of Clinical Oncology Consensus Guideline 2017*; American Society of Clinical Oncology: Alexandria, VA, USA, 2017.
3. Bensing, J.M.; Dronkers, J. Instrumental and Affective Aspects of Physician Behavior. *Med. Care* **1992**, *30*, 283–298. [CrossRef]
4. Venetis, M.; Robinson, J.D.; Turkiewicz, K.L.; Allen, M. An evidence base for patient-centered cancer care: A meta-analysis of studies of observed communication between cancer specialists and their patients. *Patient Educ. Couns.* **2009**, *77*, 379–383. [CrossRef]
5. Ong, L.M.; Visser, M.R.; Van Zuuren, F.J.; Rietbroek, R.C.; Lammes, F.B.; De Haes, J.C. Cancer patients' coping styles and doctor-patient communication. *Psychooncology* **1999**, *8*, 155–166. [CrossRef]
6. Ong, L.; De Haes, J.; Hoos, A.M.; Lammes, F.B. Doctor-patient communication: A review of the literature. *Soc. Sci. Med.* **1995**, *40*, 903–918. [CrossRef] [PubMed]
7. Butow, P.N.; Kazemi, J.N.; Beeney, L.J.; Griffin, A.M.; Dunn, S.M.; Tattersall, M.H. When the diagnosis is cancer: Patient communication experiences and preferences. *Cancer* **1996**, *77*, 2630–2637. [CrossRef]
8. Dowsett, S.; Saul, J.; Butow, P.; Dunn, S.; Boyer, M.; Findlow, R.; Dunsmore, J. Communication styles in the cancer consultation: Preferences for a patient-centred approach. *Psycho-Oncology* **2000**, *9*, 147–156. [CrossRef]
9. Epstein, R.M.; Franks, P.; Fiscella, K.; Shields, C.G.; Meldrum, S.C.; Kravitz, R.L.; Duberstein, P.R. Measuring patient-centered communication in Patient–Physician consultations: Theoretical and practical issues. *Soc. Sci. Med.* **2005**, *61*, 1516–1528. [CrossRef] [PubMed]
10. Katz, S.J.; Belkora, J.; Elwyn, G. Shared Decision Making for Treatment of Cancer: Challenges and Opportunities. *J. Oncol. Pract.* **2014**, *10*, 206–208. [CrossRef]
11. McDonagh, J.R.; Elliott, T.B.; Engelberg, R.A.; Treece, P.D.; Shannon, S.E.; Rubenfeld, G.D.; Patrick, D.L.; Curtis, J.R. Family satisfaction with family conferences about end-of-life care in the intensive care unit: Increased proportion of family speech is associated with increased satisfaction. *Crit. Care Med.* **2004**, *32*, 1484–1488. [CrossRef]
12. Ong, L.M.L.; Visser, M.R.M.; Lammes, F.B.; de Haes, J.C.J.M. Doctor–Patient communication and cancer patients' quality of life and satisfaction. *Patient Educ. Couns.* **2000**, *41*, 145–156. [CrossRef]
13. Stewart, M.A. Effective physician-patient communication and health outcomes: A review. *Can. Med. Assoc. J.* **1995**, *152*, 1423–1433.
14. Kehl, K.L.; Landrum, M.B.; Arora, N.K.; Ganz, P.A.; Van Ryn, M.; Mack, J.W.; Keating, N.L. Association of Actual and Preferred Decision Roles with Patient-Reported Quality of Care. *JAMA Oncol.* **2015**, *1*, 50–58. [CrossRef] [PubMed]
15. Orom, H.; Biddle, C.; Underwood, I.W.; Nelson, C.J.; Homish, D.L. What Is a "Good" Treatment Decision? Decisional Control, Knowledge, Treatment Decision Making, and Quality of Life in Men with Clinically Localized Prostate Cancer. *Med. Decis. Mak.* **2016**, *36*, 714–725. [CrossRef]
16. Kim, S.S.; Kaplowitz, S.; Johnston, M.V. The Effects of Physician Empathy on Patient Satisfaction and Compliance. *Eval. Health Prof.* **2004**, *27*, 237–251. [CrossRef]
17. Blatt, B.; LeLacheur, S.F.; Galinsky, A.D.; Simmens, S.J.; Greenberg, L. Does Perspective-Taking Increase Patient Satisfaction in Medical Encounters? *Acad. Med.* **2010**, *85*, 1445–1452. [CrossRef] [PubMed]
18. Lelorain, S.; Brédart, A.; Dolbeault, S.; Sultan, S. A systematic review of the associations between empathy measures and patient outcomes in cancer care. *Psycho-Oncology* **2012**, *21*, 1255–1264. [CrossRef] [PubMed]
19. Schrooten, I.; de Jong, M.D.T. If You Could Read My Mind: The Role of Healthcare Providers' Empathic and Communicative Competencies in Clients' Satisfaction with Consultations. *Health Commun.* **2017**, *32*, 111–118. [CrossRef]
20. Coulter, A.; Ellins, J. Effectiveness of strategies for informing, educating, and involving patients. *BMJ* **2007**, *335*, 24–27. [CrossRef]
21. Schofield, P.E.; Butow, P.N.; Thompson, J.F.; Tattersall, M.H.N.; Beeney, L.J.; Dunn, S.M. Psychological responses of patients receiving a diagnosis of cancer. *Ann. Oncol.* **2003**, *14*, 48–56. [CrossRef]
22. Roter, D.L.; Hall, J.A.; Katz, N.R. Patient-physician communication: A descriptive summary of the literature. *Patient Educ. Couns.* **1988**, *12*, 99–119. [CrossRef]
23. Roter, D.L.; Hall, J.A.; Katz, N.R. Relations Between Physicians' Behaviors and Analogue Patients' Satisfaction, Recall, and Impressions. *Med. Care* **1987**, *25*, 437–451. [CrossRef]
24. Roter, D.L. Communication Patterns of Primary Care Physicians. *JAMA* **1997**, *277*, 350. [CrossRef] [PubMed]
25. Fallowfield, L.; Jenkins, V. Effective communication skills are the key to good cancer care. *Eur. J. Cancer* **1999**, *35*, 1592–1597. [CrossRef]
26. Bensing, J. Bridging the gap. *Patient Educ. Couns.* **2000**, *39*, 17–25. [CrossRef] [PubMed]
27. Robinson, J.D.; Hoover, D.R.; Venetis, M.K.; Kearney, T.J.; Street, R.L. Consultations Between Patients With Breast Cancer and Surgeons: A Pathway From Patient-Centered Communication to Reduced Hopelessness. *J. Clin. Oncol.* **2013**, *31*, 351–358. [CrossRef] [PubMed]
28. Zani, B. *La Comunicazione Come Processo Sociale*; Il Mulino: Bologna, Italy, 2002.
29. Kahn, K.L.; Schneider, E.C.; Malin, J.L.; Adams, J.L.; Epstein, A.M. Patient Centered Experiences in Breast Cancer. *Med. Care* **2007**, *45*, 431–439. [CrossRef]

30. Zhang, B.; Wright, A.A.; Huskamp, H.A.; Nilsson, M.E.; Maciejewski, M.L.; Earle, C.C.; Block, S.D.; Maciejewski, P.K.; Prigerson, H.G. Health Care Costs in the Last Week of Life. *Arch. Intern. Med.* **2009**, *169*, 480. [CrossRef]
31. Fallowfield, L. The ideal consultation. *Br. J. Hosp. Med.* **1992**, *47*, 364–367. [PubMed]
32. Marino, F. Intercultural Communication in Oncological Visits: A Mixed-Methods Comparison of the PCC between Italian Patients and Patients with Migration Background. Ph.D. Thesis, Sapienza University of Rome, Rome, Italy, 2023.
33. Geraci, S.; El Hamad, I. Migranti e accessibilità ai servizi sanitari: Luci e ombre. *Ital. J. Public Health* **2011**, *8*, 14–20.
34. Pandey, M.; Maina, R.G.; Amoyaw, J.; Li, Y.; Kamrul, R.; Michaels, C.R.; Maroof, R. Impacts of English language proficiency on healthcare access, use, and outcomes among immigrants: A qualitative study. *BMC Health Serv. Res.* **2021**, *21*, 741. [CrossRef]
35. Schouten, B.C.; Meeuwesen, L.; Tromp, F.; Harmsen, H.A. Cultural diversity in patient participation: The influence of patients' characteristics and doctors' communicative behaviour. *Patient Educ. Couns.* **2007**, *67*, 214–223. [CrossRef]
36. Butow, P.N.; Sze, M.; Dugal-Beri, P.; Mikhail, M.; Eisenbruch, M.; Jefford, M.; Schofield, P.; Girgis, A.; King, M.; Goldstein, D. on behalf of the Psycho-Oncology Co-operative Research Group (PoCoG). From inside the bubble: Migrants' perceptions of communication with the cancer team. *Support. Care Cancer* **2011**, *19*, 281–290. [CrossRef] [PubMed]
37. Baraldi, C.; Gavioli, L. Dialogue interpreting as intercultural mediation: An analysis in healthcare multilingual settings. In *Dialogue and Culture*; Grein, M., Weigand, E., Eds.; John Benjamins Publishing Company: Amsterdam, The Netherlands, 2007; Volume 1, pp. 155–175.
38. Gavioli, L.; Baraldi, C. Interpreter-mediated interaction in healthcare and legal settings. *Interpret. Int. J. Res. Pract. Interpret.* **2011**, *13*, 205–233. [CrossRef]
39. Bischoff, A.; Wanner, P. The Self-reported Health of Immigrant Groups in Switzerland. *J. Immigr. Minor. Health* **2008**, *10*, 325–335. [CrossRef]
40. Jacobs, E.A.; Niels Agger-Gupta MP, P.; Chen, A.H.; Piotrowski, A.; Hardt, E.J. *Language Barriers in Health Care Settings: An Annotated Bibliography of the Research Literature*; The California Endowment: Los Angeles, CA, USA, 2003.
41. Hyatt, A.; Lipson-Smith, R.; Schofield, P.; Gough, K.; Sze, M.; Aldridge, L.; Goldstein, D.; Jefford, M.; Bell, M.L.; Butow, P. Communication challenges experienced by migrants with cancer: A comparison of migrant and English-speaking Australian-born cancer patients. *Health Expect.* **2017**, *20*, 886–895. [CrossRef]
42. Aelbrecht, K.; Pype, P.; Vos, J.; Deveugele, M. Having cancer in a foreign country. *Patient Educ. Couns.* **2016**, *99*, 1708–1716. [CrossRef]
43. Goldstein, D.; Thewes, B.; Butow, P. Communicating in a multicultural society II: Greek community attitudes towards cancer in Australia. *Intern. Med. J.* **2002**, *32*, 289–296. [CrossRef] [PubMed]
44. Van Wieringen, J.C.; Harmsen, J.A.; Bruijnzeels, M.A. Intercultural communication in general practice. *Eur. J. Public Health* **2002**, *12*, 63–68. [CrossRef] [PubMed]
45. Paternotte, E.; Scheele, F.; Seeleman, C.M.; Bank, L.; Scherpbier, A.J.J.A.; Van Dulmen, S. Intercultural doctor-patient communication in daily outpatient care: Relevant communication skills. *Perspect. Med. Educ.* **2016**, *5*, 268–275. [CrossRef]
46. Filler, T.; Jameel, B.; Gagliardi, A.R. Barriers and facilitators of patient centered care for immigrant and refugee women: A scoping review. *BMC Public Health* **2020**, *20*, 1013. [CrossRef]
47. Mitchell, J.A.; Perry, R. Disparities in patient-centered communication for Black and Latino men in the U.S.: Cross-sectional results from the 2010 health and retirement study. *PLoS ONE* **2020**, *15*, e0238356. [CrossRef] [PubMed]
48. Palmer, N.R.; Gregorich, S.E.; Livaudais-Toman, J.; Jih, J.; Kaplan, C.P. Racial and Ethnic Differences in Prostate Cancer Survivors' Perceived Engagement in Treatment Decision-Making. *J. Racial Ethn. Health Disparities* **2018**, *5*, 1273–1283. [CrossRef] [PubMed]
49. Lee, S.-Y.C.K.; Knobf, M.T. Primary Breast Cancer Decision-making among Chinese American Women. *Nurs. Res.* **2015**, *64*, 391–401. [CrossRef]
50. Lee, S.; Chen, L.; Ma, G.; Fang, C. What is lacking in patient-physician communication: Perspectives from Asian American breast cancer patients and oncologists. *J. Behav. Health* **2012**, *1*, 102–109. [CrossRef]
51. Wong, S.T.; Chen, W.; Bottorff, J.L.; Hislop, T.G. Treatment decision making among Chinese women with DCIS. *J. Psychosoc. Oncol.* **2008**, *26*, 53–73. [CrossRef]
52. Watts, K.J.; Meiser, B.; Zilliacus, E.; Kaur, R.; Taouk, M.; Girgis, A.; Butow, P.; Kissane, D.W.; Hale, S.; Perry, A.; et al. Perspectives of oncology nurses and oncologists regarding barriers to working with patients from a minority background: Systemic issues and working with interpreters. *Eur. J. Cancer Care* **2018**, *27*, e12758. [CrossRef] [PubMed]
53. Chu, J.; Wang, N.; Choi, Y.S.; Roby, D.H. The Effect of Patient-Centered Communication and Racial Concordant Care on Care Satisfaction among U.S. Immigrants. *Med. Care Res. Rev.* **2021**, *78*, 404–412. [CrossRef]
54. ISTAT. 2022. Available online: http://dati.istat.it/Index.aspx?DataSetCode=DCIS_POPSTRRES1 (accessed on 1 April 2020).
55. Council of Europe. *Common European Framework of Reference for Languages: Learning, Teaching, Assessment. Vol. Companion Volume*; Council of Europe Publishing: Strasbourg, France, 2020.
56. Alby, F.; Lauriola, M.; Marino, F.; Fatigante, M.; Zucchermaglio, C. A coding system for doctor-patient communication in oncological consultations—ONCODE. *TPM Test. Psychom. Methodol. Appl. Psychol.* **2021**, *28*, 287–311.
57. McCabe, R.; Healey, P.G.T. Miscommunication in Doctor-Patient Communication. *Top. Cogn. Sci.* **2018**, *10*, 409–424. [CrossRef]
58. Stivers, T.; Barnes, R.K. Treatment Recommendation Actions, Contingencies, and Responses: An Introduction. *Health Commun.* **2018**, *33*, 1331–1334. [CrossRef]

59. Thompson, L.; McCabe, R. How Psychiatrists Recommend Treatment and Its Relationship with Patient Uptake. *Health Commun.* **2018**, *33*, 1345–1354. [CrossRef]
60. Alby, F.; Zucchermaglio, C.; Baruzzo, M. Diagnostic Decision Making in Oncology: Creating Shared Knowledge and Managing Complexity. *Mind Cult. Act.* **2015**, *22*, 4–22. [CrossRef]
61. Alby, F.; Zucchermaglio, C.; Fatigante, M. Communicating Uncertain News in Cancer Consultations. *J. Cancer Educ.* **2017**, *32*, 858–864. [CrossRef] [PubMed]
62. Fantasia, V.; Zucchermaglio, C.; Fatigante, M.; Alby, F. 'We will take care of you': Identity categorisation markers in intercultural medical encounters. *Discourse Stud.* **2021**, *23*, 451–473. [CrossRef]
63. Fatigante, M.; Heritage, J.; Alby, F.; Zucchermaglio, C. Presenting treatment options in breast cancer consultations: Advice and consent in Italian medical care. *Soc. Sci. Med.* **2020**, *266*, 113175. [CrossRef]
64. Zucchermaglio, C.; Alby, F. Theorizing about practice: Storytelling and practical knowledge in cancer diagnoses. *J. Work. Learn.* **2016**, *28*, 174–187. [CrossRef]
65. Fatigante, M.; Alby, F.; Zucchermaglio, C.; Baruzzo, M. Formulating treatment recommendation as a logical consequence of the diagnosis in post-surgical oncological visits. *Patient Educ. Couns.* **2016**, *99*, 878–887. [CrossRef]
66. Fatigante, M.; Zucchermaglio, C.; Alby, F. Being in Place: A Multimodal Analysis of the Contribution of the Patient's Companion to "First Time" Oncological Visits. *Front. Psychol.* **2021**, *12*, 664747. [CrossRef]
67. Sterponi, L.; Zucchermaglio, C.; Fantasia, V.; Fatigante, M.; Alby, F. A room of one's own: Moments of mutual disengagement between doctor and patient in the oncology visit. *Patient Educ. Couns.* **2021**, *104*, 1116–1124. [CrossRef]
68. Sterponi, L.; Zucchermaglio, C.; Fatigante, M.; Alby, F. Structuring times and activities in the oncology visit. *Soc. Sci. Med.* **2019**, *228*, 211–222. [CrossRef] [PubMed]
69. George, D.; Mallery, P. *SPSS for Windows Step by Step: A Simple Guide and Reference 17.0 Update*; Allyn & Bacon: Boston, MA, USA, 2010.
70. MacKinnon, D.P.; Krull, J.L.; Lockwood, C.M. Equivalence of the Mediation, Confounding and Suppression Effect. *Prev. Sci.* **2000**, *1*, 173–181. [CrossRef] [PubMed]
71. Mitchell, K.-A.R.; Brassil, K.J.; Osborne, M.L.; Lu, Q.; Brown, R.F. Understanding racial-ethnic differences in patient-centered care (PCC) in oncology through a critical race theory lens: A qualitative comparison of PCC among Black, Hispanic, and White cancer patients. *Patient Educ. Couns.* **2022**, *105*, 2346–2354. [CrossRef] [PubMed]
72. Mitchell, E.; Alese, O.B.; Yates, C.; Rivers, B.M.; Blackstock, W.; Newman, L.; Davis, M.; Byrd, G.; Harris, A.E. Cancer healthcare disparities among African Americans in the United States. *J. Natl. Med. Assoc.* **2022**, *114*, 236–250. [CrossRef] [PubMed]
73. Tomai, M.; Lauriola, M. Separate but Related: Dimensions of Healthcare Provider Social Support in Day-Treatment Oncology Units. *Front. Psychol.* **2022**, *13*, 1429. [CrossRef]
74. Andrades, M.; Kausar, S.; Ambreen, A. Role and influence of the patient's companion in family medicine consultations: 'The patient's perspective'. *J. Fam. Med. Prim. Care* **2013**, *2*, 283.
75. Sheehan, O.C.; Graham-Phillips, A.L.; Wilson, J.D.; Crews, D.C.; Holt, C.L.; Gabbard, J.; Smith, K.C.; Wolff, J.L.; Roth, D.L. Non-spouse companions accompanying older adults to medical visits: A qualitative analysis. *BMC Geriatr.* **2019**, *19*, 84. [CrossRef]
76. Del Piccolo, L.; Goss, C.; Bottacini, A.; Rigoni, V.; Mazzi, M.A.; Deledda, G.; Ballarin, M.; Molino, A.; Fiorio, E.; Zimmermann, C. Asking questions during breast cancer consultations: Does being alone or being accompanied make a difference? *Eur. J. Oncol. Nurs.* **2014**, *18*, 299–304. [CrossRef]
77. Healey, A.N.; Sevdalis, N.; Vincent, C.A. Measuring intra-operative interference from distraction and interruption observed in the operating theatre. *Ergonomics* **2006**, *49*, 589–604. [CrossRef]
78. Collins, S.; Currie, L.; Patel, V.; Bakken, S.; Cimino, J.J. Multitasking by clinicians in the context of CPOE and CIS use. *Stud. Health Technol. Inform.* **2007**, *129*, 958–962.
79. Trbovich, P.; Griffin, M.; White, R.; Bourrier, V.; Dhaliwal, D.; Easty, A. The Effects of Interruptions on Oncologists' Patient Assessment and Medication Ordering Practices. *J. Health Eng.* **2013**, *4*, 127–144. [CrossRef]
80. Marino, F.; Alby, F.; Zucchermaglio, C. Interruptions or Interactive Trampolines? A Discoursive Analysis of the Interruption of the Oncological Visit with Foreign Patients. Sapienza University of Rome: Rome, Italy, 2023, *manuscript in preparation*.

*cancers*

MDPI

*Article*

# Cancer in Migrants: A Population-Based Study in Italy

**Giulia Collatuzzo [1], Margherita Ferrante [2,3], Antonella Ippolito [3], Alessia Di Prima [3], Cristina Colarossi [4], Salvatore Scarpulla [4], Paolo Boffetta [3,5,6,*] and Salvatore Sciacca [4,*]**

1 Department of Medical and Surgical Sciences, University of Bologna, 40138 Bologna, Italy; giulia.collatuzzo@studio.unibo.it
2 Department of Medical, Surgical and Advanced Technologies "G.F. Ingrassia", University of Catania, 95123 Catania, Italy
3 Integrated Cancer Registry of Catania-Messina-Siracusa-Enna, University of Catania, 95123 Catania, Italy
4 Mediterranean Institute of Oncology (IOM), 95029 Catania, Italy
5 Stony Brook Cancer Center, Stony Brook University, Stony Brook, NY 11794, USA
6 Department of Family, Population and Preventive Medicine, Renaissance School of Medicine, Stony Brook University, Stony Brook, NY 11794, USA
* Correspondence: paolo.boffetta@unibo.it (P.B.); salvatore.sciacca@grupposamed.com (S.S.)

**Simple Summary:** This study investigates cancer in migrants in Southern Italy, who represent a neglected but vulnerable population. We used data from the Eastern Sicily Cancer Registry collected between 2004 and 2019 to compare the adjusted proportionate morbidity ratio for the most common cancer types in migrants and non-migrants, and we calculated the odds of migrant status for one cancer compared to all cancers. The migrants/non-migrants odds of cancer was 2.1%, with most cancers occurring in migrant women. We observed increased proportions in cervical and lung cancer, with higher odds of cervical cancer and lower odds of colorectal cancer in migrants. Measures should be implemented to enhance the access of migrants to prevention, early diagnosis and care for cancer. These interventions should account for the migrant's country of origin. Particular attention should be given to HPV vaccination, cervical cancer screening and tobacco control to reduce the cancer burden in this population.

**Abstract:** Background: Migrants are a vulnerable and neglected population. We aimed at investigating cancer proportionate rates in migrants in Sicily, Southern Italy. Methods: We extracted data on new cancer cases diagnosed between 2004 and 2019 from the Eastern Sicily cancer registry. We compared the adjusted proportionate morbidity ratio (PMR) for the most common cancer types among migrants and non-migrants. We fitted multivariate logistic regression models comparing one cancer to all other cancers to calculate odds ratios (ORs) and 95% confidence intervals (CIs) for migration status. The analysis was stratified by region of origin. Results: Overall, 4726 new cancer cases occurred in migrants between 2004 and 2019, 63.5% of those among women and 224,211 in non-migrants, including 54.5% among men, with odds for migrants/non-migrants of 2.1%. Migrants had an increased proportion of cervical (PMR = 2.68, 95% CI = 2.29–3.10) and lung cancer (PMR = 1.20, 95% CI = 1.07–1.33). The highest OR in migrants was observed for cervical cancer (OR = 3.54, 95% CI = 2.99–4.20). Colorectal cancer was decreased among migrants (OR = 0.86, 95% CI = 0.77–0.96). Conclusions: Migrants to Sicily have higher odds of cervical cancer and a decreased risk of colorectal cancer compared to non-migrants. Increased odds were also detected for lung cancer, in particular in women. Different cancer patterns could be observed based on the region of origin. HPV-related cancers need targeted attention in migrants living in Sicily.

**Keywords:** migrants; cancer epidemiology; Italy

## 1. Introduction

Migrants represent a vulnerable subgroup of the population from multiple points of view [1], including socioeconomic condition (job position, income and educational level) [2] as well as health status (vaccination history, participation in screening programs, disease diagnosis and care). Migrants often suffer disease disparities [3,4], such as poor disease management, lack of check-ups and screening tests [5], delayed diagnosis [6] and inadequate treatments. A meta-analysis reported that foreign-born women were less likely to be diagnosed with localized-stage breast cancer compared to native women [6], including a relationship between the magnitude of the disparity and the level of development of the country of origin. On the other hand, reports have been published in which migrants registered a lower risk of cancer and lower cancer mortality compared to non-migrants [7–9], possibly due to a healthy migrant effect and low incidence of some cancers in the country of origin.

The number and proportion of cancer deaths and incident cases in migrants have been estimated in several countries, providing quantitative evidence of cancer epidemiology in this population group [8–11]. Cancer epidemiology in migrants is important for several reasons [3,4,6]. First, the description of cancer in this special population offers valuable information to understand the determinants of cancer in different ethnic groups and to disentangle the role played by environmental and genetic factors. Additionally, the investigation of cancer in migrants can highlight patterns of cancer occurrence in different ethnic groups, possibly identifying subjects to be targeted for specific preventive actions [3,12,13]. Moreover, studies on cancer in migrants may help in understanding the causes of cancer also in native populations [12]. These results may also have implications for national regulations and health policies, providing useful information derived from the comparison between the epidemiologic data of cancer in people born in different countries [14]. Indeed, migrants may acquire the same risk profile of the population of the host country [15]. An example comes from a population-based study conducted in Norway, which reported higher overall cancer incidence rates in native people than in migrants and observed higher liver cancer incidence in Asians than in Norwegians, as well as higher lung cancer incidence in male migrants from other Nordic countries and from Eastern Europe than in native men [9].

The Mediterranean countries of Europe are subject to migration from Northern Africa, Eastern Europe and West Asia, given the geographical position [14]. A recent study reported declining trends in cancer mortality in migrants in Spain between 2000 and 2016 [14]. In general, however, data on cancer incidence rates in migrants to Mediterranean countries in the last decade are scarce.

Sicily is an island in Southern Italy, which has experienced an increase in the migrant population in recent years. The official proportion of foreign subjects over the total population in Sicily in 2021 was 3.9%. The main countries of origin were Romania. Tunisia, Morocco, Sri Lanka, Albania and Bangladesh [16]. The actual number of migrants, however, is likely to be higher because of the presence of illegal and seasonal migrants. This is particularly true for Sicily, because of (i) the widespread use of seasonal migrants in agriculture and (ii) the role of Sicily as an entry point from the Mediterranean and the presence of numerous temporary transit camps for undocumented and illegal immigrants.

In order to estimate cancer proportion in migrants at a population-base level, we analyzed data of a cancer registry in Sicily, Italy. We focused on major areas of origin of the migrants and on the cancer sites with the highest occurrence in this special population.

## 2. Materials and Methods

### 2.1. Study Design and Population

This study is designed as a case–control study, where migrant status is the exposure and cancer types are the controls.

We analyzed data from the Eastern Sicily Cancer Registry covering 2.5 million people from four provinces (Catania, Enna, Messina and Syracuse) [17]. The registry is considered to be complete and is included in the Cancer Incidence in Five Continents, a collection of high-quality registries maintained by the International Agency for Research on Cancer [18]. This registry includes cases identified only from death certificates. Data are validated and periodically checked by the Associazione Italiana Registro Tumori (AIRTUM) through different programs (e.g., CheckAIRTUM and IARC CRG Tools). We selected new cases of the most frequent cancers diagnosed between 2004 and 2019 in migrants and identified new cases of the same cancers occurring among non-migrants during the same time period. The Cancer Registry collects data on cancer diagnosed mostly based on histological confirmation of the primary tumor and, for a minority of cases, clinical based on data or imaging; during 2009–2012, for only 1.6% of new cancer cases in men and 2.1% in women, the site of origin was classified as 'other or unspecified' [18].

### 2.2. Data Sources

Data derived from the Eastern Sicily Cancer Registry. We extracted the following information from the Cancer Registry: sex, age, country of birth, basis for diagnosis (histology/citology; clinical; death certificate/other), date of diagnosis and treatment (chemotherapy, radiotherapy and surgery). Information on the three treatment modalities was missing for a proportion of subjects. Since we were not able to distinguish between missing information or no therapy, we did not include these data in the analysis. Country of birth was categorized as Northern/Western Europe, Eastern Europe and Balkans, Northern Africa, Sub-Saharan Africa, Western Asia, other Asian countries excluding Japan, North America/Oceania/Japan and Latin America.

### 2.3. Statistical Analysis

Information on the total number of migrants living in the four provinces covered by the Cancer Registry was not available. We, therefore, could not calculate incidence rates and ratios directly comparing migrants and non-migrants but, rather, used the proportions of cancer occurring in the two populations. Specifically, we calculated the proportion of new cases of each cancer over total cancers among migrants and compared this with the same proportion among non-migrants. We then calculated the proportionate morbidity ratio (PMR) for each cancer type as the ratio of new observed cases in migrants over new expected cases, based on the proportion in non-migrants after adjusting for sex, age group and calendar year. Further, 95% confidence intervals (CIs) of PMR were calculated based on the Poisson distribution of new expected cases. We stratified the analyses by region of origin, sex and age. We tested heterogeneity in PIR between geographic region, sex and age categories using the Cochrane Q-test [19].

In addition, we fitted multivariate logistic regression models comparing one cancer to all other cancers to calculate ORs and 95% CIs of migration status (overall and by sex), after adjustment for sex, age category, basis of diagnosis and period of diagnosis. We repeated the analysis by geographic region of origin by fitting separate models, including migrants from one specific region and all non-migrants, and after stratification, by period of diagnosis. We tested heterogeneity between strata of sex and age period by adding interaction terms to the regression models.

For all the aforementioned analyses, $p < 0.05$ was considered statistically significant.

## 3. Results

Table 1 illustrates the main characteristics of the study population. Overall, a total of 4726 new cases of cancer were registered among migrants between 2004 and 2019, including 1724 (36.5%) new cases among men and 3002 (63.5%) new cases among women. In the same period, 224,211 new cases were registered among non-migrants, including 122,241 (54.5%) among men and 101,970 (45.5%) among women. The overall odds of new cases in migrants to non-migrants was 2.1% and increased from 1.7% in 2004–2007 to 2.5% in 2016–2019. The countries of origin with the largest number of new cases of cancer among migrants were Germany (N = 968), Libya (N = 625) and Romania (N = 442).

**Table 1.** Distribution of new cases of cancer by migrant status and selected characteristics.

| Characteristics | Migrants (%) | Non-Migrants (%) |
|---|---|---|
| Total | 4726 (100.0) | 224,211 (100.0) |
| Sex | | |
| Men | 1724 (36.5) | 122,241 (54.5) |
| Women | 3002 (63.5) | 101,970 (45.5) |
| Age group (yrs) | | |
| <55 | 2165 (45.8) | 43,294 (19.3) |
| 55–64 | 947 (20.0) | 42,317 (18.9) |
| 65–74 | 807 (17.1) | 62,606 (27.9) |
| >=75 | 807 (17.1) | 75,993 (33.9) |
| Year of diagnosis | | |
| 2004–2007 | 880 (23.2) | 52,274 (23.3) |
| 2008–2011 | 1037 (21.4) | 55,360 (24.7) |
| 2012–2015 | 1330 (28.1) | 57,930 (25.8) |
| 2016–2019 | 1479 (31.3) | 58,647 (28.2) |
| Base of diagnosis | | |
| Histology/cytology | 4183 (88.5) | 195,654 (87.3) |
| Clinical | 482 (10.2) | 25,230 (11.3) |
| Other ‡ | 61 (1.3) | 3327 (1.5) |
| Region of origin | | |
| Northern and Western Europe * | 1931 (41.1) | - |
| Eastern Europe, Balkans | 751 (16.0) | - |
| North Africa | 890 (18.9) | - |
| Sub-Saharan Africa | 216 (4.6) | - |
| West Asia | 25 (0.5) | - |
| Other Asian countries † | 207 (4.4) | - |
| North America, Oceania | 312 (6.6) | - |
| Latin America | 372 (7.9) | |

‡ Including death certificate only. * Including European Union except Bulgaria, Romania (included in Eastern Europe and Balkans). † Excluding Japan (included in North America, Oceania).

Overall and sex-specific PMR for the main cancer types is shown in Table 2. We observed an increased proportion of cervical cancer (PIR = 2.68, 95% CI = 2.29–3.10) and lung cancer (PIR = 1.20, 95% CI = 1.07–1.33) among migrants. The result of lung cancer for both sexes (PMR = 1.20, 95% CI = 1.07–1.33) was driven by the pattern in women (PMR = 1.32, 95% CI = 1.11–1.56), with no increased proportion in men ($p$-value of test of heterogeneity between sexes = 0.09). The PMR of leukemia was decreased, with a stronger result among women (PMR = 0.77, 95% CI = 0.61–0.95, $p$-heterogeneity between sexes = 0.07).

The results of the multivariate logistic regression analysis (Table 3) are consistent with the previous ones. The cancer with the highest OR in migrants was cervical cancer (OR = 3.54, 95% CI = 2.99–4.20), and an increase was also detected for lung cancer, in particular in women (OR = 1.23, 95% CI = 1.03–1.47). Colorectal cancer was the only neoplasm whose OR was decreased among migrants (OR = 0.86, 95% CI = 0.77–0.96), and a decreased OR of borderline statistical significance was observed for liver, breast and prostate cancer and NHL. Liver cancer and leukemia were the two neoplasms for which there was evidence of heterogeneity in OR between men and women ($p$ = 0.02 and 0.03, respectively).

**Table 2.** Proportionate morbidity ratios of cancer among migrants by sex.

| Cancer | N | Total PMR | 95% CI | N | Men PMR | 95% CI | N | Women PMR | 95% CI |
|---|---|---|---|---|---|---|---|---|---|
| Head and neck | 81 | 1.11 | 0.88–1.37 | 55 | 1.11 | 0.84–1.43 | 26 | 1.11 | 0.74–1.60 |
| Stomach | 94 | 1.00 | 0.81–1.21 | 46 | 1.02 | 0.75–1.34 | 48 | 0.98 | 0.72–1.28 |
| Colorectum | 361 | 0.92 | 0.82–1.01 | 144 | 0.90 | 0.76–1.05 | 217 | 0.93 | 0.81–1.05 |
| Liver | 81 | 1.09 | 0.87–1.35 | 44 | 0.99 | 0.73–1.32 | 37 | 1.24 | 0.89–1.69 |
| Lung | 331 | 1.20 | 1.07–1.33 | 194 | 1.12 | 0.97–1.28 | 137 | 1.32 | 1.11–1.56 |
| Breast | 790 | 0.94 | 0.87–1.01 | - | - | - | 790 | 0.94 | 0.87–1.01 |
| Cervix | 165 | 2.68 | 2.29–3.10 | - | - | - | 165 | 2.68 | 2.29–3.10 |
| Prostate | 165 | 0.94 | 0.80–1.09 | 165 | 0.94 | 0.80–1.09 | - | - | - |
| Bladder | 238 | 1.06 | 0.93–1.20 | 173 | 1.06 | 0.91–1.23 | 65 | 1.06 | 0.82–1.34 |
| NHL | 182 | 0.91 | 0.78–1.05 | 87 | 0.98 | 0.78–1.20 | 95 | 0.86 | 0.69–1.04 |
| Leukemia | 155 | 0.87 | 0.73–1.01 | 76 | 0.99 | 0.78–1.22 | 79 | 0.77 | 0.61–0.95 |

N, observed number of new cases among migrants; PMR, proportionate morbidity ratio; CI, confidence interval; NHL, non-Hodgkin lymphoma.

**Table 3.** Odds ratio of selected cancer for migrant status, overall and by gender—results of multivariate logistic regression analysis.

| | Total Population | Men | Women |
|---|---|---|---|
| Cancer | OR (95% CI) | OR (95% CI) | OR (95% CI) |
| Head and neck | 1.09 (0.87–1.35) | 1.14 (0.88–1.48) | 1.05 (0.71–1.45) |
| Stomach | 0.89 (0.73–1.09) | 1.01 (0.76–1.35) | 0.82 (0.62–1.09) |
| Colorectum | 0.86 (0.77–0.96) | 0.86 (0.73–1.03) | 0.89 (0.77–1.02) |
| Liver | 0.80 (0.64–1.01) | 0.68 (0.49–0.94) | 1.11 (0.80–1.55) |
| Lung | 1.12 (1.00–1.26) | 1.03 (0.88–1.20) | 1.23 (1.03–1.47) |
| Breast | 0.95 (0.88–1.04) | | 0.95 (0.88–1.04) |
| Cervix | 3.54 (2.99–4.20) | | 3.54 (2.99–4.20) |
| Prostate | 0.87 (0.74–1.03) | 0.87 (0.74–1.03) | |
| Bladder | 1.07 (0.94–1.23) | 1.10 (0.94–1.29) | 1.05 (0.82–1.35) |
| NHL | 0.86 (0.73–1.01) | 0.90 (0.71–1.16) | 0.87 (0.69–1.05) |
| Leukemia | 1.02 (0.87–1.20) | 1.26 (0.99–1.59) | 0.90 (0.71–1.13) |

OR, odds ratio adjusted for sex, age, type of diagnosis, year of diagnosis. CI, confidence interval. NHL, non-Hodgkin lymphoma.

In the analysis by region of origin in migrants (Figure 1, detailed results are available in Supplementary Table S1), migrants from Northern and Western Europe, including the European Union, showed a decreased OR for colorectal and breast cancer as well as NHL and leukemia, and an increased OR for cervical cancer. Migrants from Eastern Europe showed a decreased OR for prostate cancer and an increased OR for lung and cervical cancer. Migrants from North Africa experienced an increased OR for bladder cancer, whereas migrants from Sub-Saharan Africa experienced an increased OR of liver, breast cancer and leukemia and a decreased OR for colorectal cancer. The results on migrants from West Asia were hampered by small numbers. Migrants from other Asian countries had a decreased OR for bladder cancer and an increased OR for leukemia. Migrants from North America, Oceania and Japan did not have a statistically significant increased or decreased OR for any cancer. Finally, the OR for breast cancer was increased among migrants from Latin America.

The analysis by period of diagnosis suggested a trend in OR of liver cancer (OR increased from 0.55 (95% CI 0.30–0.98) in 2004–2007 to 1.13 (95% CI 0.78–1.65) in 2016–2019), lung cancer (OR increased from 0.89 (95% CI 0.67–1.19) to 1.22 (95% CI 1.00–1.49)) and breast cancer (OR increased from 0.84 (95% CI 0.68–1.04) to 1.08 (95% CI 0.94–1.25)), although none of these trends were statistically significant (results not shown in detail).

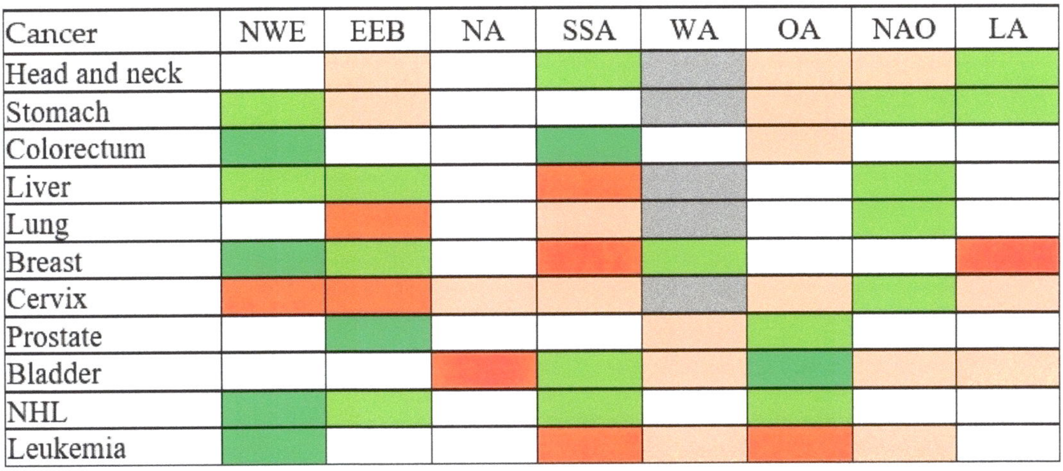


**Figure 1.** Odds ratio of selected cancer among migrants, by area of origin—results of multivariate logistic regression analysis. NWE, Northern and Western Europe and European Union, excluding Bulgaria and Romania. EEB, Eastern Europe and the Balkans. NA, North Africa. SSA, Sub-Saharan Africa. WA, West Asia. OA, Other Asia, excluding Japan. NAO, North America and Oceania, including Japan. LA, Latin America. Light green: OR < 0.8, $p > 0.05$. Dark green: OR < 1, $p < 0.05$. Light red: OR > 1.25, $p > 0.05$. Dark red: OR > 1, $p < 0.05$. Grey: Model did not converge. NHL, non-Hodgkin lymphoma. OR, odds ratio adjusted for sex, age, type of diagnosis, year of diagnosis.

## 4. Discussion

Our analysis revealed several patterns of cancer incidence among migrants in a Southern Italy population, including a higher proportion of cervical and lung cancers and a borderline statistically significant lower proportion of breast and prostate cancers compared to non-migrants. The stratification by geographical region of origin revealed that these patterns were mainly due to migration from Europe.

The results we describe are impaired by the lack of population data on the number of migrants in Sicily, thus preventing us from calculating cancer incidence rates in this population and incidence ratios in the comparisons with non-migrants. We tried to address this problem by using official data on the number of migrants present in four provinces during the study period [20] but obtained unreliable results, likely due to an undercount of migrants in official statistics. Despite this important limitation, ours remains one of the few studies to provide data on the neglected issue of cancer incidence in migrants in Italy and one of the first to provide a comprehensive analysis of different cancer types in migrants.

Although there was no increased proportion of head and neck cancer among migrants, an increase was suggested for migrants from Eastern Europe, the Balkans and from Asia, and a decrease was found among migrants from sub-Saharan Africa and Latin America. Possible explanations are relatable to the different distribution of the risk factors of head and neck cancer in Italy-born people and migrants, specifically HPV, tobacco smoking and alcohol [21]. Central and Eastern Europe is one of the regions with the highest incidence of this group of cancers [22].

Incidence of gastric cancer is elevated in Eastern European and East Asian countries [23], and migrants from these regions had a higher proportion of gastric cancer, although the difference was not statistically significant. Conversely, the incidence of colorectal cancer is relatively low in sub-Saharan Africa [24], and migrants from these countries had a non-significantly lower proportion of colorectal cancer. We observed a reduced risk of liver cancer in migrant men but not in women. Despite not having the information to assess the reason of this sex difference, we may hypothesize that it depends on sociocultural factors, leading to a better management of chronic liver disease (which can be a precursor of cancer) in men than in women, e.g., more frequent clinical visits and medical exams. However, this neoplasm was increased among migrants from Sub-Saharan Africa, a region at high risk for hepatitis B infection and liver cancer [25,26].

We observed an increased proportion of lung cancer among migrants, which was primarily related to migrants from Eastern European countries. The high proportion of lung cancer in migrants could be explained by higher exposure to risk factors, including tobacco smoking, indoor and outdoor air pollution and occupational risk factors during their lifetime. The difference between women and men is likely due to the low incidence of lung cancer among women in Southern Italy [18], which was explained by low tobacco consumption in past decades. Thus, the sex pattern observed in migrants may be an artifact rather than reflect particular risk factors in migrant women, despite the fact that we could not exclude potential confounders.

The proportion of breast cancer was reduced among migrants from Eastern Europe and the Balkans, a region with a lower incidence of these neoplasms compared to Italy [27]. A similar pattern was shown for migrants from other countries of Europe, while migrants from sub-Saharan Africa and Latin America had a higher proportion of this neoplasm. These differences by region of origin may derive from different approaches to cancer screening in addition to different exposure circumstances. In particular, among the factors which may affect breast cancer risk, oral contraceptives have been reported to be higher in women from Eastern Europe.

Cervical cancer showed the highest difference between migrants and non-migrants of all cancers, which was statistically significant for migrants from Europe. This is not unexpected, given the low incidence of this disease in Southern Italy and Sicily in particular [18]. The fact that the greatest proportion of new cases was seen among migrants from Eastern Europe might be explained by the high prevalence of HPV infection in that region [28]. An Italian study reported that 58% Eastern European and African women vs. 19% of Italy-born women to be HPV-positive [29]. Campari et al. reported a higher prevalence of preneoplastic cervical lesions and a lower participation in cervical cancer screening among migrants than Italian women [30].

The proportion of prostate cancer was lower in migrants from Eastern Europe and the Balkans and, although not significantly so, from Asian countries, excluding West Asia, which is consistent with previous findings [31,32]. This difference may be attributable to different levels of "westernization" of the lifestyle habits in different geographical areas of the Asian continent [33]; however, random fluctuation may also explain the difference we observed. Further, the results on the higher incidence rate of bladder cancer in migrants from North Africa than non-migrants are consistent with worldwide patterns of this disease [34].

These heterogeneous patterns of risk of specific cancers in migrants indicate the need for tailored cancer control programs based on the specific cancer predisposition in different populations. Overall, these results agree with a review by Arnold and colleagues, which described a higher proportion of infectious-related cancer (e.g., gastric and cervical) and a lower proportion of lifestyle-related cancer (e.g., colorectum, breast and prostate) in migrants to Europe [35].

Our results provide novel evidence on the different incidence of cancer in migrants in Italy and Sicily in particular, and they relate the pattern of cancer occurrence by geographical area [27]. The results obtained reflect lifestyle, environmental and genetic factors, which underlie the occurrence of specific cancers, such as cervical and prostate cancer in the Balkans [36] and colorectal cancer in Africa [24,37]. Compared to non-migrants, migrants from Eastern Europe and Africa may be less sedentary [38] and have a healthier lifestyle [39], including diet [40–42], and a lower prevalence of dysmetabolic diseases, such as diabetes and hypercholesterolemia [43], factors which may be associated with a lower incidence of prostate [44] and colorectal cancer [45]. Conversely, non-migrants may be less exposed than migrants to unsafe sex, resulting in a lower prevalence of HPV infection and HPV-related cancers [46–48], a pattern which has also been observed in other countries [49,50].

Migrants represent, in large part, a vulnerable group, connoted by a higher prevalence of unhealthy lifestyle habits (e.g., tobacco smoking, alcohol drinking [22], poor diet [51]), occupational disparities [2] and reduced access to healthcare services (e.g., vaccination, screening) [52,53]. These aspects are ultimately related to socioeconomic status. Most of the migrant populations, in Italy as well as in other countries, belong to low socioeconomic status. The relationship between low socioeconomic status and cancer is well described [54], especially with regard to some types of cancers, including those for which we evidenced an increased PIR, namely cervical [55,56] and lung [57–59].

Our analysis addresses the issue of cancer in migrants in Sicily through two approaches, namely PIR estimates and multivariate logistic regression analysis. This latter could account for several aspects, including treatment, which has been reported to differ between migrant and non-migrant populations. Different cancer treatment causes cancer disparities in migrants and non-migrants and is linked to barriers experienced by migrants, such as lack of language proficiency and not being familiar with the health system [60]. Our data on treatment, however, were impaired by missing data. This limitation is unlikely to have introduced bias, because even if missing data could have led to misclassification of treatment, we observed no confounding effect by this variable in the multivariate model.

When focusing on results by geographical area, an important observation is the increased proportion of breast cancer in women from sub-Saharan Africa. This result is unexpected, as African populations (incidence rates around 50/100,000) usually have lower incidence rates of breast cancer compared to European populations (incidence rates 80–90/100,000) [61]. The reason for this result is not clear. Breast cancer screening is usually associated with higher numbers of diagnoses [62]; thus, disparities in participation for cancer screening among migrants do not seem to explain our finding [63]. In addition to this, the migrant population may not precisely reflect incidence rates of the country of origin because they do not represent a random sample of that population. Interestingly, the increased proportion of breast cancer in this migrant subgroup is homogeneously distributed by age.

This study has some limitations. First, as already mentioned, the number of migrants in Sicily was not available, preventing us from calculating the incidence of cancer in migrants and comparing it with that in non-migrants. For this reason, the study design is that of a case–control study where controls are cancers in non-migrants. This approach has been used by other authors [64]. In addition, no information was available on the duration of residence of the migrants: analyses by duration of stay in the host country help to clarify the role of factors affecting cancer risk [65]. Moreover, the lack of information on lifestyle, occupational and sociodemographic factors prevented us from adjusting and stratifying for important variables. Additionally, results by area of origin of the migrant population showed patterns of risk which were not fully consistent with previous literature. Last, small numbers impaired the stratified analyses for some areas of origin.

The present study also has several strengths. We provided updated data on an under-investigated topic, focusing on a special population which is particularly vulnerable and affected by health inequalities. We identified interesting cancer patterns, and, because of the population-based nature of our data, we added valuable data to the current literature on cancer epidemiology in migrants and offered new important information on cancer incidence in different groups of migrants in Italy compared to non-migrants. Further, the data we used were from a high-quality cancer registry, increasing the reliability of our results [66,67].

## 5. Conclusions

In conclusion, migrants to Sicily appear to have an increased OR of cervical and lung cancer than non-migrants, although the comparison is based on proportionate ratios. Different cancer patterns could be observed based on the area of origin of the migrants, with lifestyle and socioeconomic factors in migrants from Centra/Eastern Europe, the Balkans and Africa possibly explaining several results. Differences were identified in particular for women, regarding HPV-related cancers as well as lung cancer and hematologic malignancies. These data may be a useful source of information for understanding cancer epidemiology in migrants in Italy. Cancer control in this special population requires public attention, despite its future trends being unpredictable given the acute nature of migration in Sicily, where most migrants move quickly to other countries.

Given the vulnerability of migrants to cancer, and the discrimination which they might be subjected to, measures should be implemented to enhance their access to prevention, diagnosis and care for cancer. Tailored intervention may be developed based on migrants' country of origin, given the different cancer risk by geographical area. Targeted attention to HPV vaccination and cervical cancer screening participation in migrant women would help to better control infection-related cancers. Tobacco control interventions targeting migrants would also be important to reduce the cancer burden in this population. Cancer control and early detection in migrants may improve, while it is difficult to establish a follow-up for such a special population, which is quickly moving from Sicily to other countries.

**Supplementary Materials:** The following supporting information can be downloaded at: https://www.mdpi.com/article/10.3390/cancers15123103/s1, Table S1: Odds ratio of selected neoplasms among migrants, by region of origin.

**Author Contributions:** Conceptualization, G.C., P.B. and S.S. (Salvatore Sciacca); methodology, G.C. and P.B.; formal analysis, A.I., A.D.P. and P.B.; resources, M.F., C.C., S.S. (Salvatore Scarpulla) and S.S. (Salvatore Sciacca); data curation, M.F., C.C., S.S. (Salvatore Scarpulla) and S.S. (Salvatore Sciacca); writing—original draft preparation, G.C. and P.B.; writing—review and editing, A.I. and A.D.P.; supervision, M.F., P.B. and S.S. (Salvatore Sciacca); project administration, M.F. and S.S. (Salvatore Sciacca). All authors have read and agreed to the published version of the manuscript.

**Funding:** The project was conducted with internal resources of the institutions involved.

**Institutional Review Board Statement:** Ethical review and approval were waived for this study due to the public nature of the de-identified data.

**Informed Consent Statement:** Not applicable.

**Data Availability Statement:** Data can be provided to external investigators upon reasonable request and agreement of the institutions involved.

**Conflicts of Interest:** The authors declare no conflict of interest.

## References

1. Bo, A.; Zinckernagel, L.; Krasnik, A.; Petersen, J.H.; Norredam, M. Coronary heart disease incidence among non-Western immigrants compared to Danish-born people: Effect of country of birth, migrant status, and income. *Eur. J. Prev. Cardiol.* **2015**, *22*, 1281–1289. [CrossRef] [PubMed]
2. Collatuzzo, G.; Teglia, F.; Boffetta, P. Role of Occupation in Shaping Cancer Disparities. *Cancers* **2022**, *14*, 4259. [CrossRef] [PubMed]
3. Taylor, V.M.; Ko, L.K.; Hwang, J.H.; Sin, M.K.; Inadomi, J.M. Gastric cancer in Asian American populations: A neglected health disparity. *Asian Pac. J. Cancer Prev.* **2014**, *15*, 10565–10571. [CrossRef] [PubMed]
4. Pruitt, S.L.; Tiro, J.A.; Xuan, L.; Lee, S.J. Hispanic and Immigrant Paradoxes in U.S. Breast Cancer Mortality: Impact of Neighborhood Poverty and Hispanic Density. *Int. J. Environ. Res. Public Health* **2016**, *13*, 1238. [CrossRef]
5. Bhargava, S.; Moen, K.; Qureshi, S.A.; Hofvind, S. Mammographic screening attendance among immigrant and minority women: A systematic review and meta-analysis. *Acta Radiol.* **2018**, *59*, 1285–1291. [CrossRef] [PubMed]
6. Herbach, E.L.; Weeks, K.S.; O'Rorke, M.; Novak, N.L.; Schweizer, M.L. Disparities in breast cancer stage at diagnosis between immigrant and native-born women: A meta-analysis. *Ann. Epidemiol.* **2021**, *54*, 64–72. [CrossRef]
7. Stevenson, J.K.; Cheung, M.C.; Earle, C.C.; Fischer, H.D.; Camacho, X.; Saskin, R.; Shah, B.R.; Austin, P.C.; Singh, S. Chinese and South Asian ethnicity, immigration status, and clinical cancer outcomes in the Ontario Cancer System. *Cancer* **2018**, *124*, 1473–1482. [CrossRef]
8. Shah, B.R.; Griffiths, R.; Hall, S.F. Thyroid cancer incidence among Asian immigrants to Ontario, Canada: A population-based cohort study. *Cancer* **2017**, *123*, 3320–3325. [CrossRef]

9. Hjerkind, K.V.; Larsen, I.K.; Aaserud, S.; Møller, B.; Ursin, G. Cancer incidence in non-immigrants and immigrants in Norway. *Acta Oncol.* **2020**, *59*, 1275–1283. [CrossRef]
10. Noel, C.W.; Sutradhar, R.; Li, Q.; Forner, D.; Hallet, J.; Cheung, M.; Singh, S.; Coburn, N.G.; Eskander, A. Association of Immigration Status and Chinese and South Asian Ethnicity with Incidence of Head and Neck Cancer. *JAMA Otolaryngol. Head Neck Surg.* **2020**, *146*, 1125–1135. [CrossRef]
11. Bates, J.H.; Hofer, B.M.; Parikh-Patel, A. Cervical cancer incidence, mortality, and survival among Asian subgroups in California, 1990–2004. *Cancer* **2008**, *113* (Suppl. 10), 2955–2963. [CrossRef] [PubMed]
12. Hemminki, K.; Mousavi, S.M.; Sundquist, J.; Brandt, A. Does the breast cancer age at diagnosis differ by ethnicity? A study on immigrants to Sweden. *Oncologist* **2011**, *16*, 146–154. [CrossRef]
13. Huang, R.J.; Sharp, N.; Talamoa, R.O.; Ji, H.P.; Hwang, J.H.; Palaniappan, L.P. One Size Does Not Fit All: Marked Heterogeneity in Incidence of and Survival from Gastric Cancer among Asian American Subgroups. *Cancer Epidemiol. Biomark. Prev.* **2020**, *29*, 903–909. [CrossRef] [PubMed]
14. Oliva-Arocas, A.; Pereyra-Zamora, P.; Copete, J.M.; Nolasco, A. Cancer Mortality Trends in Spain (2000–2016): Differences between Immigrant and Native Populations. *Int. J. Environ. Res. Public Health* **2020**, *17*, 5127. [CrossRef]
15. Benchimol, E.I.; Mack, D.R.; Guttmann, A.; Nguyen, G.C.; To, T.; Mojaverian, N.; Quach, P.; Manuel, D.G. Inflammatory bowel disease in immigrants to Canada and their children: A population-based cohort study. *Am. J. Gastroenterol.* **2015**, *110*, 553–563. [CrossRef]
16. Istat, Movimento e Calcolo Annuale Della Popolazione Straniera Residente e Struttura per Cittadinanza. Rome, ISTAT. 2021. Available online: https://noi-italia.istat.it (accessed on 5 December 2022). (In Italian)
17. Benedetto, G.; Prima, A.D.; Sciacca, S.; Grosso, G. Design, functionality, and validity of the SWInCaRe, a web-based application used to administer cancer registry records. *Health Inform. J.* **2019**, *25*, 149–160. [CrossRef]
18. Bray, F.; Colombet, M.; Mery, L.; Piñeros, M.; Znaor, A.; Zanetti, R.; Ferlay, J. (Eds.) *Cancer Incidence in Five Continents, Vol. XI (Electronic Version)*; International Agency for Research on Cancer: Lyon, France, 2017. Available online: https://ci5.iarc.fr (accessed on 5 December 2022).
19. Cochran, W.G. The comparison of percentages in matched samples. *Biometrika* **1950**, *37*, 256–266. [CrossRef] [PubMed]
20. Available online: http://dati.istat.it/Index.aspx?DataSetCode=DCIS_POPSTRRES1 (accessed on 5 December 2022). (In Italian)
21. Roman, B.R.; Aragones, A. Epidemiology and incidence of HPV-related cancers of the head and neck. *J. Surg. Oncol.* **2021**, *124*, 920–922. [CrossRef]
22. Peacock, A.; Leung, J.; Larney, S.; Colledge, S.; Hickman, M.; Rehm, J.; Giovino, G.A.; West, R.; Hall, W.; Griffiths, P.; et al. Global statistics on alcohol, tobacco and illicit drug use: 2017 status report. *Addiction* **2018**, *113*, 1905–1926. [CrossRef]
23. Karimi, P.; Islami, F.; Anandasabapathy, S.; Freedman, N.D.; Kamangar, F. Gastric cancer: Descriptive epidemiology, risk factors, screening, and prevention. *Cancer Epidemiol. Biomark. Prev.* **2014**, *23*, 700–713. [CrossRef]
24. Bray, F.; Parkin, D.M.; African Cancer Registry Network. Cancer in sub-Saharan Africa in 2020: A review of current estimates of the national burden, data gaps, and future needs. *Lancet Oncol.* **2022**, *23*, 719–728. [CrossRef] [PubMed]
25. D'Angelo, F.; Ferrigno, L.; Mele, A.; Alfonsi, V.; Declich, S.; De Ponte, G.; Crateri, S.; Burgio, A.; Caminada, S.; Tosti, M.E.; et al. Differences in Incidence of Acute Viral Hepatitis between Foreigners and Autochthonous Population in Italy. *Int. J. Environ. Res. Public Health* **2021**, *18*, 7944. [CrossRef] [PubMed]
26. Coppola, N.; Alessio, L.; Gualdieri, L.; Pisaturo, M.; Sagnelli, C.; Minichini, C.; Di Caprio, G.; Starace, M.; Onorato, L.; Signoriello, G.; et al. Hepatitis B virus infection in undocumented immigrants and refugees in Southern Italy: Demographic, virological, and clinical features. *Infect. Dis. Poverty* **2017**, *6*, 33. [CrossRef]
27. Ferlay, J.; Ervik, M.; Lam, F.; Colombet, M.; Mery, L.; Piñeros, M.; Znaor, A.; Soerjomataram, I.; Bray, F. *Global Cancer Observatory: Cancer Today*; International Agency for Research on Cancer: Lyon, France, 2020. Available online: https://gco.iarc.fr/today (accessed on 5 December 2022).
28. Bruni, L.; Diaz, M.; Castellsagué, X.; Ferrer, E.; Bosch, F.X.; de Sanjosé, S. Cervical human papillomavirus prevalence in 5 continents: Meta-analysis of 1 million women with normal cytological findings. *J. Infect. Dis.* **2010**, *202*, 1789–1799. [CrossRef]
29. Tornesello, M.L.; Cassese, R.; De Rosa, N.; Buonaguro, L.; Masucci, A.; Vallefuoco, G.; Palmieri, S.; Schiavone, V.; Piccoli, R.; Buonaguro, F.M. High prevalence of human papillomavirus infection in Eastern European and West African women immigrants in South Italy. *APMIS* **2011**, *119*, 701–709. [CrossRef] [PubMed]
30. Campari, C.; Fedato, C.; Petrelli, A.; Zorzi, M.; Cogo, C.; Caprioglio, A.; Gallo, F.; Giordano, L.; Domenighini, S.; Pasquale, L.; et al. HPV prevalence and risk of pre-cancer and cancer in regular immigrants in Italy: Results from HPV DNA test-based screening pilot programs. *Infect. Agent Cancer* **2015**, *10*, 14. [CrossRef]
31. Culp, M.B.; Soerjomataram, I.; Efstathiou, J.A.; Bray, F.; Jemal, A. Recent Global Patterns in Prostate Cancer Incidence and Mortality Rates. *Eur. Urol.* **2020**, *77*, 38–52. [CrossRef]
32. Roshandel, G.; Boreiri, M.; Sadjadi, A.; Malekzadeh, R. A diversity of cancer incidence and mortality in West Asian populations. *Ann. Glob. Health* **2014**, *80*, 346–357. [CrossRef]
33. Kimura, T.; Egawa, S. Epidemiology of prostate cancer in Asian countries. *Int. J. Urol.* **2018**, *25*, 524–531. [CrossRef]
34. Antoni, S.; Ferlay, J.; Soerjomataram, I.; Znaor, A.; Jemal, A.; Bray, F. Bladder Cancer Incidence and Mortality: A Global Overview and Recent Trends. *Eur. Urol.* **2017**, *71*, 96–108. [CrossRef]

35. Arnold, M.; Razum, O.; Coebergh, J.W. Cancer risk diversity in non-western migrants to Europe: An overview of the literature. *Eur. J. Cancer* **2010**, *46*, 2647–2659. [CrossRef] [PubMed]
36. Rebbeck, T.R. Prostate Cancer Genetics: Variation by Race, Ethnicity, and Geography. *Semin. Radiat. Oncol.* **2017**, *27*, 3–10. [CrossRef] [PubMed]
37. Katsidzira, L.; Gangaidzo, I.; Thomson, S.; Rusakaniko, S.; Matenga, J.; Ramesar, R. The shifting epidemiology of colorectal cancer in sub-Saharan Africa. *Lancet Gastroenterol. Hepatol.* **2017**, *2*, 377–383. [CrossRef]
38. Guthold, R.; Stevens, G.A.; Riley, L.M.; Bull, F.C. Worldwide trends in insufficient physical activity from 2001 to 2016: A pooled analysis of 358 population-based surveys with 1.9 million participants. *Lancet Glob. Health* **2018**, *6*, e1077–e1086. [CrossRef] [PubMed]
39. Kerr, J.; Anderson, C.; Lippman, S.M. Physical activity, sedentary behaviour, diet, and cancer: An update and emerging new evidence. *Lancet Oncol.* **2017**, *18*, e457–e471. [CrossRef]
40. Roswall, N.; Olsen, A.; Boll, K.; Christensen, J.; Halkjær, J.; Sørensen, T.I.; Dahm, C.C.; Overvad, K.; Clavel-Chapelon, F.; Boutron-Ruault, M.C.; et al. Consumption of predefined 'Nordic' dietary items in ten European countries—An investigation in the European Prospective Investigation into Cancer and Nutrition (EPIC) cohort. *Public Health Nutr.* **2014**, *17*, 2650–2659. [CrossRef] [PubMed]
41. Ghosh, T.S.; Rampelli, S.; Jeffery, I.B.; Santoro, A.; Neto, M.; Capri, M.; Giampieri, E.; Jennings, A.; Candela, M.; Turroni, S.; et al. Mediterranean diet intervention alters the gut microbiome in older people reducing frailty and improving health status: The NU-AGE 1-year dietary intervention across five European countries. *Gut* **2020**, *69*, 1218–1228. [CrossRef]
42. Vitale, M.; Masulli, M.; Calabrese, I.; Rivellese, A.A.; Bonora, E.; Signorini, S.; Perriello, G.; Squatrito, S.; Buzzetti, R.; Sartore, G.; et al. Impact of a Mediterranean Dietary Pattern and Its Components on Cardiovascular Risk Factors, Glucose Control, and Body Weight in People with Type 2 Diabetes: A Real-Life Study. *Nutrients* **2018**, *10*, 1067. [CrossRef]
43. Cena, H.; Calder, P.C. Defining a Healthy Diet: Evidence for the Role of Contemporary Dietary Patterns in Health and Disease. *Nutrients* **2020**, *12*, 334. [CrossRef]
44. Oczkowski, M.; Dziendzikowska, K.; Pasternak-Winiarska, A.; Włodarek, D.; Gromadzka-Ostrowska, J. Dietary Factors and Prostate Cancer Development, Progression, and Reduction. *Nutrients* **2021**, *13*, 496. [CrossRef]
45. Schwingshackl, L.; Schwedhelm, C.; Galbete, C.; Hoffmann, G. Adherence to Mediterranean Diet and Risk of Cancer: An Updated Systematic Review and Meta-Analysis. *Nutrients* **2017**, *9*, 1063. [CrossRef] [PubMed]
46. Liivlaid, H.; Uusküla, A. Changes in high-risk sexual behaviour among Estonian adults between 1996 and 2006. *Sex. Transm. Infect.* **2013**, *89*, 91–97. [CrossRef] [PubMed]
47. Panatto, D.; Amicizia, D.; Lugarini, J.; Sasso, T.; Sormani, M.P.; Badolati, G.; Gasparini, R. Sexual behaviour in Ligurian (Northern Italy) adolescents and young people: Suggestions for HPV vaccination policies. *Vaccine* **2009**, *27* (Suppl. 1), A6–A10. [CrossRef]
48. Panatto, D.; Amicizia, D.; Trucchi, C.; Casabona, F.; Lai, P.L.; Bonanni, P.; Boccalini, S.; Bechini, A.; Tiscione, E.; Zotti, C.M.; et al. Sexual behaviour and risk factors for the acquisition of human papillomavirus infections in young people in Italy: Suggestions for future vaccination policies. *BMC Public Health* **2012**, *12*, 623. [CrossRef] [PubMed]
49. Bhattacharya, M.; Reiter, P.L.; McRee, A.L. Nativity status and genital HPV infection among adults in the U.S. *Hum. Vaccin. Immunother.* **2019**, *15*, 1897–1903. [CrossRef]
50. Causevic, S.; Salazar, M.; Orsini, N.; Kågesten, A.; Ekström, A.M. Sexual risk-taking behaviors among young migrant population in Sweden. *BMC Public Health* **2022**, *22*, 625. [CrossRef]
51. Gilbert, P.A.; Khokhar, S. Changing dietary habits of ethnic groups in Europe and implications for health. *Nutr. Rev.* **2008**, *66*, 203–215. [CrossRef]
52. Bao, H.; Zhang, L.; Wang, L.; Zhang, M.; Zhao, Z.; Fang, L.; Cong, S.; Zhou, M.; Wang, L. Significant variations in the cervical cancer screening rate in China by individual-level and geographical measures of socioeconomic status: A multilevel model analysis of a nationally representative survey dataset. *Cancer Med.* **2018**, *7*, 2089–2100. [CrossRef]
53. Kurani, S.; MacLaughlin, K.L.; Jacobson, R.M.; St Sauver, J.L.; Jenkins, G.D.; Fan, C.; Jacobson, D.J.; Inselman, J.; Zhu, X.; Griffin, J.M.; et al. Socioeconomic disadvantage and human papillomavirus (HPV) vaccination uptake. *Vaccine* **2022**, *40*, 471–476. [CrossRef]
54. Vaccarella, S.; Lortet-Tieulent, J.; Saracci, R.; Conway, D.I.; Straif, K.; Wild, C.P. (Eds.) *Reducing Social Inequalities in Cancer: Evidence and Priorities for Research*; International Agency for Research on Cancer: Lyon, France, 2019.
55. Morriscey, C.; Hajizadeh, M. Income and education inequalities in cervical cancer incidence in Canada, 1992–2010. *J. Public Health* **2021**, *43*, 814–823. [CrossRef]
56. Froment, M.A.; Gomez, S.L.; Roux, A.; DeRouen, M.C.; Kidd, E.A. Impact of socioeconomic status and ethnic enclave on cervical cancer incidence among Hispanics and Asians in California. *Gynecol. Oncol.* **2014**, *133*, 409–415. [CrossRef] [PubMed]
57. Hajizadeh, M.; Johnston, G.M.; Manos, D. Socio-economic inequalities in lung cancer incidence in Canada, 1992–2010: Results from the Canadian Cancer Registry. *Public Health* **2020**, *185*, 189–195. [CrossRef] [PubMed]
58. Hovanec, J.; Siemiatycki, J.; Conway, D.I.; Olsson, A.; Stücker, I.; Guida, F.; Jöckel, K.-H.; Pohlabeln, H.; Ahrens, W.; Brüske, I.; et al. Lung cancer and socioeconomic status in a pooled analysis of case-control studies. *PLoS ONE* **2018**, *13*, e0192999. [CrossRef] [PubMed]
59. Sidorchuk, A.; Agardh, E.E.; Aremu, O.; Hallqvist, J.; Allebeck, P.; Moradi, T. Socioeconomic differences in lung cancer incidence: A systematic review and meta-analysis. *Cancer Causes Control* **2009**, *20*, 459–471. [CrossRef] [PubMed]

60. Scanlon, B.; Brough, M.; Wyld, D.; Durham, J. Equity across the cancer care continuum for culturally and linguistically diverse migrants living in Australia: A scoping review. *Global Health* **2021**, *17*, 87. [CrossRef]
61. Sung, H.; Ferlay, J.; Siegel, R.L.; Laversanne, M.; Soerjomataram, I.; Jemal, A.; Bray, F. Global Cancer Statistics 2020: GLOBOCAN Estimates of Incidence and Mortality Worldwide for 36 Cancers in 185 Countries. *CA Cancer J. Clin.* **2021**, *71*, 209–249. [CrossRef]
62. Independent UK Panel on Breast Cancer Screening. The benefits and harms of breast cancer screening: An independent review. *Lancet* **2012**, *380*, 1778–1786. [CrossRef]
63. Petrelli, A.; Giorgi Rossi, P.; Francovich, L.; Giordani, B.; Di Napoli, A.; Zappa, M.; Mirisola, C.; Gargiulo, L. Geographical and socioeconomic differences in uptake of Pap test and mammography in Italy: Results from the National Health Interview Survey. *BMJ Open* **2018**, *8*, e021653. [CrossRef]
64. Siemiatycki, J.; Day, N.E.; Fabry, J.; Cooper, J.A. Discovering carcinogens in the occupational environment: A novel epidemiologic approach. *J. Natl. Cancer Inst.* **1981**, *66*, 217–225.
65. Parkin, D.M. *Studies of Cancer in Migrant Populations*; International Agency for Research on Cancer: Lyon, France, 1993.
66. Ragusa, R.; Torrisi, A.; Di Prima, A.A.; Torrisi, A.A.; Ippolito, A.; Ferrante, M.; Madeddu, A.; Guardabasso, V. Cancer Prevention for Survivors: Incidence of Second Primary Cancers and Sex Differences—A Population-Based Study from an Italian Cancer Registry. *Int. J. Environ. Res. Public Health* **2022**, *19*, 12201. [CrossRef]
67. AIRTUM Working Group. Italian cancer figures, report 2013: Multiple tumours. *Epidemiol. Prev.* **2013**, *37* (Suppl. 1), 1–152.

*cancers* MDPI

*Article*

# The Risk of Colorectal Polyps after Weight Loss Therapy Versus Obesity: A Propensity-Matched Nationwide Cohort Study

**Hisham Hussan [1,*], Eric McLaughlin [2], Chienwei Chiang [2], Joseph G. Marsano [1] and David Lieberman [3]**

[1] Division of Gastroenterology and Hepatology, Department of Internal Medicine, University of California Davis, Sacramento, CA 95616, USA
[2] Department of Biomedical Informatics, College of Medicine, The Ohio State University, Columbus, OH 43210, USA
[3] Division of Gastroenterology and Hepatology, Department of Internal Medicine, Oregon Health and Science University, Portland, OR 97239, USA
* Correspondence: hhussan@ucdavis.edu

**Simple Summary:** Obesity is a strong risk factor for the development of colorectal cancer, with a higher risk in men compared to women. Bariatric surgery is the most effective weight loss method. However, studies suggest a lower risk of colorectal cancer in women but not in men after bariatric surgery. In this study, we find that bariatric surgery mitigates the effect of obesity on the risk of colorectal polyps in both men and women. Future studies are needed to understand why men remain at higher risk of colorectal cancer despite a lower risk of polyps after bariatric surgery.

**Abstract:** Background: A fundamental understanding of the impact of bariatric surgery (BRS) on mechanisms of colorectal carcinogenesis is limited. For instance, studies report a reduced risk of colorectal cancer in females but not in males after BRS. We examined whether this sex-specific difference existed at the earlier polyp development stage. Methods: This retrospective cohort study included 281,417 adults from the 2012–2020 MarketScan database. We compared polyps rates on colonoscopy in four groups: post- vs. pre-BRS (treatment) to post- vs. pre-severe obesity (SO) diagnosis (control). We focused our main analysis on a propensity-matched sample that yielded a balanced distribution of covariates in our four groups ($n$ = 9680 adults, 21.9% males). We also adjusted for important covariates. Results: Metabolic syndrome parameters improved after bariatric surgery and worsened after severe obesity diagnosis ($p < 0.05$). The rate of polyps was 46.7% at a median of 0.5 years pre-BRS and 47.9% at a median of 0.6 years pre-SO diagnosis. The polyps rate was 45.4% at a median (range) of 3.2 (1.0–8.5) years post-BRS. Conversely, 53.8% of adults had polyps at 3.0 (1.0–8.6) years post-SO. There was no change in the risk of colorectal polyps in males or females post- vs. pre-BRS. However, the risk of polyps was higher in males (OR = 1.32, 95% CI: 1.02–1.70) and females (OR = 1.29, 95% CI: 1.13–1.47) post- vs. pre-SO. When compared to the control group (SO), the odds ratios for colorectal polyps were lower for males and females after bariatric surgery (OR = 0.63, 95% CI: 0.44–0.90, and OR = 0.79, 95% CI: 0.66–0.96, respectively). Conclusions: Obesity is associated with an increased risk of colorectal polyps, an effect that is ameliorated after bariatric surgery. These data are relevant for studies investigating colorectal carcinogenesis mechanisms.

**Keywords:** bariatric surgery; gastric bypass; sleeve gastrectomy; colorectal cancer; risk factor

## 1. Introduction

Obesity will soon surpass smoking and alcohol as a leading cause of preventable cancer in the United States and worldwide [1,2]. Obesity is a substantial risk factor for the development of colorectal cancer (CRC), the most frequent gastrointestinal cancer, affecting 2 million adults annually [3,4]. Notably, the risk of CRC is higher in males when compared to females with obesity [5,6]. Therefore, targeting obesity should help reduce the burden of

CRC, especially in males. In that regard, bariatric surgery (BRS) offers the most impactful and sustained weight loss treatment for individuals with medically complicated obesity [7]. For instance, the weight loss conferred by Roux-en-Y gastric bypass is 21% higher at 10 years than non-surgical controls [8]. Metabolic parameters are also drastically improved after bariatric surgery [7,9]. Thus, through the lens of bariatric surgery, investigators will gain insight into the biology and impact of weight loss interventions on colorectal carcinogenesis.

Indeed, multiple studies investigated CRC after bariatric surgery. Yet, despite a suggested lower risk of CRC in females after bariatric surgery, prior epidemiological data do not confirm a reduction in CRC risk in males [10–13]. The lack of a response in males is despite a more pronounced weight loss than in females after bariatric surgery [14]. Understanding this biological effect of sex on the risk of colorectal neoplasia after bariatric surgery is critical for generalizability and informing future mechanistic and interventional studies investigating the interaction between sex, energy balance, and the risk of CRC. Notably, colorectal polyps can serve as early, intermediate surrogates of CRC risk. However, most prior studies examining the risk of colorectal polyps after bariatric surgery had a small sample size and did not assess if the risk of polyps varied by sex [10,15–17]. Therefore, we aimed to fill this knowledge gap by employing a propensity-score-matched, sex-stratified analysis using a nationwide database. We hypothesized that in adults with severe obesity, bariatric surgery is associated with a lower risk of colorectal polyps in both males and females when compared to no surgery.

## 2. Materials and Methods

### 2.1. The MarketScan Database

This was a retrospective cohort study using the IBM® MarketScan Insurance Claims Research Databases, which has healthcare data for more than 39.7 million covered individuals and is one of the longest-running and largest collections of proprietary de-identified claims data for privately and publicly insured people in the U.S. [18]. Our study is based on automated claims data, which include confirmed age and sex. The MarketScan insurance claims are collected for reimbursement purposes. Therefore, we defined diagnoses and medications entered as billing claims as present. In contrast, in the absence of a diagnosis or medication insurance claim, we defined the disease or medication as absent. As a result, there were no missing data in our database, similar to other studies using MarketScan [19]. Data from MarketScan are de-identified and, thus, do not meet the federal definition of "human subject" per 45 Code of the Federal Regulation (CFR 46.101). Therefore, our study did not require review or approval by the Ohio State University Institutional Review Board.

### 2.2. Study Cohort

Details of our study design, inclusion, and exclusion criteria are in Figure 1. The 2012–2020 MarketScan database was queried using validated billing codes as published elsewhere [12]. First, we included adults $\geq$ 18 years of age with a colonoscopy and the diagnosis of severe obesity (SO). Severe obesity was defined as (1) a body mass index (BMI) $\geq 40\ kg/m^2$ or (2) BMI $\geq 35\ kg/m^2$ with obesity-related comorbidities. The above-mentioned definition of severe obesity is what is typically indicated for bariatric surgery and has been used in prior studies [11,20,21]. Then, we divided our cohort into a treatment and a control group. Our treatment group was defined as adults with SO who underwent either Roux-en-Y gastric bypass or vertical sleeve gastrectomy. Our control group was defined as adults with SO and no prior bariatric surgery. We further classified our treatment and control groups depending on the timing of colonoscopy, leading to 4 cross-sectional groups: adults with colonoscopy post-BRS or post-SO and adults with a baseline colonoscopy pre-BRS or pre-SO diagnosis [11,20]. We excluded patients with CRC risk factors other than severe obesity (e.g., personal history of CRC or polyps). We also excluded other less commonly used bariatric surgeries or gastric surgeries performed for reasons other than weight loss (e.g., gastric outlet obstruction or upper gastrointestinal ulcers). Finally, we did not include adults with colonoscopies performed within one year after BRS or SO to allow time for SO and BRS-induced weight change to take effect on the colon.

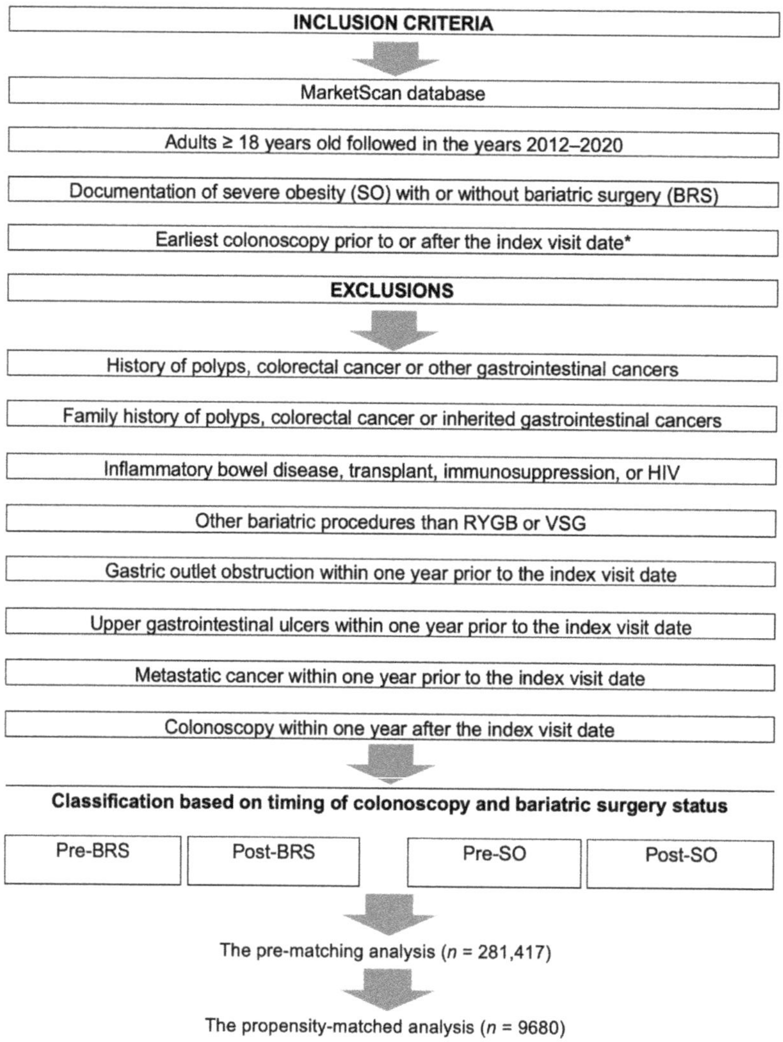


**Figure 1.** Study schema. * Index visit is earliest documentation of severe obesity for controls or date of bariatric surgery for cases.

### 2.3. Outcomes

Our primary outcome was the difference in the rate of colorectal polyps post- vs. pre-BRS compared to post- vs. pre-SO. We investigated this outcome in the pre-matching and post-propensity-matching cohorts. A colonoscopy with a polyp was defined as a colonoscopy with polypectomy using cold forceps, snare, or mucosal resection, and an associated polyp diagnosis within 3 months after colonoscopy as previously defined [22]. A colonoscopy without polyp detection was defined as a complete colonoscopy without polypectomy and no polyps. In a sub-analysis, we assessed the risk of rectal polyps, which can be performed by restricting ICD codes to rectal polyps. Due to the absence of specific

ICD-9-CM codes for colon polyps, it was not possible to specifically narrow the outcome to colon polyps or other anatomic locations.

### 2.4. Definition of Covariates

The Charlson comorbidity index (CCI) score, which accounted for number and severity of comorbidities, was used in our multivariable adjustment as was done in prior studies [10,11]. Alcohol or tobacco were defined by the presence of their respective billing codes at or prior to index visit. We also adjusted for colonoscopy screening versus diagnostic indications, which can confound the risk or detection of polyps on colonoscopy [23]. Type 2 diabetes and hyperlipidemia are components of metabolic syndrome, independently associated with an increased risk of CRC [24,25]. Therefore, we adjusted for the use of diabetes and cholesterol medications at or prior to the index visit, which can be done using MarketScan [26]. We defined being on diabetes or cholesterol medications as having at least two prescriptions belonging to these medications, at least 6 months apart, with one prescription date falling within 1 year prior to index visit date in the post-index date bariatric and control cohorts and prior to the pre-index colonoscopy in the pre-index cohorts [27].

### 2.5. Statistical Analysis

#### 2.5.1. The Pre-Matching Cohort

Our pre-matching cohort is described in Supplementary Table S1. Multivariable logistic regression was used to compare the odds of polyps post- vs. pre-BRS and post- vs. pre-SO in the unmatched cohort. Interactions were also utilized to compare post- vs. pre-BRS odds ratios to post- vs. pre-SO. Our multivariable model adjusted for age at colonoscopy, sex, Charlson comorbidity index, tobacco use, alcohol use, screening/non-screening colonoscopy, and colonoscopy performed < or ≥10/1/2015.

#### 2.5.2. The Propensity-Matched Analysis

Our matching flow is described in Supplementary Figure S1. We propensity matched our four cross-sectional groups (post-BRS, post-SO, pre-BRS, and pre-SO) without replacement and using the greedy nearest neighbor methods to create a final analytical cohort matched 1:1:1:1. Propensity scores were calculated for each unique individual from the following variables: age at time of colonoscopy (within 2 years match, required), sex (exact match, required), Charlson comorbidity index individual components (diabetes without complications, diabetes with complications, myocardial infarction, congestive heart failure, peripheral vascular disease, cerebrovascular disease, dementia, chronic pulmonary disease, connective tissue disease-rheumatic disease, mild liver disease, paraplegia and hemiplegia, renal disease, cancer after excluding CRC and metastatic cancer, and moderate to severe liver disease), and colonoscopy performed < or ≥10/1/2015 (exact match, in order to account for potential coding bias related to transitioning from ICD-9CM to ICD-10CM codes) [28]. In the pre-BRS and pre-SO groups, length of time from colonoscopy to index was included in the propensity-matching between those groups, as were the times from index to colonoscopy in the post-BRS and post-SO groups. A caliper of 0.3 was used for matching, and standardized mean differences of the propensity score logit were assessed throughout the matching process to ensure adequate balance was generated. Chi-square and Kruskal–Wallis tests were reported to display the differences across groups in the cohort eligible prior to matching and the final cohort after matching was performed. Multivariable weighted logistic regression was used to compare the odds of polyps post- vs. pre-BRS and post- vs. pre-SO. Interactions were also utilized to compare post- vs. pre-BRS odds ratios to that post- vs. pre-SO. Our multivariable model adjusted for age at colonoscopy, sex, Charlson comorbidity index, tobacco use, alcohol use, screening/non-screening colonoscopy, colonoscopy performed < or ≥10/1/2015, and use of diabetes/cholesterol medications. Chi-square tests were used to compare diabetes and cholesterol medication use at index visit date and time of colonoscopy in the post-surgery patients and post-index controls. Multivariable logistic regression was also used to assess the odds of polyps in relation to diabetes medications. All statistical analyses were performed using SAS version 9.4 (SAS Institute, Inc., Cary, NC, USA).

## 3. Results

### 3.1. The Pre-Matching Population Analysis

#### 3.1.1. General Characteristics

Our pre-matching cohort included 281,417 adults (characteristics are described in Supplementary Table S1). In the pre-matched cohort, the SO adults were older than the BRS subjects (median of 55–56 vs. 52 years, respectively), with almost twice as many males and a slightly shorter follow-up post-index visit (median of 2.3 vs. 2.7 years, respectively); all statistically significant ($p < 0.001$). Tobacco and alcohol use trended towards higher frequencies pre-BRS and pre-SO, while screening colonoscopy indication trended to be higher in the post-index visit cohort ($p < 0.001$).

#### 3.1.2. The Risk of Polyps in Adults with or without Bariatric Surgery (the Pre-Matching Cohort)

In our 281,417 adults, the rates of polyps on colonoscopy were 47.3% pre-BRS and 51.8% pre-SO. At post-index colonoscopy, the rates of polyps were 45.9% post-BRS while 56.9% post-SO (polyp rates in males and females at pre- and post-colonoscopies are in Supplementary Table S2). Our unadjusted odds ratios are included in Supplementary Table S3. Our multivariable analysis (Table 1) showed reduced odds of colorectal polyps post- vs. pre-BRS (14% in males and 10% in females), while the odds of polyps increased post- vs. pre-SO (10% in males and 22% in females). As a result, the risk of colorectal polyps post-BRS was 22% lower in males and 27% lower in females than that of SO. However, in our sub-analysis, there was no change in the odds of rectal polyps pre- or post-SO or BRS, as in Supplementary Table S4.

**Table 1.** The full pre-matched cohort. Comparison of colorectal polyp odds ratios by sex pre- and post-bariatric surgery, pre- and post-severe obesity.

| Post- vs. Pre- Colonoscopy | | Males | Females |
|---|---|---|---|
| Adjusted* OR (95% CI) | BRS | 0.86 (0.77–0.97) | 0.90 (0.84–0.96) |
| | SO | 1.10 (1.06–1.14) | 1.22 (1.19–1.26) |
| | BRS vs. SO | 0.78 (0.70–0.88) | 0.73 (0.69–0.78) |

* Models adjusted for age at colonoscopy, tobacco use, alcohol use, Charlson comorbidity index, screening colonoscopy, and date of colonoscopy (before/after 1 October 2015)

### 3.2. The Matched Cohort Analysis

#### 3.2.1. General Characteristics

Our final propensity-matched cohort included 9680 adults (2420 in each cross-sectional group, Table 2). Our propensity-matched groups had the same age median (52 years) and male distribution (21.9%). The number of comorbidities was also clinically similar between our groups (median CCI score of 3). Comparable time elapsed between pre- and post-colonoscopy in the treatment and control groups. Differences in the unmatched covariates (screening colonoscopy indication, tobacco, and alcohol use) remained statistically significant between our matched groups, with a trend towards higher frequencies pre-BRS and pre-SO ($p < 0.001$).

**Table 2.** Demographics of propensity-matched cohort.

| Variable | | Colonoscopy Pre-BRS ($n$ = 2420) | Colonoscopy Post-BRS ($n$ = 2420) | Colonoscopy Pre-SO ($n$ = 2420) | Colonoscopy Post-SO ($n$ = 2420) | $p$-Value |
|---|---|---|---|---|---|---|
| Age at Time of Colonoscopy | | 52 [49–57] | 52 [49–57] | 52 [49–57] | 52 [49–57] | 0.99 |
| Sex<br>Male<br>Female | | 530 (21.9)<br>1890 (78.1) | 530 (21.9)<br>1890 (78.1) | 530 (21.9)<br>1890 (78.1) | 530 (21.9)<br>1890 (78.1) | 0.99 |
| Charlson Comorbidity Index | | 3 [2–5] | 3 [2–4] | 3 [[2–4] | 3 [1–4] | <0.001 |
| Years from Pre-BRS or Pre-SO Colonoscopy to Index Visit Date * | Median [IQR] | 0.5 [0.2–1.1] | N/A | 0.6 [0.2–1.2] | N/A | 0.003 |
| | Range | 0–6 | N/A | 0–6 | N/A | |
| Years from Index Visit Date to Post-BRS or Post-SO Colonoscopy | Median [IQR] | N/A | 3.2 [2.0–4.7] | N/A | 3.0 [1.9–4.6] | 0.19 |
| | Range | N/A | 1–8.5 | N/A | 1–8.6 | |
| Screening Colonoscopy Indication | | 1475 (61.0) | 1420 (58.7) | 1380 (57.0) | 1335 (55.2) | <0.001 |
| Alcohol Use | | 39 (1.6) | 11 (0.5) | 34 (1.4) | 23 (1.0) | <0.001 |
| Tobacco Use | | 458 (18.9) | 237 (9.8) | 380 (15.7) | 233 (9.6) | <0.001 |

Results are presented as count (column percentage) or median (first-third quartiles) BRS: Bariatric Surgery; SO: Severe Obesity. * Index visit date is earliest documentation of severe obesity for controls or date of bariatric surgery for cases.

### 3.2.2. The Propensity-Matched Analysis Comparing the Risk of Colorectal Polyps in Adults with or without Bariatric Surgery

In our propensity-matched cohort of 9680 adults, the rate of colorectal polyps on colonoscopy was 46.7% at a median of 0.5 years pre-BRS and 47.9% at 0.6 years pre-SO (Figure 2). At the end of follow-up, the rate of polyps was 45.4% at a median (range) of 3.2 (1.0–8.5) years post-BRS. Conversely, 53.8% of adults had polyps at a median (range) of 3.0 (1.0–8.6) years post-SO. Our unadjusted odds ratios are included in Supplementary Table S5. After adjustment for all the variables in Table 2, date of colonoscopy, and also medication use at baseline, there was no change in the risk of colorectal polyps in males or females post- vs. pre-BRS (Table 3). Conversely, the risk of polyps was higher in SO controls after a similar follow-up period (OR = 1.32, 95% CI: 1.02–1.70 for males and OR = 1.29, 95% CI: 1.13–1.47 for females). As a result, the risk of colorectal polyps post-BRS was lower than that of severe obesity and no bariatric surgery (OR = 0.63, 95% CI: 0.44–0.90 for males and OR = 0.79, 95% CI: 0.66–0.96 for females).

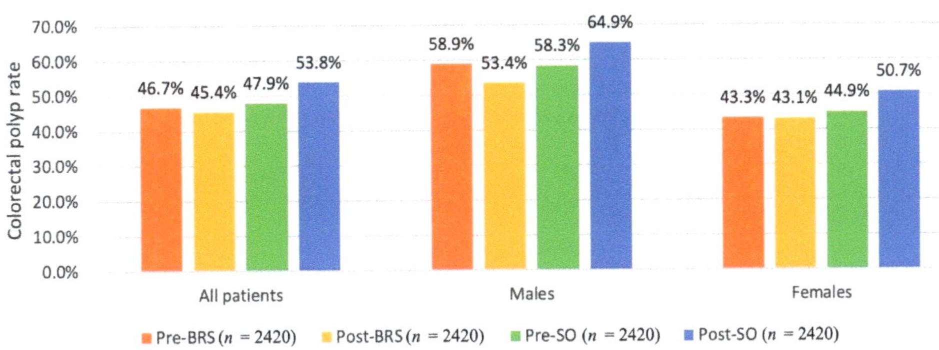


**Figure 2.** The propensity-matched analysis. Colorectal polyp rates by group and sex. BRS: Bariatric Surgery; SO: Severe Obesity.

**Table 3.** The propensity-matched analysis. Comparison of colorectal polyp odds ratios by sex pre- and post-bariatric surgery, pre- and post-severe obesity.

| Post- vs. Pre- Colonoscopy | | Males | Females |
|---|---|---|---|
| Adjusted* OR (95% CI) | BRS | 0.83 (0.65–1.07) | 1.02 (0.89–1.17) |
| | SO | 1.32 (1.02–1.70) | 1.29 (1.13–1.47) |
| | BRS vs. SO | 0.63 (0.44–0.90) | 0.79 (0.66–0.96) |

BRS: Bariatric Surgery; SO: Severe Obesity. * Models adjusted for age at colonoscopy, tobacco use, alcohol use, Charlson comorbidity index, screening colonoscopy, date of colonoscopy (before/after 1 October 2015), diabetes medication use, and cholesterol medication use (medications in pre-index/BRS are at time of colonoscopy, medications in post-index/BRS are at time of index).

#### 3.2.3. The Propensity-Matched Analysis Comparing the Risk of Rectal Polyps in Adults with or without Bariatric Surgery

Rectal polyps rates ranged between 7.9 and 8.9% in our propensity-matched cohort (Supplementary Table S6). When stratified by sex, the risk of rectal polyps was lower post- vs. pre-BRS in males but not in females as in Table 4 (OR = 0.66, 95% CI: 0.43–0.99 vs. OR = 1.11, 95% CI: 0.86–1.42, respectively). In controls with SO, there was no difference in the adjusted risk of rectal polyps during a similar follow-up. When compared to adults with bariatric surgery, there was a trend towards a reduction in rectal polyps in males, although that was not statistically significant.

**Table 4.** The propensity-matched analysis. Comparison of rectal polyp odds ratios by sex pre- and post-bariatric surgery, pre- and post-severe obesity and in an interaction model.

| Post- vs. Pre- Colonoscopy | | Males | Females |
|---|---|---|---|
| Adjusted* OR (95% CI) | BRS | 0.66 (0.43–0.99) | 1.11 (0.86–1.42) |
| | SO | 1.08 (0.72–1.61) | 0.86 (0.68–1.09) |
| | BRS vs. SO | 0.61 (0.34–1.08) | 1.29 (0.92–1.81) |

BRS: Bariatric Surgery; SO: Severe Obesity. * Models adjusted for age at colonoscopy, tobacco use, alcohol use, Charlson comorbidity index, screening colonoscopy, date of colonoscopy (before/after 1 October 2015), diabetes medication use, and cholesterol medication use (medications in pre-index/BRS are at time of colonoscopy, medications in post-index/BRS are at time of index).

### 3.3. *The Impact of Bariatric Surgery on Metabolic Markers and Relation to Polyp Outcomes*

We identify a reduction in diabetes and cholesterol medications' usage at the time of post-BRS colonoscopy (e.g., a 24.3% reduction in males vs. 16.5% in females for diabetes medications as in Table 5, $p < 0.001$). In contrast, controls with SO were on more diabetes and cholesterol medications at the time of the post-SO colonoscopy ($p < 0.001$). Supplementary Table S7 stratifies the rate of diabetes at index visits and changes in diabetes medications by sex post-bariatric surgery. When compared to our outcomes, we do not see an association between the odds of polyps and diabetes medications at index visits or at the time of colonoscopy, as in Table 6.

**Table 5.** Analysis restricted to the propensity-matched post-index cohort. Medication usage from index visit to post-BRS or post-SO colonoscopy, stratified by sex.

| Diabetes Medications' Changes | | | | | |
|---|---|---|---|---|---|
| Group | N | Index Visit * | Post-BRS or Post-SO Colonoscopy | Difference | *p*-Value |
| **Male, BRS** | 530 | 44.7% | 20.4% | −24.3% | <0.001 |
| **Male, SO** | 530 | 24.2% | 34.9% | +10.7% | <0.001 |
| **Female, BRS** | 1890 | 30.1% | 13.6% | −16.5% | <0.001 |
| **Female, SO** | 1890 | 16.1% | 28.2% | +12.1% | <0.001 |

**Table 5.** *Cont.*

| Cholesterol Medications' Changes | | | | | |
|---|---|---|---|---|---|
| **Group** | **N** | **Index Visit *** | **Post-BRS or Post-SO Colonoscopy** | **Difference** | ***p*-Value** |
| **Male, BRS** | 530 | 41.3% | 29.3% | −12.0% | <0.001 |
| **Male, SO** | 530 | 26.6% | 37.2% | +10.6% | <0.001 |
| **Female, BRS** | 1890 | 25.4% | 17.6% | −7.8% | <0.001 |
| **Female, SO** | 1890 | 15.5% | 25.0% | +9.5% | <0.001 |

BRS: Bariatric Surgery; SO: Severe Obesity. * Index visit date is earliest documentation of severe obesity for controls or date of bariatric surgery for cases

**Table 6.** Adjusted odds ratios for polyps post-BRIS stratified by gender in relation to diabetes mellitus *.

| Variable | Post-BRS Males ($n$ = 530) | Post-BRS Females ($n$ = 1890) |
|---|---|---|
| **Diabetes medications at index (Reference = No)** | 0.80 (0.54–1.17) $p = 0.25$ | 0.88 (0.71–1.10) $p = 0.26$ |
| **Cessation of diabetes medications at post-index colonoscopy (Reference = Still use medication)** | 0.83 (0.48–1.42) $p = 0.50$ | 0.91 (0.63–1.29) $p = 0.59$ |
| **Began diabetes medication after index (Reference = No)** | 1.04 (0.26–4.14) $p = 0.96$ | 1.00 (0.54–1.86) $p = 0.99$ |
| **Diabetes medications at colonoscopy (Reference = No)** | 1.04 (0.66–1.64) $p = 0.86$ | 0.98 (0.74–1.29) $p = 0.86$ |

* Models adjusted for age at colonoscopy, tobacco use, alcohol use, Charlson comorbidity index, screening colonoscopy, and date of colonoscopy (before/after 1 October 2015).

## 4. Discussion

This nationally representative, propensity-matched cohort study is the largest and first to evaluate sex-based differences in the risk of colorectal polyps after bariatric surgery as compared to persistent obesity. Per our propensity-matched analysis, the persistence of obesity was associated with an increased risk of polyps in both males and females—an expected result of worsening metabolic parameters. In contrast, the risk of colorectal polyps remained the same post- vs. pre-bariatric surgery, similar to our prior institutional data [29]. This finding is consistent with a recent meta-analysis showing an increased risk of CRC with weight gain but no conclusive change with weight loss [30]. Still, when compared to persistent obesity, bariatric surgery was associated with a lower risk of polyps, like a prior study that compared bariatric surgery to obesity controls [16]. Furthermore, our large sample size allowed us to stratify our sample by sex, where we noted a more pronounced effect in males who also had a lower risk of rectal polyps when comparing post- vs. pre-bariatric surgery in our propensity-matched analysis. We conclude that the persistence of obesity can increase the risk of colorectal polyps, an effect that can be ameliorated with bariatric surgery, especially in males, where the risk of rectal polyps is also suggestively reduced. These data strengthen the evidence for the deleterious effect of obesity on the risk of colorectal cancer in both males and females and the potentially protective effect of bariatric surgery.

In this study, we also investigated the change in diabetes and hyperlipidemia after bariatric surgery as compared to controls in both males and females. In this analysis, we used the change in the usage of diabetes medications to define new-onset diabetes (or its resolution) instead of disease codes since bariatric surgery can reduce weight and metabolic syndrome, making disease billing codes less precise after surgery. Our results show an improvement in diabetes and hyperlipidemia after bariatric surgery, while it worsened in controls with severe obesity. Nevertheless, we identified no relationship between metabolic improvement after bariatric surgery and the risk of polyps in males and females.

Our polyp data are consistent with accumulating evidence showing a lower risk of colorectal cancer in females undergoing bariatric surgery compared to controls with severe obesity [10–13]. Males also had lower odds of colorectal polyps compared to adults with persistent obesity. However, this finding in males does not conform with the epidemiological literature showing no change in CRC risk in males after bariatric surgery [13]. An explanation for a discrepancy between the risk of colorectal polyps and that of CRC in males after bariatric surgery compared to controls could be due to the lack of power or follow-up duration to detect a reduction of CRC in males. However, a recent meta-analysis with a supposably sufficient sample size shows a reduction in CRC in females but not in males followed for a similar amount of years [13]. Another theory is the beneficial effect of bariatric surgery on the colon but not rectosigmoid cancer [12]. This would be consistent with a known stronger effect of obesity on colon but not rectosigmoid cancer [31,32]. However, in this current study, there was a suggestive lower risk of rectal polyps in males post- vs. pre-bariatric surgery in our propensity-matched analysis, consistent with a more profound weight loss after bariatric surgery in males than females [33]. There was also an almost significantly lower risk of rectal polyps after bariatric surgery compared to severe obesity in males. This is, again, against data showing an almost increased risk of rectosigmoid cancer in males compared to controls [12]. Therefore, further data are needed to understand the impact of bariatric surgery on colon and rectosigmoid cancer risk in males.

One possible theory for a persistently increased risk of CRC in males compared to controls despite a lower prevalence of polyps may be due to increased acceleration of colorectal carcinogenesis due to colitis-associated carcinogenesis, a distinct pathway from adenoma-associated carcinogenesis [34–37]. Indeed, murine and human studies also report an increased colorectal inflammation after bariatric surgery for unknown mechanisms [38–40]. Furthermore, the diagnosis of de novo colitis after bariatric surgery has been reported [41–43]. These phenomena are likely due to a reduced colonic butyrate, a fiber fermentation product of colon bacteria that suppresses colonic NF-κB activity inflammatory cytokines and can modulate Wnt signaling, the most activated pathway in CRC [44–62]. Certainly, fiber intake drops by 45% post-bariatric surgery to 6–17 g/day—below the recommended intake of 25–30 g/day [63–72]. In parallel, studies observe a reduction in fecal butyrate levels and the abundance of butyrate-producing bacteria after bariatric surgery [73–79]. We suspect a lower butyrate would be more pronounced in males, who are reported to consume 20% less fiber per kcal/day than females after bariatric surgery [80]. As a result, an altered colonic milieu with lower butyrate could counteract the beneficial effect of weight loss on the colorectum. Data are limited; therefore, future mechanistic studies need to assess this theory and the impact of bariatric surgery on adenoma- and colitis-associated carcinogenesis.

Strengths and limitations: An ideal method to examine our hypothesis would be to prospectively measure the risk of neoplastic polyps on colonoscopy in males and females randomized to bariatric surgery vs. no surgery [81]. However, this design would be cumbersome and likely yield a small sample size to detect sex-based differences. As an alternative, our study used a propensity score, which allows for quasi-randomization depending on the status of bariatric surgery and the timing of colonoscopy. By comparing bariatric surgery to controls with severe obesity, we accounted for the effect of obesity or weight loss during a similar follow-up period on the risk of colorectal polyps. Our propensity-matched pre- and post-cohorts had similar characteristics except for the timing of colonoscopy, either pre- or post-BRS or SO. We also used thorough exclusions when choosing appropriate controls without bariatric surgery in order to minimize confounding and isolate the effect of obesity/bariatric surgery. As a result, our matched pre-SO cohort had a comparable rate of polyps to the pre-BRS cohort (47.9% vs. 46.7%, respectively, $p = 0.42$). Despite our comprehensive analysis, we report a few limitations due to the nature of the MarketScan database. For instance, we are limited by our retrospective design and use of billing codes despite using previously validated codes. Our cohort also remains a convenience sample, limited to patients with commercial insurance who received colonoscopies either pre- or post-surgery. Our stringent exclusions may also limit the generalizability of this study to adults who were excluded from our study. Also, we could not assess the pathology of polyps in MarketScan, which can be either precancerous (adenoma or serrated polyps) or completely benign (hyperplastic). Still, there is a strong correlation between adenoma detection rate (ADR) and polyp detection rate, which is used as a surrogate of ADR in some countries [22,82]. Furthermore, there is no association between hyperplastic polyps and adipokines/obesity, unlike adenomas, which makes hyperplastic polyps less likely to be altered after surgical weight loss to confound our findings [83–86]. Finally, we could not account for the exact BMI values or duration of obesity prior to surgery or prior to documentation of obesity in our controls. However, we adjusted for markers of metabolic syndrome that correlate with the duration and severity of obesity [87]. Future prospective studies also need to account for other risk factors such as diet, exercise, and race/ ethnicity, which we could not include using the MarketScan administrative database.

## 5. Conclusions

In summary, obesity is becoming the number one healthcare concern in the world. The study using a nationwide database is designed to provide descriptive data addressing the differential impact of bariatric surgery on the risk of colorectal polyps according to sex. This information sheds light on the natural history of the adenoma–carcinoma pathway of colorectal carcinogenesis with obesity and after bariatric surgery. These data also provide sex-based data for mechanistic studies and the design of future interventional studies using bariatric surgery. These studies are specifically needed to understand why men remain at higher risk of colorectal cancer despite a lower risk of polyps after bariatric surgery, which would be pivotal for public efforts aimed at reducing the risk of CRC.

**Supplementary Materials:** The following supporting information can be downloaded at https://www.mdpi.com/article/10.3390/cancers15194820/s1. Table S1: Demographics of eligible cohort prior to matching; Table S2: Polyp rates in the pre-matching cohort; Table S3: The full pre-matched cohort. Comparison of colorectal/rectal polyps' unadjusted odds ratios by sex pre- and post-BRS, pre- and post-SO; Table S4: The full pre-matched cohort. Comparison of rectal polyp odds ratios by sex pre- and post-bariatric surgery, pre- and post-severe obesity in full cohort prior to matching; Table S5: The propensity-matched analysis. Comparison of colorectal/rectal polyps' unadjusted odds ratios by sex pre- and post-BRS, pre- and post-SO; Table S6: The propensity-matched cohort. Rectal polyps' rates by group and sex—the propensity-matched analysis; Table S7: The propensity-matched cohort. Diabetes at index visit date, defined as date of bariatric surgery. Diabetes medications' cessation or new usage at time of colonoscopy; Figure S1: Flowchart of 1:1:1:1 propensity matching algorithm (LPS SD: Logit of propensity score standardized difference).

**Author Contributions:** H.H. was involved in the conception, design, funding acquisition, and interpretation of data, as well as in the drafting and critical revision of the manuscript; C.C. was involved in acquiring the data and the study design; E.M. was involved in the study methodology, statistical analysis of the data, and drafting of the manuscript. The above authors had full access to all the data in the study and take responsibility for the integrity and accuracy of the data and analyses. D.L. and J.G.M. were involved in the methodology, editing, and revisions of the manuscript. All authors have read and agreed to the published version of the manuscript.

**Funding:** The MarketScan database analysis was supported by an award (UL1TR002733) from the National Center for Advancing Translational Sciences. Additional support for the tertiary center dietary data was obtained from the Molecular Carcinogenesis and Chemo-prevention program at the Ohio State University Comprehensive Cancer Center. The content is solely the responsibility of the authors and does not necessarily represent the official views of the National Center for Advancing Translational Sciences or the National Institutes of Health.

**Institutional Review Board Statement:** Data from MarketScan are de-identified and, thus, do not meet the federal definition of "human subject" per 45 Code of the Federal Regulation (CFR 46.101). Therefore, our study did not require review or approval by the Ohio State University Institutional Review Board.

**Informed Consent Statement:** Not applicable due to using a de-identified database.

**Data Availability Statement:** Our detailed methods and codes are described in our paper. Patient-level, de-identified data were obtained from IBM MarketScan as part of a data agreement with the Ohio State University. Our investigators will make the analytical files available to any researchers for non-commercial purposes after the researcher obtains approval for third-party access from IBM MarketScan. Any researcher requesting access to the raw patient-level de-identified data that were used to generate the analytical files can access the data directly through IBM MarketScan under a license agreement with IBM MarketScan.

**Conflicts of Interest:** The authors have no relevant conflict of interest, including relevant financial interests, activities, relationships, or affiliations.

## References


1. Tran, K.B.; Lang, J.J.; Xu, R.; Compton, k.; Acheson, A.R.; Henrikson, H.J.; Kocarnik, J.M.; Penberthy, L.; Aali, A.; Abbas, Q. The global burden of cancer attributable to risk factors, 2010–19: A systematic analysis for the Global Burden of Disease Study 2019. *Lancet* **2022**, *400*, 563–591. [CrossRef] [PubMed]
2. Ward, Z.J.; Bleich, S.N.; Cradock, A.L.; Barrett, J.L.; Giles, C.M.; Flax, C.; Long, M.W.; Gortmaker, S.L. Projected U.S. State-Level Prevalence of Adult Obesity and Severe Obesity. *N. Engl. J. Med.* **2019**, *381*, 2440–2450. [CrossRef] [PubMed]
3. Lauby-Secretan, B.; Scoccianti, C.; Loomis, D.; Grosse, Y.; Bianchini, F.; Straif, K. Body Fatness and Cancer—Viewpoint of the IARC Working Group. *N. Engl. J. Med.* **2016**, *375*, 794–798. [CrossRef] [PubMed]
4. Morgan, E.; Arnold, M.; Gini, A.; Lorenzoni, V.; Cabasag, C.J.; Laversanne, M.; Vignat, J.; Ferlay, J.; Murphy, N.; Bray, F. Global burden of colorectal cancer in 2020 and 2040: Incidence and mortality estimates from GLOBOCAN. *Gut* **2023**, *72*, 338–344. [CrossRef] [PubMed]
5. Loosen, S.H.; Roderburg, C.; Jördens, M.S.; Fluegen, G.; Luedde, T.; Kostev, K. Overweight and Obesity Determine the Risk for Gastrointestinal Cancer in a Sex-Dependent Manner: A Retrospective Cohort Study of 287,357 Outpatients in Germany. *Cancers* **2022**, *14*, 931. [CrossRef]
6. Demb, J.; Earles, A.; Martínez, M.E.; Bustamante, R.; Bryant, A.K.; Murphy, J.D.; Liu, L.; Gupta, S. Risk factors for colorectal cancer significantly vary by anatomic site. *BMJ Open Gastroenterol.* **2019**, *6*, e000313. [CrossRef]
7. Maciejewski, M.L.; Arterburn, D.E.; Van Scoyoc, L.; Smith, V.A.; Yancy, W.S., Jr.; Weidenbacher, H.J.; Livingston, E.H.; Olsen, M.K. Bariatric Surgery and Long-term Durability of Weight Loss. *JAMA Surg.* **2016**, *151*, 1046–1055. [CrossRef]
8. Kennedy-Dalby, A.; Adam, S.; Ammori, B.J.; Syed, A.A. Weight loss and metabolic outcomes of bariatric surgery in men versus women—A matched comparative observational cohort study. *Eur. J. Intern. Med.* **2014**, *25*, 922–925. [CrossRef]
9. Katsogiannos, P.; Kamble, P.G.; Wiklund, U.; Sundbom, M.; Espes, D.; Hammar, U.; Karlsson, F.A.; Pereira, M.J.; Eriksson, J.W. Rapid changes in neuroendocrine regulation may contribute to reversal of type 2 diabetes after gastric bypass surgery. *Endocrine* **2020**, *67*, 344–353. [CrossRef]
10. Bailly, L.; Fabre, R.; Pradier, C.; Iannelli, A. Colorectal Cancer Risk Following Bariatric Surgery in a Nationwide Study of French Individuals with Obesity. *JAMA Surg.* **2020**, *155*, 395–402. [CrossRef]
11. Schauer, D.P.; Feigelson, H.S.; Koebnick, C.; Caan, B.; Weinmann, S.; Leonard, A.C.; Powers, J.D.; Yenumula, P.R.; Arterburn, D.E. Bariatric Surgery and the Risk of Cancer in a Large Multisite Cohort. *Ann. Surg.* **2019**, *269*, 95–101. [CrossRef] [PubMed]
12. Hussan, H.; Akinyeye, S.; Mihaylova, M.; McLaughlin, E.; Chiang, C.; Clinton, S.K.; Lieberman, D. Colorectal Cancer Risk Is Impacted by Sex and Type of Surgery after Bariatric Surgery. *Obes. Surg.* **2022**, *32*, 2880–2890. [CrossRef] [PubMed]
13. Chierici, A.; Amoretti, P.; Drai, C.; De Fatico, S.; Barriere, J.; Schiavo, L.; Iannelli, A. Does Bariatric Surgery Reduce the Risk of Colorectal Cancer in Individuals with Morbid Obesity? A Systematic Review and Meta-Analysis. *Nutrients* **2023**, *15*, 467. [CrossRef] [PubMed]
14. Risi, R.; Rossini, G.; Tozzi, R.; Pieralice, S.; Monte, L.; Masi, D.; Castagneto-Gissey, L.; Gallo, I.F.; Strigari, L.; Casella, G. Sex difference in the safety and efficacy of bariatric procedures: A systematic review and meta-analysis. *Surg. Obes. Relat. Dis.* **2022**, *18*, 983–996. [CrossRef]
15. Kedrin, D.; Gandhi, S.-C.C.; Wolf, M.; Roper, J.; Yilmaz, O.; Corey, K.; Khalili, H.; Stanford, F.C.; Gala, M. Bariatric Surgery Prior to Index Screening Colonoscopy Is Associated with a Decreased Rate of Colorectal Adenomas in Obese Individuals. *Clin. Transl. Gastroenterol.* **2017**, *8*, e73. [CrossRef]
16. Droney, A.C.; Sellers, W.; Gupta, A.; Johnson, K.R.; Fluck, M.; Petrick, A.; Bannon, J.; Erchinger, T.; Protyniak, B. Incidence of polyp formation following bariatric surgery. *Surg. Obes. Relat. Dis.* **2021**, *17*, 1773–1779. [CrossRef]
17. Peleg, N.; Sapoznikov, S.; Levi, Z.; Dotan, I.; Shamah, S. Incidence of Colorectal Adenomas after Bariatric Surgery: Pre-operative Super Morbid Obesity Is Independently Associated with Increased Risk. *Obes. Surg.* **2021**, *31*, 4220–4226. [CrossRef]

18. IBM. IBM MarketScan Research Databases. Available online: https://www.ibm.com/watson-health/about/truven-health-analytics (accessed on 21 April 2021).
19. Gill, K.; Chia, V.M.; Hernandez, R.K.; Navetta, M. Rates of Vascular Events in Patients with Migraine: A MarketScan® Database Retrospective Cohort Study. *Headache J. Head Face Pain* **2020**, *60*, 2265–2280. [CrossRef]
20. Arterburn, D.; Wellman, R.; Emiliano, A.; Smith, S.R.; Odegaard, A.O.; Murali, S.; Williams, N.; Coleman, K.J.; Courcoulas, A.; Coley, R.Y. Comparative Effectiveness and Safety of Bariatric Procedures for Weight Loss: A PCORnet Cohort Study. *Ann. Intern. Med.* **2018**, *169*, 741–750. [CrossRef]
21. Wolfe, B.M.; Kvach, E.; Eckel, R.H. Treatment of Obesity: Weight Loss and Bariatric Surgery. *Circ. Res.* **2016**, *118*, 1844–1855. [CrossRef]
22. Gandhi, S.K.; Reynolds, M.W.; Boyer, J.G.; Goldstein, J.L. Recurrence and malignancy rates in a benign colorectal neoplasm patient cohort: Results of a 5-year analysis in a managed care environment. *Am. J. Gastroenterol.* **2001**, *96*, 2761–2767. [CrossRef] [PubMed]
23. Ahmed, S.; Naumann, D.N.; Karandikar, S. Differences in screening vs non-screening colonoscopy: Scope for improvement? *Color. Dis.* **2016**, *18*, 903–909. [CrossRef]
24. Ma, Y.; Yang, W.; Song, M.; Smith-Warner, S.A.; Yang, J.; Li, Y.; Ma, W.; Hu, Y.; Ogino, S.; Hu, F.B. Type 2 diabetes and risk of colorectal cancer in two large U.S. prospective cohorts. *Br. J. Cancer* **2018**, *119*, 1436–1442. [CrossRef] [PubMed]
25. Yao, X.; Tian, Z. Dyslipidemia and colorectal cancer risk: A meta-analysis of prospective studies. *Cancer Causes Control* **2015**, *26*, 257–268. [CrossRef] [PubMed]
26. Liu, G.; Sterling, N.W.; Kong, L.; Lewis, M.M.; Mailman, R.B.; Chen, H.; Leslie, D.; Huang, X. Statins may facilitate Parkinson's disease: Insight gained from a large, national claims database. *Mov. Disord.* **2017**, *32*, 913–917. [CrossRef]
27. Cho, I.-J.; Shin, J.-H.; Jung, M.-H.; Kang, C.Y.; Hwang, J.; Kwon, C.H.; Kim, W.; Kim, D.-H.; Lee, C.J.; Kang, S.-H. Antihypertensive Drugs and the Risk of Cancer: A Nationwide Cohort Study. *J. Clin. Med.* **2021**, *10*, 771. [CrossRef]
28. Sabatino, M.J.; Burroughs, P.J.; Moore, H.G.; Grauer, J.N. Spine coding transition from ICD-9 to ICD-10: Not taking advantage of the specificity of a more granular system. *N. Am. Spine Soc. J.* **2020**, *4*, 100035. [CrossRef]
29. Hussan, H.; Drosdak, A.; Le Roux, M.; Patel, K.; Porter, K.; Clinton, S.K.; Focht, B.; Noria, S. The Long-term Impact of Roux-en-Y Gastric Bypass on Colorectal Polyp Formation and Relation to Weight Loss Outcomes. *Obes. Surg.* **2019**, *30*, 407–415. [CrossRef]
30. Karahalios, A.; English, D.R.; Simpson, J.A. Weight change and risk of colorectal cancer: A systematic review and meta-analysis. *Am. J. Epidemiol.* **2015**, *181*, 832–845. [CrossRef]
31. Ben, Q.; An, W.; Jiang, Y.; Zhan, X.; Du, Y.; Cai, Q.C.; Gao, J.; Li, Z. Body mass index increases risk for colorectal adenomas based on meta-analysis. *Gastroenterology* **2012**, *142*, 762–772. [CrossRef]
32. Bardou, M.; Barkun, A.N.; Martel, M. Obesity and colorectal cancer. *Gut* **2013**, *62*, 933–947. [CrossRef]
33. Larsson, S.C.; Wolk, A. Obesity and colon and rectal cancer risk: A meta-analysis of prospective studies. *Am. J. Clin. Nutr.* **2007**, *86*, 556–565. [CrossRef]
34. Baker, A.-M.; Cross, W.; Curtius, K.; Bakir, I.A.; Choi, C.-H.R.; Davis, H.L.; Temko, D.; Biswas, S.; Martinez, P.; Williams, M.J. Evolutionary history of human colitis-associated colorectal cancer. *Gut* **2019**, *68*, 985–995. [CrossRef] [PubMed]
35. Huang, L.C.; Merchea, A. Dysplasia and Cancer in Inflammatory Bowel Disease. *Surg. Clin. N. Am.* **2017**, *97*, 627–639. [CrossRef] [PubMed]
36. Rutter, M.D.; Saunders, B.P.; Wilkinson, K.H.; Rumbles, S.; Schofield, G.; Kamm, M.A.; Williams, C.B.; Price, A.B.; Talbot, I.C.; Forbes, A. Thirty-year analysis of a colonoscopic surveillance program for neoplasia in ulcerative colitis. *Gastroenterology* **2006**, *130*, 1030–1038. [CrossRef]
37. Itzkowitz, S.H.; Harpaz, N. Diagnosis and management of dysplasia in patients with inflammatory bowel diseases. *Gastroenterology* **2004**, *126*, 1634–1648. [CrossRef]
38. Sainsbury, A.; Goodlad, R.A.; Perry, S.L.; Pollard, S.G.; Robins, G.G.; Hull, M.A. Increased colorectal epithelial cell proliferation and crypt fission associated with obesity and roux-en-Y gastric bypass. *Cancer Epidemiol. Biomark. Prev.* **2008**, *17*, 1401–1410. [CrossRef]
39. Kant, P.; Sainsbury, A.; Reed, K.R.; Pollard, S.G.; Scott, N.; Clarke, A.R.; Coletta, P.L.; Hull, M.A. Rectal epithelial cell mitosis and expression of macrophage migration inhibitory factor are increased 3 years after Roux-en-Y gastric bypass (RYGB) for morbid obesity: Implications for long-term neoplastic risk following RYGB. *Gut* **2011**, *60*, 893–901. [CrossRef]
40. Garibay, D.; Zaborska, K.E.; Shanahan, M.; Zheng, Q.; Kelly, K.M.; Montrose, D.C.; Dannenberg, A.J.; Miller, A.D.; Sethupathy, P.; Cummings, B.P. TGR5 Protects against Colitis in Mice, but Vertical Sleeve Gastrectomy Increases Colitis Severity. *Obes. Surg.* **2019**, *29*, 1593–1601. [CrossRef] [PubMed]
41. Braga Neto, M.B.; Gregory, M.; Ramos, G.P.; Loftus, E.V., Jr.; Ciorba, M.A.; Bruining, D.H.; Bazerbachi, F.; Abu Dayyeh, B.K.; Kushnir, V.M.; Shah, M. De-novo Inflammatory Bowel Disease after Bariatric Surgery: A Large Case Series. *J. Crohn's Colitis* **2018**, *12*, 452–457. [CrossRef]
42. Ungaro, R.; Fausel, R.; Chang, H.L.; Chang, S.; Chen, L.A.; Nakad, A.; El Nawar, A.; Prytz Berset, I.; Axelrad, J.; Lawlor, G. Bariatric surgery is associated with increased risk of new-onset inflammatory bowel disease: Case series and national database study. *Aliment. Pharmacol. Ther.* **2018**, *47*, 1126–1134. [CrossRef]
43. Allin, K.H.; Jacobsen, R.K.; Ungaro, R.C.; Colombel, J.F.; Egeberg, A.; Villumsen, M.; Jess, T. Bariatric Surgery and Risk of New-onset Inflammatory Bowel Disease: A Nationwide Cohort Study. *J. Crohn's Colitis* **2021**, *15*, 1474–1480. [CrossRef]

44. Jiang, L.; Wang, J.; Liu, Z.; Jiang, A.; Li, S.; Wu, D.; Zhang, Y.; Zhu, X.; Zhou, E.; Wei, Z. Sodium Butyrate Alleviates Lipopolysaccharide-Induced Inflammatory Responses by Down-Regulation of NF-κB, NLRP3 Signaling Pathway, and Activating Histone Acetylation in Bovine Macrophages. *Front. Vet. Sci.* **2020**, *7*, 579674. [CrossRef] [PubMed]
45. Segain, J.-P.; de la Blétière, D.R.; Bourreille, A.; Leray, V.; Gervois, N.; Rosales, C.; Ferrier, L.; Bonnet, C.; Blottière, H.M.; Galmiche, J.-P. Butyrate inhibits inflammatory responses through NFκB inhibition: Implications for Crohn's disease. *Gut* **2000**, *47*, 397–403. [CrossRef] [PubMed]
46. Wang, N.; Liang, H.; Zen, K. Molecular mechanisms that influence the macrophage m1-m2 polarization balance. *Front. Immunol.* **2014**, *5*, 614. [CrossRef]
47. Karin, M.; Greten, F.R. NF-κB: Linking inflammation and immunity to cancer development and progression. *Nat. Rev. Immunol.* **2005**, *5*, 749–759. [CrossRef] [PubMed]
48. Tong, X.; Yin, L.; Joshi, S.; Rosenberg, D.W.; Giardina, C. Cyclooxygenase-2 Regulation in Colon Cancer Cells: Modulation of RNA Polymerase II Elongation by Histone Deacetylase Inhibitors *. *J. Biol. Chem.* **2005**, *280*, 15503–15509. [CrossRef]
49. Tong, X.; Yin, L.; Giardina, C. Butyrate suppresses Cox-2 activation in colon cancer cells through HDAC inhibition. *Biochem. Biophys. Res. Commun.* **2004**, *317*, 463–471. [CrossRef] [PubMed]
50. Carretta, M.D.; Quiroga, J.; López, R.; Hidalgo, M.A.; Burgos, R.A. Participation of Short-Chain Fatty Acids and Their Receptors in Gut Inflammation and Colon Cancer. *Front. Physiol.* **2021**, *12*, 662739. [CrossRef]
51. Kurata, N.; Tokashiki, N.; Fukushima, K.; Misao, T.; Hasuoka, N.; Kitagawa, K.; Mashimo, M.; Regan, J.W.; Murayama, T.; Fujino, H. Short chain fatty acid butyrate uptake reduces expressions of prostanoid EP4 receptors and their mediation of cyclooxygenase-2 induction in HCA-7 human colon cancer cells. *Eur. J. Pharmacol.* **2019**, *853*, 308–315. [CrossRef]
52. Zhang, Z.H.; Ouyang, Q.; Gan, H.T. Targeting cyclooxygenase-2 with sodium butyrate and NSAIDs on colorectal adenoma/carcinoma cells. *World J. Gastroenterol.* **2004**, *10*, 2954–2957. [CrossRef] [PubMed]
53. Jahns, F.; Wilhelm, A.; Jablonowski, N.; Mothes, H.; Radeva, M.; Wölfert, A.; Greulich, K.O.; Glei, M. Butyrate suppresses mRNA increase of osteopontin and cyclooxygenase-2 in human colon tumor tissue. *Carcinogenesis* **2011**, *32*, 913–920. [CrossRef]
54. Krawczyk, M.; Emerson, B.M. p50-associated COX-2 extragenic RNA (PACER) activates COX-2 gene expression by occluding repressive NF-κB complexes. *eLife* **2014**, *3*, e01776. [CrossRef] [PubMed]
55. Shi, G.; Li, D.; Fu, J.; Sun, Y.; Li, Y.; Qu, R.; Jin, X.; Li, D. Upregulation of cyclooxygenase-2 is associated with activation of the alternative nuclear factor kappa B signaling pathway in colonic adenocarcinoma. *Am. J. Transl. Res.* **2015**, *7*, 1612–1620. [PubMed]
56. Yamamoto, K.; Arakawa, T.; Ueda, N.; Yamamoto, S. Transcriptional roles of nuclear factor kappa B and nuclear factor-interleukin-6 in the tumor necrosis factor alpha-dependent induction of cyclooxygenase-2 in MC3T3-E1 cells. *J. Biol. Chem.* **1995**, *270*, 31315–31320. [CrossRef]
57. Tan, J.; McKenzie, C.; Potamitis, M.; Thorburn, A.N.; Mackay, C.R.; Macia, L. Chapter Three—The Role of Short-Chain Fatty Acids in Health and Disease. In *Advances in Immunology*; Alt, F.W., Ed.; Academic Press: Cambridge, MA, USA, 2014; pp. 91–119.
58. Schwitalla, S.; Fingerle, A.; Cammareri, P.; Nebelsiek, T.; Göktuna, S.I.; Ziegler, P.K.; Canli, O.; Heijmans, J.; Huels, D.J.; Moreaux, G. Intestinal Tumorigenesis Initiated by Dedifferentiation and Acquisition of Stem-Cell-like Properties. *Cell* **2013**, *152*, 25–38. [CrossRef]
59. Bordonaro, M.; Lazarova, D.L.; Sartorelli, A.C. Butyrate and Wnt signaling: A possible solution to the puzzle of dietary fiber and colon cancer risk? *Cell Cycle* **2008**, *7*, 1178–1183. [CrossRef]
60. Cray, N.; Zhao, Y.; Fang, Y.; Liu, P.; Pollak, L.; Duvick, S.; Birt, D.F.; Whitley, E.M. Effects of Dietary Resistant Starch on the Wnt Signaling Pathway and Preneoplastic Cells in the Colons of Azoxymethane-Treated Rats. *Nutr. Cancer* **2017**, *69*, 632–642. [CrossRef]
61. Malcomson, F.C.; Willis, N.D.; McCallum, I.; Xie, L.; Shivappa, N.; Wirth, M.D.; Hébert, J.R.; Kocaadam-Bozkurt, B.; Özturan-Sirin, A.; Kelly, S.B. Diet-Associated Inflammation Modulates Inflammation and WNT Signaling in the Rectal Mucosa, and the Response to Supplementation with Dietary Fiber. *Cancer Prev. Res.* **2021**, *14*, 337–346. [CrossRef]
62. Malcomson, F.C.; Willis, N.D.; Mathers, J.C. Is resistant starch protective against colorectal cancer via modulation of the WNT signalling pathway? *Proc. Nutr. Soc.* **2015**, *74*, 282–291. [CrossRef]
63. American, D.G.F. Dietary Guidelines for Americans 2015–2020. Available online: https://health.gov/sites/default/files/2019-09/2015-2020_Dietary_Guidelines.pdf (accessed on 15 May 2023).
64. World Cancer Research Fund. Diet, Nutrition, Physical Activity and Cancer: A Global Perspective. Cancer prevention guidelines. Available online: https://www.wcrf.org/dietandcancer. (accessed on 20 May 2023).
65. Farias, G.; Silva, R.M.O.; da Silva, P.P.P.; Vilela, R.M.; Bettini, S.C.; Dâmaso, A.R.; Netto, B.D.M. Impact of dietary patterns according to NOVA food groups: 2 y after Roux-en-Y gastric bypass surgery. *Nutrition* **2020**, *74*, 110746. [CrossRef] [PubMed]
66. Johnson, L.K.; Andersen, L.F.; Hofsø, D.; Aasheim, E.T.; Holven, K.B.; Sandbu, R.; Røislien, J.; Hjelmesæth, J. Dietary changes in obese patients undergoing gastric bypass or lifestyle intervention: A clinical trial. *Br. J. Nutr.* **2013**, *110*, 127–134. [CrossRef]
67. Ziadlou, M.; Hosseini-Esfahani, F.; Mozaffari Khosravi, H.; Hosseinpanah, F.; Barzin, M.; Khalaj, A.; Valizadeh, M. Dietary macro- and micro-nutrients intake adequacy at 6th and 12th month post-bariatric surgery. *BMC Surg.* **2020**, *20*, 232. [CrossRef] [PubMed]
68. Golzarand; Toolabi, K.; Djafarian, K. Changes in Body Composition, Dietary Intake, and Substrate Oxidation in Patients Underwent Laparoscopic Roux-en-Y Gastric Bypass and Laparoscopic Sleeve Gastrectomy: A Comparative Prospective Study. *Obes. Surg.* **2019**, *29*, 406–413. [CrossRef] [PubMed]

69. Carvalho, A.C.; Mota, M.C.; Marot, L.P.; Mattar, L.A.; de Sousa, J.A.G.; Araújo, A.C.T.; da Costa Assis, C.T.; Crispim, C.A. Circadian Misalignment Is Negatively Associated with the Anthropometric, Metabolic and Food Intake Outcomes of Bariatric Patients 6 Months after Surgery. *Obes. Surg.* **2021**, *31*, 159–169. [CrossRef]
70. Novais, P.F.S.; Rasera, I.; Leite, C.V.d.S.; Marin, F.A.; de Oliveira, M.R.M. Food intake in women two years or more after bariatric surgery meets adequate intake requirements. *Nutr. Res.* **2012**, *32*, 335–341. [CrossRef] [PubMed]
71. Verger, E.O.; Aron-Wisnewsky, J.; Dao, M.C.; Kayser, B.D.; Oppert, J.-M.; Bouillot, J.-L.; Torcivia, A.; Clément, K. Micronutrient and Protein Deficiencies after Gastric Bypass and Sleeve Gastrectomy: A 1-year Follow-up. *Obes. Surg.* **2016**, *26*, 785–796. [CrossRef]
72. Jeffreys, R.M.; Hrovat, K.; Woo, J.G.; Schmidt, M.; Inge, T.H.; Xanthakos, S.A. Dietary assessment of adolescents undergoing laparoscopic Roux-en-Y gastric bypass surgery: Macro- and micronutrient, fiber, and supplement intake. *Surg. Obes. Relat. Dis.* **2012**, *8*, 331–336. [CrossRef]
73. Farup, P.G.; Valeur, J. Changes in Faecal Short-Chain Fatty Acids after Weight-Loss Interventions in Subjects with Morbid Obesity. *Nutrients* **2020**, *12*, 802. [CrossRef]
74. Meijer, J.L.; Roderka, M.N.; Chinburg, E.L.; Renier, T.J.; McClure, A.C.; Rothstein, R.I.; Barry, E.L.; Billmeier, S.; Gilbert-Diamond, D. Alterations in Fecal Short-Chain Fatty Acids after Bariatric Surgery: Relationship with Dietary Intake and Weight Loss. *Nutrients* **2022**, *14*, 4243. [CrossRef]
75. Tremaroli, V.; Karlsson, F.; Werling, M.; Ståhlman, M.; Kovatcheva-Datchary, P.; Olbers, T.; Fändriks, L.; le Roux, C.W.; Nielsen, J.; Bäckhed, F. Roux-en-Y Gastric Bypass and Vertical Banded Gastroplasty Induce Long-Term Changes on the Human Gut Microbiome Contributing to Fat Mass Regulation. *Cell Metab.* **2015**, *22*, 228–238. [CrossRef]
76. Juárez-Fernández, M.; Román-Sagüillo, S.; Porras, D.; García-Mediavilla, M.V.; Linares, P.; Ballesteros-Pomar, M.D.; Urioste-Fondo, A.; Álvarez-Cuenllas, B.; González-Gallego, J.; Sánchez-Campos, S. Long-Term Effects of Bariatric Surgery on Gut Microbiota Composition and Faecal Metabolome Related to Obesity Remission. *Nutrients* **2021**, *13*, 2519. [CrossRef]
77. Ou, J.; DeLany, J.P.; Zhang, M.; Sharma, S.; O'Keefe, S.J.D. Association between low colonic short-chain fatty acids and high bile acids in high colon cancer risk populations. *Nutr. Cancer* **2012**, *64*, 34–40. [CrossRef] [PubMed]
78. Graessler, J.; Qin, Y.; Zhong, H.; Zhang, J.; Licinio, J.; Wong, M.L.; Xu, A.; Chavakis, T.; Bornstein, A.B.; Ehrhart-Bornstein, M. Metagenomic sequencing of the human gut microbiome before and after bariatric surgery in obese patients with type 2 diabetes: Correlation with inflammatory and metabolic parameters. *Pharmacogenom. J.* **2013**, *13*, 514–522. [CrossRef]
79. Sowah, S.A.; Riedl, L.; Damms-Machado, A.; Johnson, T.S.; Schübel, R.; Graf, M.; Kartal, E.; Zeller, G.; Schwingshackl, L.; Stangl, G.I. Effects of Weight-Loss Interventions on Short-Chain Fatty Acid Concentrations in Blood and Feces of Adults: A Systematic Review. *Adv. Nutr.* **2019**, *10*, 673–684. [CrossRef] [PubMed]
80. Kanerva, N.; Larsson, I.; Peltonen, M.; Lindroos, A.K.; Carlsson, L.M. Sociodemographic and lifestyle factors as determinants of energy intake and macronutrient composition: A 10-year follow-up after bariatric surgery. *Surg. Obes. Relat. Dis.* **2017**, *13*, 1572–1583. [CrossRef] [PubMed]
81. Schauer, P.R.; Kashyap, S.R.; Wolski, K.; Brethauer, S.A.; Kirwan, J.P.; Pothier, C.E.; Thomas, S.; Abood, B.; Nissen, S.E.; Bhatt, D.L. Bariatric surgery versus intensive medical therapy in obese patients with diabetes. *N. Engl. J. Med.* **2012**, *366*, 1567–1576. [CrossRef]
82. Murphy, B.; Myers, E.; O'Shea, T.; Feeley, K.; Waldron, B. Correlation between adenoma detection rate and polyp detection rate at endoscopy in a non-screening population. *Sci. Rep.* **2020**, *10*, 2295. [CrossRef]
83. Comstock, S.S.; Hortos, K.; Kovan, B.; McCaskey, S.; Pathak, D.R.; Fenton, J.I. Adipokines and obesity are associated with colorectal polyps in adult males: A cross-sectional study. *PLoS ONE* **2014**, *9*, e85939. [CrossRef]
84. Wernli, K.J.; Newcomb, P.A.; Wang, Y.; Makar, K.W.; Shadman, M.; Chia, V.M.; Burnett-Hartman, A.; Wurscher, M.A.; Zheng, Y.; Mandelson, M.T. Body size, IGF and growth hormone polymorphisms, and colorectal adenomas and hyperplastic polyps. *Growth Horm. IGF Res.* **2010**, *20*, 305–309. [CrossRef]
85. Lieberman, D.A.; Prindiville, S.; Weiss, D.G.; Willett, W. Risk Factors for Advanced Colonic Neoplasia and Hyperplastic Polyps in Asymptomatic Individuals. *JAMA* **2003**, *290*, 2959–2967. [CrossRef] [PubMed]
86. Omata, F.; Brown, W.R.; Tokuda, Y.; Takahashi, O.; Fukui, T.; Ueno, F.; Mine, T. Modifiable risk factors for colorectal neoplasms and hyperplastic polyps. *Intern. Med.* **2009**, *48*, 123–128. [CrossRef] [PubMed]
87. Mongraw-Chaffin, M.; Foster, M.C.; Kalyani, R.R.; Vaidya, D.; Burke, G.L.; Woodward, M.; Anderson, C.A. Obesity Severity and Duration Are Associated with Incident Metabolic Syndrome: Evidence against Metabolically Healthy Obesity from the Multi-Ethnic Study of Atherosclerosis. *J. Clin. Endocrinol. Metab.* **2016**, *101*, 4117–4124. [CrossRef] [PubMed]

*cancers*

MDPI

*Article*

# The Incidence of Rectal Neuroendocrine Tumors Is Increasing in Younger Adults in the US, 2001–2020

**Yazan Abboud [1,*], Navya Pendyala [1], Alexander Le [1], Anmol Mittal [1], Saqr Alsakarneh [2], Fouad Jaber [2] and Kaveh Hajifathalian [3]**

1 Department of Internal Medicine, Rutgers New Jersey Medical School, Newark, NJ 07103, USA; np726@njms.rutgers.edu (N.P.); al1424@njms.rutgers.edu (A.L.); am1777@njms.rutgers.edu (A.M.)
2 Department of Internal Medicine, University of Missouri-Kansas City, Kansas City, MO 64108, USA; s.alsakarneh@umkc.edu (S.A.); fouad.jaber@umkc.edu (F.J.)
3 Division of Gastroenterology and Hepatology, Rutgers New Jersey Medical School, Newark, NJ 07103, USA; kh852@njms.rutgers.edu
* Correspondence: yazanabboud.md@gmail.com

**Simple Summary:** Prior data showed an increasing incidence of rectal neuroendocrine tumors (RNET) in the US. There are limited comprehensive recent data on RNET incidence and time-trends among demographic-specific populations. The aim of this study was to evaluate recent age-specific RNET incidence rates and time-trends in demographic- and tumor-specific populations, using the United States Cancer Statistics (USCS) data covering ~98% of the US population between 2001 and 2020. Our nationwide analysis including 59,846 patients diagnosed with RNET shows a significantly increasing incidence of RNET in younger adults. An age-specific comparative analysis showed a significantly greater increase in younger adults compared to older adults. A sex-specific analysis showed that the increase was mostly driven by younger women and by tumors diagnosed at an early stage. The age-specific difference in RNET incidence was noted in various races. A sensitivity analysis of microscopically confirmed RNET cases showed similar results to the overall analysis. Our study provides comprehensive epidemiological data aiming to guide further investigations on this emerging topic.

**Abstract:** Prior non-comparative data showed increasing incidence of rectal neuroendocrine tumors (RNET) in the US. We aimed to evaluate age-specific RNET incidence rates and time-trends in demographic- and tumor-specific populations. The RNET age-adjusted incidence rates were calculated from the United States Cancer Statistics (USCS) database between 2001 and 2020. The population was stratified by age into older ($\geq$55 years) and younger adults (<55 years), as well as by sex and race. The tumors were categorized by their stage at diagnosis into early and late. The annual percentage change (APC) and average APC (AAPC) were estimated using joinpoint regression and Monte Carlo permutation analysis. Pairwise comparison assessed for parallelism and coincidence. There were 59,846 patients diagnosed with RNET between 2001 and 2020 (50.3% women). Overall, the RNET incidence rates during this period were increasing in younger but not older adults (AAPC = 3.12 vs. −1.10; AAPC difference = 4.22, $p < 0.001$), with non-identical non-parallel data ($p$-values < 0.001). While similar results were seen in men, a greater age-specific difference was noted in women (AAPC = 3.31 vs. −1.10; AAPC difference = 4.41, $p = 0.003$). The difference between younger and older adults was seen in non-Hispanic White (AAPC-difference = 4.89; $p < 0.001$) and non-Hispanic Black (AAPC-difference = 3.33; $p = 0.03$) patients, and, in most years, among Hispanic and Non-Hispanic Asian/Pacific Islander patients, and it was mostly driven by early-stage tumors (AAPC-difference = 3.93; $p < 0.001$). The nationwide data show a significantly increasing RNET incidence in younger adults, most notably in younger women and in early-stage tumors, seen in various races. Future studies should evaluate RNET risk factors and outcomes in demographic-specific populations.

**Keywords:** rectal neuroendocrine tumors; incidence; epidemiology; rectal cancer; health disparity; neuroendocrine tumors

## 1. Introduction

Neuroendocrine tumors are a group of neoplasms that can exhibit dichotomous functions mimicking both the characteristics of nerve cells and the hormone-secreting capabilities of endocrine cells [1]. The incidence of neuroendocrine tumors was shown to be increasing in a previous analysis of the Surveillance Epidemiology and End Results (SEER) database in multiple body organs, including several parts of the gastrointestinal tract [2]. Prior theories suggested that the increase in incidence could be the result of the improvement in detection modalities, including imaging and endoscopic procedures. The small intestine has been considered the most common site for neuroendocrine tumors in the past; however, after the implementation of the new colonoscopy screening recommendations by the American College of Gastroenterology, rectal neuroendocrine tumors (RNET) are at least as prevalent as small intestine carcinoid tumors [3]. RNET are mostly asymptomatic and found incidentally [4], with an incidence rate of 0.17% during screening colonoscopies [5]. A previous nationwide analysis evaluating 4918 RNET cases showed an increasing RNET incidence between 1992 and 2015. However, the study was limited in such that it only covered 13.4% of the US population, which may limit the generalizability of the findings. Furthermore, the study did not provide comparative data of age-specific trends, nor evaluated the rates or trends by race or tumor characteristics [6]. Despite the growing literature investigating RNET, there are limited data on recent RNET age- and sex-specific incidence rates. Therefore, the aim of this study was to evaluate recent RNET incidence rates and time-trends among population-specific demographics and tumor-specific characteristics using a nationwide comprehensive database, the United States Cancer Statistics (USCS) database [7]. We aimed to evaluate the following:

- The RNET incidence rates and time-trends in age- and sex-specific populations;
- The impact of race on RNET incidence rates and time-trends in different age groups;
- The impact of a tumor's stage at diagnosis on the RNET incidence rates and time-trends in different age groups.

The findings of this study were presented in part as a lecturer presentation at the Digestive Diseases Week (DDW) 2023 conference at the "AGA Colorectal Cancer Screening and Surveillance: High-Risk Populations, Including Hereditary Syndromes and Inflammatory Bowel Disease" session on the 6th of May 2023 (10:45 A.M. to 11:00 A.M.), in Chicago, IL. Other findings of this study were accepted at the American College of Gastroenterology Annual Scientific Meeting & Postgraduate Course and were presented on the 22nd of October 2023 in Vancouver, Canada.

## 2. Materials and Methods

This is a nationwide population-based time-trend analysis of RNET incidence rates in the US between 2001 and 2020, using the USCS database. The data were de-identified and publicly available, and, therefore, based on the National Human Research Protections Advisory Committee Policy, the data were exempted from review by the institutional review board.

### 2.1. Data Collection

The RNET incidence rates between the 1st of January 2001 and the 31st of December 2020 were collected from the USCS database, a comprehensive source of cancer incidence statistics in the US, which nearly covers 98% of the US population [7]. The USCS database has data from the Centers for Disease Control and Prevention (CDC)'s National Program of Cancer Registries (NPCR) and from the National Cancer Institute (NCI)'s Surveillance, Epidemiology, and End Results (SEER) program. It covers all 50 states, the District of Columbia, and Puerto Rico, providing data on nearly 33 million cancer cases [7]. All collected data by the US cancer registries get implemented into automated software programs to maintain high-quality standardization and coding as per the North American Association of Central Cancer Registries' data standards [8].

### 2.2. Definitions

The RNET incidence rate was defined as the number of patients diagnosed with RNET per 100,000 population each year. The annual percentage change (APC) was defined as the percentage change in the RNET incidence rates between two years. The average APC (AAPC) was defined as the average percentage change in the RNET incidence rates between 2001 and 2020. Increasing and decreasing trends were defined as the statistically significant positive and negative values of the AAPC, respectively, while the non-statistically significant changes in the AAPC were identified as stable trends. The tumors' location was specified as being in the "Rectum and Rectosigmoid Junction", with a malignant behavior. The *International Classification of Diseases for Oncology*, Third Edition, Site Record ICD-O-3/WHO 2008, was used to identify RNET codes as follows: 8240, 8241, 8245, 8246, and 8249 [9]. The population was divided using a cutoff age of 55 years into the following two pre-specified age groups, as defined in prior studies [10,11]: older adults, i.e., patients aged 55 years or older, and younger adults, i.e., patients aged 15–54 years (<55 years). The population was also categorized by sex and by race into the following groups, as defined in the database: Hispanic (H), Non-Hispanic Black (NHB), Non-Hispanic White (NHW), Non-Hispanic Asian/Pacific Islander (NHAPI), and Non-Hispanic American Indian/Alaska Native (NHAIAN). The tumors' stage at diagnosis was defined as early stage, including in situ and localized tumors, and late stage, including tumors with regional or distant site/nodes' involvements.

### 2.3. Statistical Analysis

The RNET incidence rates were calculated and adjusted for age based on the 2000 standard US population using the SEER*Stat software (v.8.4.1.2, National Cancer Institute "NCI"). The Joinpoint Regression Software (v.4.9.0.1, NCI) was used to analyze the time-trends, which were estimated as the APC and the AAPC. This software uses Monte Carlo permutation analysis to identify the simplest trend that reflects the change in rates over time [12,13]. Using tests of parallelism and coincidence, a pairwise comparison was conducted between the age-specific trends, and the absolute AAPC difference was evaluated [14]. Further analysis was conducted in sex- and race-specific populations and, also, after categorizing the tumors by their stage at diagnosis. Lastly, a sensitivity analysis was conducted using microscopically confirmed cases only. A two-sided $p$-value cutoff at 0.05 was utilized for statistical significance.

## 3. Results

### 3.1. RNET Incidence Rates and Time-Trends in Age- and Sex-Specific Populations

From 2001 to 2020, there were 59,846 cases of RNET diagnosed in the US. Notably, RNET incidence rates have been significantly increasing in younger adults in contrast to the stable trend that has been maintained in older adults (AAPC = 3.12 vs. −1.10; AAPC difference = 4.22, $p < 0.001$). The age-specific trends during this period were not uniform ($p < 0.001$), nor parallel ($p < 0.001$), suggesting that the RNET incidence rates in younger adults are distinct and rising at a greater rate compared to older adults (Table 1). This trend was replicated in men (29,772 patients), with a greater increase in RNET incidence rates among younger adults compared to older adults (AAPC = 3.08 vs. −0.02; AAPC difference = 3.10, $p = 0.01$). While similar results were seen in women (30,074 patients), a greater AAPC difference between younger and older adults was noted (AAPC = 3.31 vs. −1.10; AAPC difference = 4.41, $p = 0.003$), with non-parallel ($p < 0.001$) non-identical ($p < 0.001$) data. This underscores women as the population exhibiting the greatest disparity between the RNET incidence trends between age-specific groups (Figure 1).

**Table 1.** Age-specific trends for rectal neuroendocrine tumors (RNET) incidence rates among men and women.

| Age Group, y | Cancer Cases (N = 59,846) [a] | Trends [b] | | | Age-Specific AAPC Difference [c] (95% CI) | Pairwise Comparison $p$-Values | | |
|---|---|---|---|---|---|---|---|---|
| | | Time Period | APC (95% CI) | AAPC (95% CI) | | Age-Specific AAPC Difference | Coincidence [d] | Parallelism [e] |
| Both Sexes | | | | | | | | |
| Younger Adults | 28,963 (48.4%) | 2001–2008 | 8.48 (7.56 to 9.41) | 3.12 (2.14 to 4.11) | 4.22 (2.33 to 6.10) | <0.001 | <0.001 | <0.001 |
| | | 2008–2011 | −1.44 (−6.55 to 3.96) | | | | | |
| | | 2011–2018 | 4.19 (3.30 to 5.08) | | | | | |
| | | 2018–2020 | −10.85 (−15.41 to −6.05) | | | | | |
| Older Adults | 30,869 (51.6%) | 2001–2018 | 0.64 (0.05 to 1.23) | −1.10 (−2.69 to 0.52) | | | | |
| | | 2018–2020 | −14.70 (−27.34 to 0.13) | | | | | |
| Men | | | | | | | | |
| Younger Men | 13,898 (23.2%) | 2001–2007 | 8.03 (5.43 to 10.70) | 3.08 (1.67 to 4.51) | 3.10 (0.65 to 5.55) | 0.01 | <0.001 | <0.001 |
| | | 2007–2018 | 2.94 (2.04 to 3.84) | | | | | |
| | | 2018–2020 | −9.79 (−19.66 to 1.30) | | | | | |
| Older Men | 15,865 (26.5%) | 2001–2003 | 14.76 (−2.56 to 35.15) | −0.02 (−2.00 to 2.00) | | | | |
| | | 2003–2018 | 0.28 (−0.32 to 0.87) | | | | | |
| | | 2018–2020 | −14.81 (−24.87 to −3.41) | | | | | |
| Women | | | | | | | | |
| Younger Women | 15,065 (25.2%) | 2001–2008 | 8.58 (6.29 to 10.93) | 3.31 (0.98 to 5.70) | 4.41 (1.53 to 7.30) | 0.003 | <0.001 | <0.001 |
| | | 2008–2011 | −1.93 (−14.16 to 12.05) | | | | | |
| | | 2011–2017 | 4.78 (1.82 to 7.84) | | | | | |
| | | 2017–2020 | −5.80 (−11.78 to 0.59) | | | | | |
| Older Women | 15,004 (25.1%) | 2001–2018 | 0.30 (−0.26 to 0.87) | −1.10 (−2.75 to 0.57) | | | | |

[a] The data are presented as count numbers followed by their respective percentages relative to the total cases of RNET cancer in the database. [b] The time-trends were analyzed using the Joinpoint Regression Program (v4.9.0.1, NCI), with a maximum of three joinpoints allowed (four-line segments). [c] A positive value demonstrates a higher AAPC in younger adults compared to older adults. [d] Tests whether the age-specific trends were identical. A significant $p$-value demonstrates that the trends were not equivalent (i.e., they had varying incidence rates and coincidence was rejected). [e] Tests whether the age-specific trends were parallel. A significant $p$-value indicates non-parallel trends (i.e., parallelism was rejected).

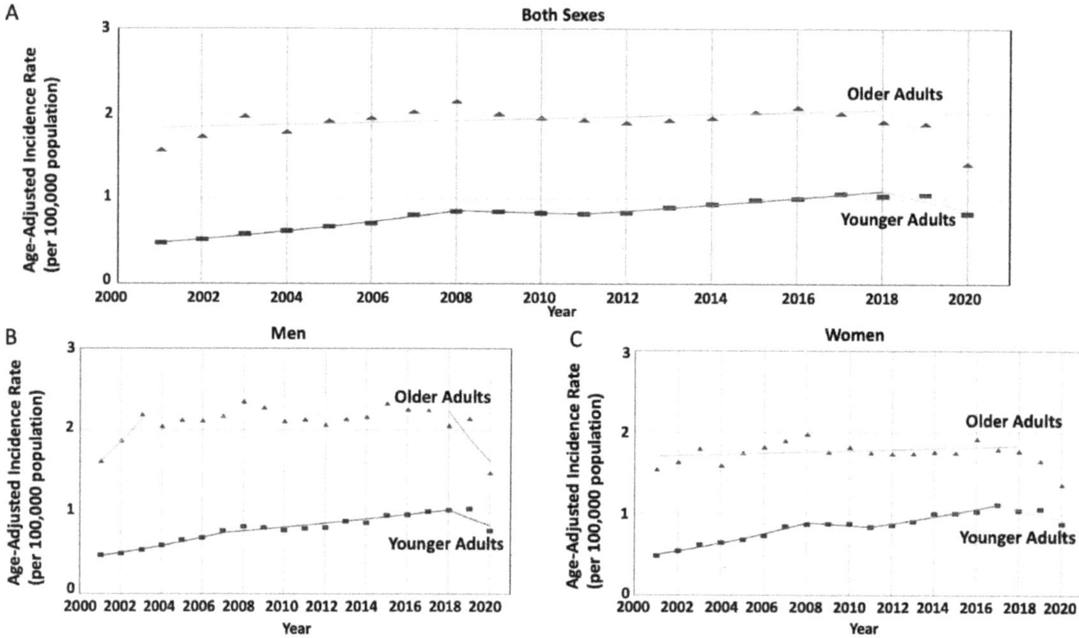


**Figure 1.** Age-specific time-trends of incidence rates per 100,000 population for rectal neuroendocrine tumors (RNET) among men and women. (**A**) The average annual percentage change (AAPC) is increasing in younger adults at a greater rate compared to the stable trend in older adults, with a significant difference (3.12 vs. −1.10, $p < 0.001$). (**B**) The average annual percentage change (AAPC) is increasing in younger men at a greater rate compared to the stable trend in older men, with a significant difference (3.08 vs. −0.02, $p = 0.01$). (**C**) The average annual percentage change (AAPC) is increasing in younger women at a greater rate compared to the stable trend in older men, with a significant difference (3.31 vs. −1.10, $p = 0.003$).

### *3.2. RNET Incidence Rates and Time-Trends in Age- and Race-Specific Populations*

In NHW patients (29,720 patients), the RNET incidence rates were significantly increasing in younger adults and decreasing in older adults (AAPC = 2.83 vs. −2.06; AAPC difference = 4.89, $p < 0.001$). In NHB patients (16,025 patients), the incidence rates were also increasing in younger adults but not in older adults (AAPC = 2.90 vs. −0.43; AAPC difference = 3.33, $p = 0.03$). In H patients (6903 patients), while the RNET incidence rates were increasing only in younger adults between 2001 and 2018 (APC = 3.77 vs. 0.95), the rates were stable in both age groups between 2018 and 2020. The AAPCs were non-identical ($p < 0.001$) and non-parallel ($p < 0.001$), with an AAPC difference of 3.62 ($p = 0.05$), suggesting that the rates in younger adults were different than older adults and that the absolute difference was trending to be statistically significant. In NHAPI patients (4577 patients), while the rates were increasing in younger adults between 2001 and 2018 (AAPC = 3.16) and stabilized afterward, older adults experienced stable trends during the study period, with parallel data ($p = 0.15$) and a non-significant difference ($p = 0.36$). Lastly, in NHAIAN patients, there were 425 patients who were diagnosed with RNET, but the number of yearly cases was too small to estimate a trend (Table 2 and Figure 2).

**Table 2.** Age-Specific Time-Trends for Rectal Neuroendocrine Tumors (RNET) Incidence Rates Among Different Race Groups and per Stage at Diagnosis. [a] Data are presented as count numbers followed by percentages of the count numbers from the total cases of RNET cancer in the database. [b] Time-trends were computed using Joinpoint Regression Program (v4.9.0.1, NCI) with 3 maximum joinpoints allowed (4-line segments). [c] A positive value indicates a greater AAPC in younger adults compared to older adults. [d] Tests whether age-specific trends were identical. A significant P-value indicates that the trends were not identical (i.e., they had different incidence rates and coincidence was rejected). [e] Tests whether age-specific trends were parallel. A significant P-value indicates that the trends were not parallel (i.e., parallelism was rejected).

| Age Group, y | Cancer Cases (N = 53,188) [a] | Trends [b] | | | Age-Specific AAPC Difference [c] (95% CI) | Pairwise Comparison *p*-Values | | |
|---|---|---|---|---|---|---|---|---|
| | | Time Period | APC (95% CI) | AAPC (95% CI) | | Age-Specific AAPC Difference | Coincidence [d] | Parallelism [e] |
| Race | | | | | | | | |
| Non-Hispanic White | | | | | | | | |
| Younger Adults | 13,827 (23.1%) | 2001–2007 | 7.12 (4.81 to 9.47) | 2.83 (1.47 to 4.21) | 4.89 (2.47 to 7.32) | <0.001 | <0.001 | <0.001 |
| | | 2007–2018 | 2.29 (1.42 to 3.16) | | | | | |
| | | 2018–2020 | −6.33 (−16.55 to 5.13) | | | | | |
| Older Adults | 15,886 (26.5%) | 2001–2018 | −0.55 (−1.22 to 0.14) | −2.06 (−4.05 to −0.04) | | | | |
| | | 2018–2020 | −14.06 (−29.85 to 5.30) | | | | | |
| Non-Hispanic Black | | | | | | | | |
| Younger Adults | 7963 (12.9%) | 2001–2009 | 8.43 (6.39 to 10.49) | 2.90 (0.28 to 5.58) | 3.33 (0.25 to 6.40) | 0.03 | <0.001 | <0.001 |
| | | 2009–2012 | −2.97 (−15.54 to 11.48) | | | | | |
| | | 2012–2017 | 5.63 (1.39 to 10.04) | | | | | |
| | | 2017–2020 | −8.31 (−19.80 to 4.84) | | | | | |
| Older Adults | 8330 (14.0%) | 2001–2007 | 3.69 (0.33 to 7.17) | −0.43 (−1.99 to 1.15) | | | | |
| | | 2007–2017 | −0.09 (−1.48 to 1.33) | | | | | |
| | | 2017–2020 | −9.25 (−15.91 to −2.06) | | | | | |
| Hispanic | | | | | | | | |
| Younger Adults | 3640 (6.1%) | 2001–2018 | 3.77 (2.67 to 4.90) | 2.03 (−0.44 to 4.56) | 3.62 (−0.08 to 7.31) | 0.05 | <0.001 | <0.001 |
| | | 2018–2020 | −11.68 (−30.25 to 11.83) | | | | | |
| Older Adults | 3160 (5.3%) | 2001–2018 | 0.95 (−0.17 to 2.08) | −1.59 (−4.28 to 1.18) | | | | |
| | | 2018–2020 | −20.73 (−39.48 to 3.83) | | | | | |

**Table 2.** *Cont.*

| Age Group, y | Cancer Cases (N = 53,188) [a] | Trends [b] | | | Age-Specific AAPC Difference [c] (95% CI) | Pairwise Comparison p-Values | | |
|---|---|---|---|---|---|---|---|---|
| | | Time Period | APC (95% CI) | AAPC (95% CI) | | Age-Specific AAPC Difference | Coincidence [d] | Parallelism [e] |
| Race | | | | | | | | |
| Non-Hispanic Asian/Pacific Islander | | | | | | | | |
| Younger Adults | 2287 (3.8%) | 2001–2018 | 3.16 (1.87 to 4.48) | 0.81 (−2.28 to 4.00) | 3.49 (1.22 to 5.76) | 0.36 | <0.001 | 0.15 |
| | | 2018–2020 | −17.11 (−38.80 to 12.26) | | | | | |
| Older Adults | 2289 (3.8%) | 2001–2016 | 1.60 (−0.36 to 3.59) | −1.14 (−3.90 to 1.70) | | | | |
| | | 2016–2020 | −10.75 (−21.37 to 1.32) | | | | | |
| Stage at Diagnosis | | | | | | | | |
| Early Stage | | | | | | | | |
| Younger Adults | 22,371 (37.4%) | 2001–2007 | 9.68 (7.48 to 11.93) | 3.47 (2.31 to 4.64) | 3.93 (1.82 to 6.05) | <0.001 | <0.001 | <0.001 |
| | | 2007–2018 | 2.54 (1.81 to 3.27) | | | | | |
| | | 2018–2020 | −8.70 (−16.93 to 0.36) | | | | | |
| Older Adults | 22,763 (38.0%) | 2001–2007 | 4.46 (1.36 to 7.66) | −0.46 (−2.21 to 1.32) | | | | |
| | | 2007–2018 | −0.41 (−1.52 to 0.71) | | | | | |
| | | 2018–2020 | −14.16 (−26.26 to −0.07) | | | | | |
| Late Stage | | | | | | | | |
| Younger Adults | 1300 (2.2%) | 2001–2020 | 3.43 (1.96 to 4.92) | 3.43 (1.96 to 4.92) | 2.44 (0.79 to 4.10) | 0.004 | <0.001 | 0.001 |
| Older Adults | 2712 (4.5%) | 2001–2020 | 0.99 (0.02 to 1.97) | 0.99 (0.02 to 1.97) | | | | |

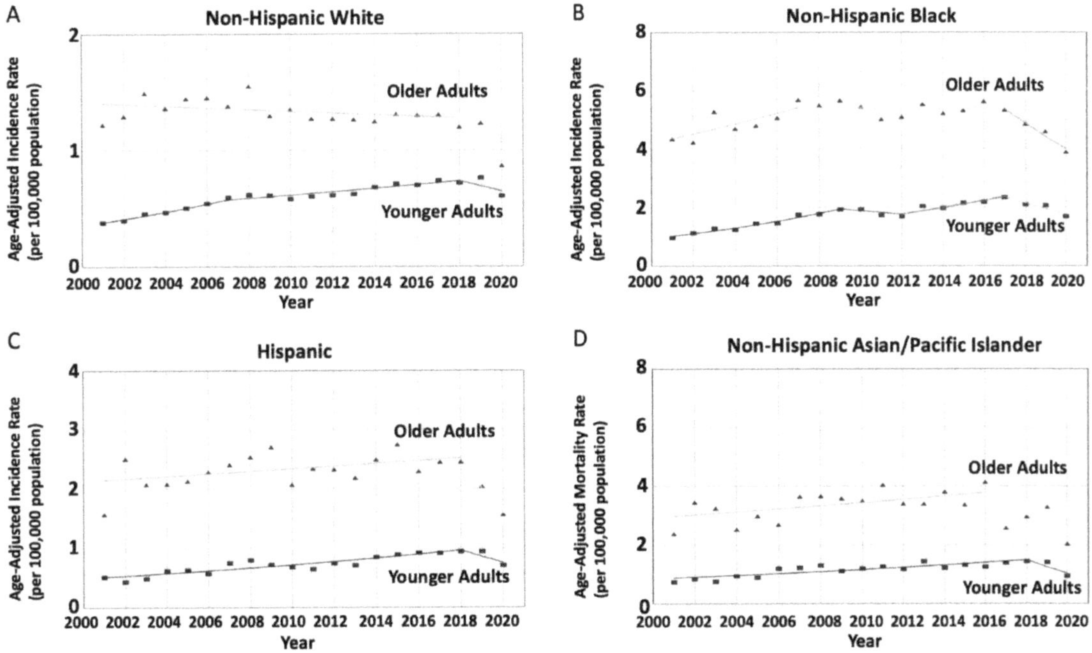


**Figure 2.** Age-specific time-trends of incidence rates per 100,000 population for rectal neuroendocrine tumors (RNET) among different race groups. (**A**) The average annual percentage change (AAPC) is increasing in younger NHW patients while decreasing in older NHW patients, with a significant difference (2.83 vs. −2.06; $p < 0.001$) and non-parallel ($p < 0.001$) non-identical ($p < 0.001$) trends. (**B**) The average annual percentage change (AAPC) is increasing in younger NHB patients while remaining stable in older NHB patients, with a significant difference (2.90 vs. −0.43; $p = 0.03$) and non-parallel ($p < 0.001$) non-identical ($p < 0.001$) trends. (**C**) The average annual percentage change (AAPC) is stable in younger H patients and older H patients (2.03 vs. −1.59; $p = 0.005$), with non-parallel ($p < 0.001$) non-identical ($p < 0.001$) trends. (**D**) The average annual percentage change (AAPC) is increasing in younger NHAPI patients while remaining stable in older NHAPI patients, with a significant difference (0.81 vs. −1.14; $p = 0.36$) and parallel ($p = 0.15$) non-identical ($p < 0.001$) trends.

### *3.3. RNET Incidence Rates and Time-Trends in Age-Specific Populations Characterized by Tumors' Stage at Diagnosis*

In tumors diagnosed at an early stage (45,146 patients), the RNET incidence rates were increasing in younger adults but not in older adults (AAPC = 3.47 vs. −0.46; AAPC difference= 3.93, $p < 0.001$). The age-specific trends were non-identical ($p < 0.001$) and non-parallel ($p < 0.001$), suggesting that the rates in younger adults were increasing at a greater rate compared to older adults. In tumors diagnosed at a late stage (4012 patients), the RNET incidence rates were increasing in younger adults at a greater rate compared to older adults (AAPC = 3.43 vs. 0.99; AAPC difference = 2.44, $p = 0.004$), with non-identical ($p < 0.001$) non-parallel data ($p < 0.001$) as well (Table 2 and Figure 3).

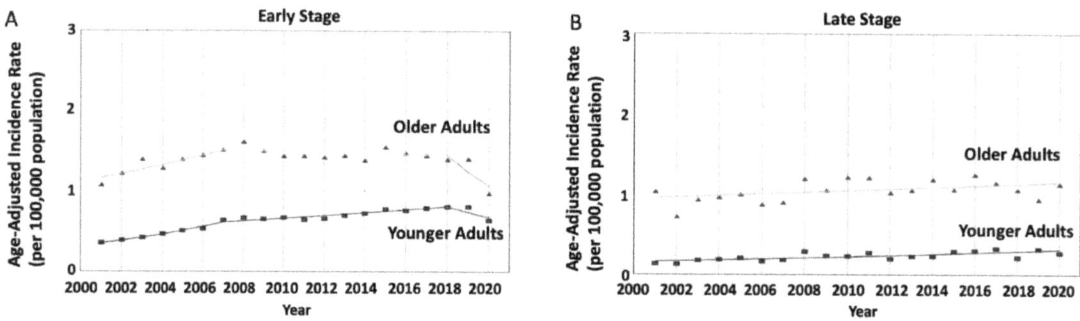


**Figure 3.** Age-specific time-trends of incidence rates per 100,000 population for rectal neuroendocrine tumors (RNET) characterized by tumors' stage at diagnosis. (**A**) For tumors diagnosed at an early stage, the average annual percentage change (AAPC) is increasing in younger adults but not in older adults, with a significant difference (3.47 vs. −0.46; $p < 0.001$) and non-parallel ($p < 0.001$) non-identical ($p < 0.001$) trends. (**B**) For tumors diagnosed at a late stage, the average annual percentage change (AAPC) is increasing in younger adults at a significantly greater rate compared to older adults (3.43 vs. 0.99; $p = 0.004$) with non-parallel ($p < 0.001$) non-identical ($p < 0.001$) trends.

### 3.4. Sensitivity Analysis

Our sensitivity analysis of microscopically confirmed RNET cases shows similar results to the overall analysis, showing a greater increase in the RNET incidence rates in younger adults compared to older adults (AAPC = 3.10 vs. −1.10; AAPC difference = 4.20; $p < 0.001$) (Table 3 and Figure 4).

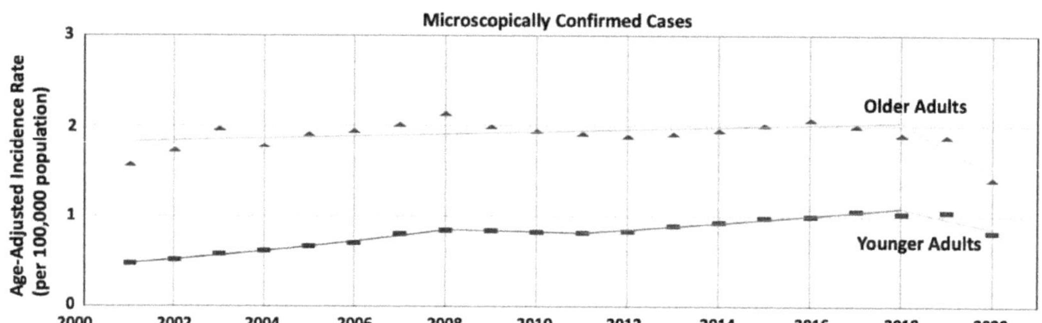


**Figure 4.** Age-specific time-trends of incidence rates per 100,000 population for microscopically confirmed rectal neuroendocrine tumors (RNET). The average annual percentage change (AAPC) is increasing in younger adults at a greater rate compared to the stable trend in older adults, with a significant difference (3.10 vs. −1.10, $p < 0.001$).

**Table 3.** Age-specific time-trends for microscopically confirmed rectal neuroendocrine tumors (RNET) incidence rates among men and women. [a] Count numbers followed by percentages from the total cases of RNET cancer. [b] The Joinpoint Regression Program (v4.9.0.1, NCI) was used to estimate time-trends with three maximum joinpoints allowed (four-line segments). [c] A positive value suggests a greater AAPC in younger adults. [d] Evaluates whether the age-specific trends were identical. [e] Evaluates whether the age-specific trends were parallel.

| Age Group, y | Cancer Cases (N = 59,846) [a] | Trends [b] | | | Age-Specific AAPC Difference [c] (95% CI) | Pairwise Comparison *p*-Values | | |
|---|---|---|---|---|---|---|---|---|
| | | Time Period | APC (95% CI) | AAPC (95% CI) | | Age-Specific AAPC Difference | Coincidence [d] | Parallelism [e] |
| Both Sexes | | | | | | | | |
| Younger Adults | 28,890 (48.3%) | 2001–2008 | 8.48 (7.53 to 9.43) | 3.10 (2.10 to 4.12) | 4.20 (2.29 to 6.10) | <0.001 | <0.001 | <0.001 |
| | | 2008–2011 | −1.44 (−6.70 to 4.12) | | | | | |
| | | 2011–2018 | 4.20 (3.29 to 5.12) | | | | | |
| | | 2018–2020 | −11.02 (−15.71 to −6.07) | | | | | |
| Older Adults | 30,772 (51.4%) | 2001–2018 | 0.63 (0.04 to 1.23) | −1.10 (−2.70 to 0.53) | | | | |
| | | 2018–2020 | −14.62 (−27.31 to 0.28) | | | | | |

## 4. Discussion

Our nationwide study evaluating nearly all patients diagnosed with RNET in the US between 2001 and 2020 showed a significant increase in the RNET incidence rates in younger adults aged <55 years when compared to older adults aged ≥55 years. Our analysis by sex and by race showed that the largest disparity between younger and older adults was arising from women's rates and was seen in NHW and NHB patients, as well as in H and NHAPI patients in most years. When characterizing the tumors by stage at diagnosis, the greatest difference between the age-specific trends was seen in the tumors diagnosed at an early stage.

The rising incidence of NETs has been widely established in the literature, with a 6-fold increase in the US over the last three decades [15]. However, there are limited data evaluating the increased incidence of rectal NETs in recent years while also identifying differences in the incidence rates across different sexes, age groups, and racial populations. A previous non-comparative SEER-based analysis found that there has been a rising incidence of RNETs from 1975 to 2015 [6] While the previous study shows similar findings to our current study, there are several differences. Our study offers a significantly larger sample size (59,846 patients vs. 4918 patients), provides an age-specific comparative analysis, evaluates updated data between 2001 and 2020, and provides a sensitivity analysis of microscopically confirmed cases. We also categorized the age-specific analysis by sex and showed that the largest difference between younger and older adults was arising from women.

This increase in RNET incidence may in part be ascribed to an increase in the breadth of knowledge known about GI NETs, as demonstrated by new classifications of the tumors defined by the WHO as recently as 2019 [16]. Although there has been little research on the role of more developed imaging techniques, such as PET radiography using gallium-based tracers which act as somatostatin analogs for RNET diagnosis specifically, these techniques have been proven to be effective and a contributing factor to the rising incidence of numerous GI NETs, including RNET [17,18]. This could also be a possible reason driving the increase in RNET in recent years. Another possible explanation for the increased RNET incidence has been attributed to growing awareness of these tumors and advancements in endoscopy utilization for cancer screening, and, thus, diagnosing a wider population range [19]. Procedural advancements in recent years have allowed for increased detection of smaller lesions or precursor lesions, potentially explaining the increased AAPC in younger adults when compared to older adults [6]. It was hypothesized that this effect would eventually plateau, as it can be seen from our data showing a stable trend of RNET incidence in older adults [20]. Having said that, prior data showed that women are less likely to obtain screening colonoscopies compared to men [21,22], which does not align with the prior theories of increased detection of RNET, given that the greater increase was seen in younger women. Considering the differences in AAPC between men and women, it is crucial to further investigate the reasoning behind this, while also identifying the differences in risk factors which may contribute to missed diagnoses.

There is a growing body of literature showing racial disparities in RNET incidence rates. Previous data showed that the most common location of NET in African American, American Indian/Alaskan Native, and Asian/Pacific Islander patients was the rectum [23]. Prior data also showed that the increasing incidence of RNET was more prominent in the African American population [9]. Our findings show that the RNET incidence rates were highest in all racial minorities (NHB, H, and NHAPI patients) compared to the NHW population, consistent with the literature [3]. However, our study provides an age-specific analysis of different race groups and shows that the greatest AAPC in different age- and race-specific cohorts was found in younger NHB patients (AAPC = 2.90). We also show that younger Hispanic patients and younger NHAPI patients experienced a significant increase in RNET incidence rates between 2001 and 2018, with an AAPC of 3.77 and 3.16, respectively. Our findings suggest an overall greater increase in younger adults compared to older adults in NHW, NHB, and H patients. Our study also shows that the RNET incidence rates in older adults were decreasing in NHW patients and remained stable in all the other racial groups. Many may attribute the increase in RNET incidence in the various population groups to the increase in colonoscopy screening, but this seems to only hold true for age and population as a whole. It has been found that ethnic minorities are less likely to obtain screening colonoscopies [24], suggesting that there must be another reason for the disparities within the various demographic characteristics which must be further investigated [3].

With regard to the stage at diagnosis, prior nationwide data from Canada suggested that the increasing incidence of RNET was driven by tumors diagnosed at an early stage [25]. Our study adds to the existing literature by providing comprehensive US data on RNET incidence categorized by the stage at diagnosis in different age groups. We demonstrate an increasing incidence of early- and late-stage RNET, with the most significant increase in tumors diagnosed at an early stage in younger adults and significant differences between age-specific groups. This could be the result of the increased detection of those tumors due to improvements in diagnostic modalities such as computed tomography and endoscopic procedures. It has also been postulated that these findings may partly reflect changes in the diagnostic criteria or changes in tumor biology [6]. However, the data on these theories are very limited, and, ultimately, a true increase in the tumors' incidence cannot be ruled out.

Some of the strengths of our study include the large sample size in the USCS database (59,846 patients; ~98% of the US population) and the use of joinpoint regression to conduct time-trend analysis, which is recommended in large databases [26]. Furthermore, we demonstrated an age-specific comparative analysis of RNET incidence rates between older and younger adults. We also provided an analysis categorized by patients' race and tumors' stage at diagnosis, with the goal of better understanding the epidemiology of RNET in different populations. In addition, we performed a sensitivity analysis of microscopically confirmed cases and found similar results to the overall analysis. With that in mind, our study suffers from several limitations. First, our study is observational in nature and hypothesis-generating, which limited us from identifying any risk factors for the revealed findings. Second, the coding reliability and possible loss of records are some inherent limitations of the SEER database that can be implied for the NPCR database, given the similar methodology utilized for collecting data between the two databases [27]. Therefore, those limitations can be generalized to the USCS database. However, the USCS database is the official source of federal cancer statistics in the US. It is a high-quality database and undergoes rigorous quality checks and reviews before publication to minimize any human errors [7]. Similar to much of the new literature establishing an increasing incidence of gastrointestinal cancers, such as colorectal cancer [28], gastric cancer [29], and pancreatic cancer [10,11], in younger adults in the US, we hope that our current findings of an increasing incidence of RNET in younger adults will help guide health care screening guidelines and policies toward further investigations on this topic. Future studies are needed to assess the risk factors associated with the revealed trends and to evaluate the RNET mortality and outcomes in demographic-specific populations.

## 5. Conclusions

Our nationwide analysis of the USCS database, covering approximately 98% of the US population, has found that RNET incidence trends have been steady over the past two decades in older adults, while the rates have been increasing in younger adults. The greatest difference between older and younger adults seemed to be arising from younger women and was seen in NHW and NHB patients, as well as in H and NHAPI patients in most years. The increasing trend of RNET in younger adults was mostly driven by tumors diagnosed at an early stage. While this increase can be partially attributed to the increased detection of RNET due to improvements in screening modalities, it can also be a true increase, especially with growing data showing an increase in a variety of gastrointestinal malignancies in younger adults. The exact causes of the revealed trend are unclear. It may be driven by age-specific exposure or response to risk factors that are disproportionally affecting younger adults. The study outlines the imperative need for future studies to investigate the risk factors associated with the increasing incidence of RNET in younger adults, especially in younger women.

**Author Contributions:** Y.A.: Substantial contributions to the conception and design of the work; the acquisition, analysis, and interpretation of data for the work; drafting the work; final approval of the version to be published; and agreement to be accountable for all aspects of the work in ensuring that questions related to the accuracy or integrity of any part of the work are appropriately investigated and resolved. N.P.: Substantial contributions to the interpretation of data; revising the work critically for important intellectual content; final approval of the version to be published; and agreement to be accountable for all aspects of the work in ensuring that questions related to the accuracy or integrity of any part of the work are appropriately investigated and resolved. A.L.: Substantial contributions to the interpretation of data; revising the work critically for important intellectual content; final approval of the version to be published; and agreement to be accountable for all aspects of the work in ensuring that questions related to the accuracy or integrity of any part of the work are appropriately investigated and resolved. A.M.: Substantial contributions to the interpretation of data; revising the work critically for important intellectual content; final approval of the version to be published; and agreement to be accountable for all aspects of the work in ensuring that questions related to the accuracy or integrity of any part of the work are appropriately investigated and resolved. S.A.: Substantial contributions to the interpretation of data; revising the work critically for important intellectual content; final approval of the version to be published; and agreement to be accountable for all aspects of the work in ensuring that questions related to the accuracy or integrity of any part of the work are appropriately investigated and resolved. F.J.: Substantial contributions to the interpretation of data; revising the work critically for important intellectual content; final approval of the version to be published; and agreement to be accountable for all aspects of the work in ensuring that questions related to the accuracy or integrity of any part of the work are appropriately investigated and resolved. K.H.: Substantial contributions to the interpretation of data; revising the work critically for important intellectual content; final approval of the version to be published; and agreement to be accountable for all aspects of the work in ensuring that questions related to the accuracy or integrity of any part of the work are appropriately investigated and resolved. All authors have read and agreed to the published version of the manuscript.

**Funding:** This research received no external funding.

**Institutional Review Board Statement:** The data were de-identified and publicly available, and, therefore, based on the National Human Research Protections Advisory Committee Policy, the data were exempted from review by the institutional review board.

**Informed Consent Statement:** Not applicable.

**Data Availability Statement:** The data used in this study are publicly available and can be obtained from the United States Cancer Statistics' website.

**Conflicts of Interest:** The authors declare no conflict of interest.

## References

1. Cives, M.; Strosberg, J.R. Gastroenteropancreatic Neuroendocrine Tumors. *CA Cancer J. Clin.* **2018**, *68*, 471–487. [CrossRef]
2. Dasari, A.; Shen, C.; Halperin, D.; Zhao, B.; Zhou, S.; Xu, Y.; Shih, T.; Yao, J.C. Trends in the Incidence, Prevalence, and Survival Outcomes in Patients With Neuroendocrine Tumors in the United States. *JAMA Oncol.* **2017**, *3*, 1335–1342. [CrossRef] [PubMed]
3. Taghavi, S.; Jayarajan, S.N.; Powers, B.D.; Davey, A.; Willis, A.I. Examining rectal carcinoids in the era of screening colonoscopy: A surveillance, epidemiology, and end results analysis. *Dis. Colon Rectum.* **2013**, *56*, 952–959. [CrossRef] [PubMed]
4. Basuroy, R.; Haji, A.; Ramage, J.K.; Quaglia, A.; Srirajaskanthan, R. Review article: The investigation and management of rectal neuroendocrine tumours. *Aliment. Pharmacol. Ther.* **2016**, *44*, 332–345. [CrossRef] [PubMed]
5. Wang, X.Y.; Chai, N.L.; Linghu, E.Q.; Li, H.K.; Zhai, Y.Q.; Feng, X.X.; Zhang, W.G.; Zou, J.L.; Li, L.S.; Xiang, J.Y. Efficacy and safety of hybrid endoscopic submucosal dissection compared with endoscopic submucosal dissection for rectal neuroendocrine tumors and risk factors associated with incomplete endoscopic resection. *Ann. Transl. Med.* **2020**, *8*, 368. [CrossRef]
6. Lumsdaine, C.T.; Liu-Smith, F.; Li, X.; Zell, J.A.; Lu, Y. Increased incidence of early onset colorectal adenocarcinoma is accompanied by an increased incidence of rectal neuroendocrine tumors. *Am. J. Cancer Res.* **2020**, *10*, 1888–1899.
7. National Program of Cancer Registries and Surveillance. 2022 Submission (2001–2020). United States Department of Health and Human Services, Centers for Disease Control and Prevention and National Cancer Institute. Available online: www.cdc.gov/cancer/uscs/public-use (accessed on 1 June 2023).

8. Software and Tools for Cancer Registries and Surveillance. Centers for Disease Control and Prevention. Available online: https://www.cdc.gov/cancer/npcr/tools/index.htm (accessed on 1 June 2023).
9. Tsikitis, V.L.; Wertheim, B.C.; Guerrero, M.A. Trends of incidence and survival of gastrointestinal neuroendocrine tumors in the United States: A seer analysis. *J. Cancer* **2012**, *3*, 292–302. [CrossRef]
10. Abboud, Y.; Samaan, J.S.; Oh, J.; Jiang, Y.; Randhawa, N.; Lew, D.; Ghaith, J.; Pala, P.; Leyson, C.; Watson, R.; et al. Increasing Pancreatic Cancer Incidence in Young Women in the United States: A Population-Based Time-Trend Analysis, 2001–2018. *Gastroenterology* **2023**, *164*, 978–989.e6. [CrossRef]
11. Gaddam, S.; Abboud, Y.; Oh, J.; Samaan, J.S.; Nissen, N.N.; Lu, S.C.; Lo, S.K. Incidence of Pancreatic Cancer by Age and Sex in the US, 2000–2018. *JAMA* **2021**, *326*, 2075–2077. [CrossRef]
12. Statistical Research and Applications Branch NCI. Joinpoint Regression Program, V.M. 2021. Available online: https://surveillance.cancer.gov/joinpoint/ (accessed on 1 June 2023).
13. Clegg, L.X.; Hankey, B.F.; Tiwari, R.; Feuer, E.J.; Edwards, B.K. Estimating average annual per cent change in trend analysis. *Stat. Med.* **2009**, *28*, 3670–3682. [CrossRef]
14. Kim, H.J.; Fay, M.P.; Yu, B.; Barrett, M.J.; Feuer, E.J. Comparability of segmented line regression models. *Biometrics* **2004**, *60*, 1005–1014. [CrossRef] [PubMed]
15. Chauhan, A.; Yu, Q.; Ray, N.; Farooqui, Z.; Huang, B.; Durbin, E.B.; Tucker, T.; Evers, M.; Arnold, S.; Anthony, L.B. Global burden of neuroendocrine tumors and changing incidence in Kentucky. *Oncotarget* **2018**, *9*, 19245–19254. [CrossRef] [PubMed]
16. Nagtegaal, I.D.; Odze, R.D.; Klimstra, D.; Paradis, V.; Rugge, M.; Schirmacher, P.; Washington, K.M.; Carneiro, F.; Cree, I.A.; WHO Classification of Tumours Editorial Board. The 2019 WHO classification of tumours of the digestive system. *Histopathology* **2020**, *76*, 182–188. [CrossRef] [PubMed]
17. Paiella, S.; Landoni, L.; Tebaldi, S.; Zuffante, M.; Salgarello, M.; Cingarlini, S.; D'Onofrio, M.; Parisi, A.; Deiro, G.; Manfrin, E.; et al. Dual-Tracer (68Ga-DOTATOC and 18F-FDG-)-PET/CT Scan and G1-G2 Nonfunctioning Pancreatic Neuroendocrine Tumors: A Single-Center Retrospective Evaluation of 124 Nonmetastatic Resected Cases. *Neuroendocrinology* **2022**, *112*, 143–152. [CrossRef] [PubMed]
18. Fortunati, E.; Argalia, G.; Zanoni, L.; Fanti, S.; Ambrosini, V. New PET Radiotracers for the Imaging of Neuroendocrine Neoplasms. *Curr. Treat. Options Oncol.* **2022**, *23*, 703–720. [CrossRef] [PubMed]
19. Scherübl, H. Rectal carcinoids are on the rise: Early detection by screening endoscopy. *Endoscopy* **2009**, *41*, 162–165. [CrossRef] [PubMed]
20. Cope, J.; Srirajaskanthan, R. Rectal Neuroendocrine Neoplasms: Why Is There a Global Variation? *Curr. Oncol. Rep.* **2022**, *24*, 257–263. [CrossRef]
21. Denberg, T.D.; Melhado, T.V.; Coombes, J.M.; Beaty, B.L.; Berman, K.; Byers, T.E.; Marcus, A.C.; Steiner, J.F.; Ahnen, D.J. Predictors of nonadherence to screening colonoscopy. *J. Gen. Intern. Med.* **2005**, *20*, 989–995. [CrossRef]
22. Shavers, V.L.; Jackson, M.C.; Sheppard, V.B. Racial/ethnic patterns of uptake of colorectal screening, National Health Interview Survey 2000–2008. *J. Natl. Med. Assoc.* **2010**, *102*, 621–635. [CrossRef]
23. Yao, J.C.; Hassan, M.; Phan, A.; Dagohoy, C.; Leary, C.; Mares, J.E.; Abdalla, E.K.; Fleming, J.B.; Vauthey, J.N.; Rashid, A.; et al. One hundred years after "carcinoid": Epidemiology of and prognostic factors for neuroendocrine tumors in 35,825 cases in the United States. *J. Clin. Oncol.* **2008**, *26*, 3063–3072. [CrossRef]
24. McLeod, M.R.; Galoosian, A.; May, F.P. Racial and Ethnic Disparities in Colorectal Cancer Screening and Outcomes. *Hematol. Oncol. Clin. N. Am.* **2022**, *36*, 415–428. [CrossRef] [PubMed]
25. Hallet, J.; Law, C.H.; Cukier, M.; Saskin, R.; Liu, N.; Singh, S. Exploring the rising incidence of neuroendocrine tumors: A population-based analysis of epidemiology, metastatic presentation, and outcomes. *Cancer* **2015**, *121*, 589–597. [CrossRef] [PubMed]
26. Gillis, D.; Edwards, B.P.M. The utility of joinpoint regression for estimating population parameters given changes in population structure. *Heliyon* **2019**, *5*, e02515. [CrossRef]
27. Park, H.S.; Lloyd, S.; Decker, R.H.; Wilson, L.D.; Yu, J.B. Limitations and biases of the Surveillance, Epidemiology, and End Results database. *Curr. Probl. Cancer* **2012**, *36*, 216–224. [CrossRef] [PubMed]
28. Bailey, C.E.; Hu, C.Y.; You, Y.N.; Bednarski, B.K.; Rodriguez-Bigas, M.A.; Skibber, J.M.; Cantor, S.B.; Chang, G.J. Increasing disparities in the age-related incidences of colon and rectal cancers in the United States, 1975–2010. *JAMA Surg.* **2015**, *150*, 17–22. [CrossRef] [PubMed]
29. Oh, J.; Abboud, Y.; Burch, M.; Gong, J.; Waters, K.; Ghaith, J.; Jiang, Y.; Park, K.; Liu, Q.; Watson, R.; et al. Rising Incidence of Non-Cardia Gastric Cancer among Young Women in the United States, 2000–2018: A Time-Trend Analysis Using the USCS Database. *Cancers* **2023**, *15*, 2283. [CrossRef]

*cancers*

MDPI

*Hypothesis*

# Association between Environmental Temperature and Survival in Gastroesophageal Cancers: A Population Based Study

**Kush Gupta [1], Anthony George [2], Kristopher Attwood [2], Ashish Gupta [3], Arya Mariam Roy [3], Shipra Gandhi [3], Beas Siromoni [4], Anurag Singh [3], Elizabeth Repasky [3] and Sarbajit Mukherjee [3,*]**

1 Department of Internal Medicine, Umass Chan Medical School—Baystate, Springfield, MA 01199, USA; kush.gupta@baystatehealth.org
2 Department of Biostatistics and Bioinformatics, Roswell Park Comprehensive Cancer Center, Buffalo, NY 14263, USA; kristopher.attwood@roswellpark.org (K.A.)
3 Department of Hematology and Oncology, Roswell Park Comprehensive Cancer Center, Buffalo, NY 14263, USA; arya.roy@roswellpark.org (A.M.R.)
4 School of Health Sciences, University of South Dakota, Vermillion, SD 57069, USA
* Correspondence: sarbajit.mukherjee@roswellpark.org

**Simple Summary:** Recent animal studies have shown a correlation between environmental temperature and tumor growth. Based on these studies, we hypothesized that esophageal cancer and gastric cancer patients living in warmer climates have improved survival as compared to patients living in colder climates. We conducted a study using the SEER (Surveillance, Epidemiology, and End Results) database and analyzed the cancer outcomes with the county-level average annual temperature in which those patients resided. We analyzed 17,408 esophageal cancer and 20,533 gastric cancer patients. We noted for the first time that higher environmental temperatures were associated with significant improvements in survival in patients with esophageal and gastric cancers. Further confirmatory population-based studies as well as mechanistic-bench studies are needed to support our findings.

**Abstract:** Background: Cold stress suppresses antitumor response in animal models, leading to tumor growth. Recent studies have also shown a negative correlation between the average annual temperature (AAT) and cancer incidence. We hypothesized that esophageal cancer (EC) and gastric cancer (GC) patients living in warmer climates have improved survival outcomes than those living in colder climates. Methods: We conducted a retrospective analysis using the Surveillance, Epidemiology, and End Results (SEER) database from 1996 to 2015. We retrieved the National Centers for Environmental Information data to calculate the county-level AAT. Cox multivariate regression models were performed to measure the association between temperature (measured continuously at diagnosis and in 5-degree increments) and OS/DSS, adjusting for variables. All associations were compared at a significance level of 0.05. The OS and DSS were summarized using Kaplan–Meier methods. All statistics were performed using SAS version 9.4 (SAS Institute Inc., Cary, NC, USA). Results: A total of 17,408 EC patients were analyzed. The average age of the cohort was 65 years, 79% of which were males and 21% were females. Of them, 61.6% had adenocarcinoma, and 37.6% were squamous. After adjusting for covariates, patients in regions with an AAT > 53.5 °F had an 11% improvement in OS [HR 0.89 (95% CI 0.86–0.92), $p < 0.0001$] and 13% in DSS [HR 0.87 (95% CI 0.84–0.90), $p < 0.0001$]. When the temperature was analyzed in 5 °F increments, with each increment, there was a 3% improvement in OS [HR 0.97 (95% CI 0.96–0.98), $p < 0.0001$] and 4% in DSS [HR 0.96 (95% CI 0.95–0.97), $p < 0.0001$]. Subgroup analysis of squamous and adenocarcinoma showed similar results. These findings were validated in 20,553 GC patients. After adjusting for covariates, patients in regions with an AAT > 53.5 had a 13% improvement in OS [HR 0.87 (95% CI 0.85–0.90), $p < 0.0001$] and 14% in DSS [HR 0.86 (95% CI 0.83–0.89), $p < 0.0001$]. When analyzed in 5 °F increments, with each increment, there was a 4% improvement in OS [HR 0.96 (95% CI 0.952–0.971), $p < 0.0001$] and 4% in DSS [HR 0.96 (95% CI 0.945–0.965), $p < 0.0001$]. Conclusion: We showed for the first time that higher environmental temperatures are associated with significant improvements in OS and DSS in patients with gastro-esophageal cancers, notwithstanding the limitations of a retrospective database analysis. Further confirmatory and mechanistic studies are required to implement specific interventional strategies.

**Keywords:** esophageal cancer; gastric cancer; environmental temperature; cold stress; overall survival; disease-specific survival

## 1. Introduction

Gastroesophageal cancers (GEC) are highly aggressive malignancies and leading causes of cancer-related mortality. According to GLOBOCAN 2020 statistics, esophageal (EC) and gastric cancers (GC) were the fourth and sixth leading causes of cancer-related deaths globally, with 768,793 and 544,076 new deaths reported, respectively [1]. In the United States (US), the estimated annual new cases of EC and GC were 26,380 and 20,640, respectively, in 2022 [2]. Unfortunately, majority of the patients are diagnosed at advanced stages, and the prognosis of EC and GC remains poor (5-year overall survival [OS] in 2022 ranged between 20–32%) [3–5]. In addition, patients with GEC may suffer from a wide range of morbidities, such as bleeding, obstruction, and worsened quality of life [6,7]. Therefore, GECs are a global public health concern that substantially burdens patients and healthcare resource utilization.

Several environmental risk factors are implicated in developing GEC, which vary according to the underlying histology and biological characteristics. Tobacco smoking and alcohol consumption are predominantly associated with esophageal squamous cell carcinoma, while gastroesophageal reflux, obesity, and low fruit/vegetable intake are associated with the esophageal adenocarcinoma subtype [8]. Additionally, *H. pylori* infection, Epstein–Barr virus (EBV), and dietary factors increase the risk of GC [9,10]. Several prognostic factors affect survival in GECs, such as advanced age, location, histological type, stage and lymph node status, and genetic biomarkers [11–14]. However, patient, disease, and management-specific factors were not found to fully explain the geographical disparities of GE outcomes [15,16]. Therefore, further research is needed to evaluate potential environmental and social prognostic factors for GEC.

Acute and chronic stressors are well-established modulators of the tumor microenvironment and significantly promote cancer invasion and progression through cascades of signaling pathways and adaptive immune responses [17]. Chronic cold stress has been found to prompt genetic and pre-genetic alterations and immunosuppressive responses, creating a pro-tumorigenic microenvironment [18,19]. Previous animal models have shown that chronic cold temperatures alter murine physiology and dysregulate immune response, leading to overexpression of immunosuppressive M2 macrophages, excessive release of pro-inflammatory cytokines and regulatory T cells (Tregs), and myeloid-derived suppressor cells (MDSCs)-mediated suppression of immune effector T cells [20,21]. It has also been found that sub-thermoneutral housing temperature (22 °C/71.6 °F) promotes tumor cell proliferation, pro-metastatic effects, and cancer progression [22–24].

Such findings led epidemiological studies to investigate the "cancer-cold" hypothesis, a term that denotes higher cancer risk in areas with colder temperatures. In a previous retrospective study, patients from the coldest countries were found to have the highest cancer incidence [25]. Likewise, data from the US found that lower environmental temperature/average annual temperature (AAT) was a significant predictor of higher cancer risk, including GEC and EC [26,27]. Notably, colder temperatures were found to have prognostic implications and significantly affected cancer survival. In a study by Sharma et al., most countries with the coldest AAT were among the top 50 countries with the highest cancer-related mortality, indicating a negative predictive value of colder AAT on cancer outcomes [28]. More recently, it was found that lower environmental temperatures were significantly associated with worse OS in patients with breast cancer [29].

Although there is an increasing body of evidence associating environmental temperature with cancer incidence, there remains a distinct lack of focused research examining the impact of climate on survival outcomes, particularly in GEC patients. Prior research primarily has stratified cancer incidence according to county-specific temperatures, and while it has established a potential relationship between colder temperatures and increased cancer risk, the specific implications of cold temperatures on survival outcomes remain largely unexplored. This study analyzed the data of the Surveillance, Epidemiology, and End Results (SEER) to investigate the predictive value of AAT on the overall (OS) and disease-specific survival (DSS) of GEC patients in the US.

## 2. Materials and Methods

### 2.1. Data Source and Population

The present study was a population-based retrospective analysis that retrieved data of all patients with EC and GE from the SEER database, covering nearly one-third of the US population. Data of all adult patients diagnosed between 1996 and 2017 were retrieved. There were no restrictions regarding the tumor stage. We used the 3rd edition of the WHO International Classification of Diseases for Oncology for tumor site identification. Patients with missing survival follow-up data were excluded. We extracted data regarding demographic characteristics, tumor histology, histological stage, grade and stage, history of surgery, and survival outcomes.

Data regarding the AAT were obtained from the National Centers for Environmental Information (NCEI; https://www.ncei.noaa.gov/, accessed on 20 July 2022), which provides county- and time-specific data regarding the average temperature [30]. We retrieved the county-specific monthly average temperatures at diagnosis to calculate the AAT. As the present study was based on a publicly available de-identified database, the need for ethics committee approval was waived.

### 2.2. Statistical Analysis

All statistical analyses were performed using SAS version 9.4 (SAS Institute Inc., Cary, NC, USA). The mean, median, and standard deviation were reported for continuous variables, with comparisons made using the Kruskal–Wallis and Mann– Whitney U tests. The frequencies and relative frequencies were reported and compared for categorical variables using the chi-square and Fisher's exact tests. The temperature was treated as continuous, categorized by quantiles (<q1, q1–q3, and >q3), and binary (dichotomized at the optimal cut-point by the maximal log-rank criterion). The OS and DSS were summarized using standard Kaplan–Meier methods. The median survival rates were reported, and log-rank $p$-values were provided. Utilizing Cox univariate regression models, the relationship between AAT (continuously assessed at diagnosis in 5-degree intervals) and OS/DSS was evaluated. The outcomes of this analysis were expressed as hazard ratios (HR) along with their respective 95% confidence intervals (CI). Cox multivariate regression modeling was performed to measure the association between AAT and survival after adjusting for age (continuous), sex, race, stage, histology, and grade. A $p$-value of less than 5% was considered statistically significant.

The relationship between temperature at diagnosis and survival outcomes was assessed for both EC and GC. In addition, a subgroup analysis was conducted according to the histological subtype of malignancy. To validate the findings and compare the survivability between EC and GC, the esophageal cut point was used for secondary analyses of stomach cancer. Survival summaries and results from multivariate analyses were reported.

## 3. Results

A. Patients with esophageal cancer

1. Characteristics of the included patients

A total of 17,408 patients with stage I–IV EC patients from the SEER database were included in the analysis, with a mean age of 65 ± 11.6 years and male predominance

(79.4%). Overall, 80% of the patients were non-Hispanic white, and 85.3% lived in urban areas. The most common primary site of malignancy was the lower third of the esophagus (58.7%), followed by the middle third (16.5%). Adenocarcinoma was noted in 61.6% of the patients, while squamous carcinoma was noted in 37.6%. Overall, 41% of the patients had grade I/II disease, and 42% had grade III/IV disease. According to the maximal log-rank criterion, an AAT of 53.5 °F was defined as an optimal cut-off value. Patients living in warmer temperatures (>53.5 °F) had significantly older age ($p < 0.001$) and were more likely to be Hispanic ($p < 0.001$), insured ($p = 0.037$), and higher grade ($p < 0.001$). Table 1 shows the demographic and clinical characteristics of the patients categorized by the AAT.

**Table 1.** Characteristics of esophageal cancer cohort according to temperature groups ($n$ = 17,408 patients).

| | | **AAT ≤ 53.5 °F** | **AAT > 53.5 °F** | ***p*-Value** |
|---|---|---|---|---|
| | N | 7637 (43.9) | 9771 (56.1) | |
| Age | Mean/Std/N | 64.27/11.52/7637 | 65.68/11.62/9771 | <0.001 |
| Sex | Male | 6099 (79.9%) | 7719 (79.0%) | 0.163 |
| | Female | 1538 (20.1%) | 2052 (21.0%) | |
| Race | Non-Hispanic White | 6111 (80.0%) | 7809 (79.9%) | <0.001 |
| | Non-Hispanic Black | 1286 (16.8%) | 1420 (14.5%) | |
| | Hispanic | 240 (3.1%) | 542 (5.5%) | |
| Marital Status | Married | 4183 (54.8%) | 5299 (54.2%) | 0.477 |
| | Single | 3454 (45.2%) | 4472 (45.8%) | |
| Insurance Status | Insured | 3959 (51.8%) | 5239 (53.6%) | 0.037 |
| | Uninsured | 231 (3.0%) | 259 (2.7%) | |
| | Unknown | 3447 (45.1%) | 4273 (43.7%) | |
| Primary Site | C150 Cervical esophagus | 144 (1.9%) | 196 (2.0%) | <0.001 |
| | C151 Thoracic esophagus | 264 (3.5%) | 353 (3.6%) | |
| | C152 Abdominal esophagus | 47 (0.6%) | 82 (0.8%) | |
| | C153 Upper third of the esophagus | 397 (5.2%) | 463 (4.7%) | |
| | C154 Middle third of esophagus | 1282 (16.8%) | 1593 (16.3%) | |
| | C155 Lower third of esophagus | 4573 (59.9%) | 5642 (57.7%) | |
| | C158 Overlapping lesion of the esophagus | 299 (3.9%) | 405 (4.1%) | |
| | C159 Esophagus, NOS | 631 (8.3%) | 1037 (10.6%) | |
| Histology | Adenocarcinoma | 4768 (62.4%) | 5957 (61.0%) | 0.104 |
| | Squamous | 2811 (36.8%) | 3726 (38.1%) | |
| | Adenosquamous | 58 (0.8%) | 88 (0.9%) | |
| Stage | Localized | 1931 (25.3%) | 2325 (23.8%) | 0.076 |
| | Regional | 2716 (35.6%) | 3539 (36.2%) | |
| | Distant | 2990 (39.2%) | 3907 (40.0%) | |
| Grade | I/II | 3195 (41.8%) | 3914 (40.1%) | <0.001 |
| | III/IV | 3046 (39.9%) | 4223 (43.2%) | |
| | Unknown | 1396 (18.3%) | 1634 (16.7%) | |

°F: Fahrenheit; Std: Standard deviation; NOS: Not otherwise specified.

2. Impact of AAT at diagnosis on survival outcomes

EC patients' median OS and DSS were 10.0 (95% CI 10.0, 11.0) and 12 (95% CI not defined) months, respectively. Patients living at an AAT > 53.5 °F had significantly longer

OS (11 [95% CI not defined] versus 10.0 [95% CI 9.0, 10.0] months; $p < 0.001$) and DSS (13 [95% CI 12, 13] versus 11.0 (95% CI 10.0, 11.0) months; $p < 0.001$) than patients living at a temperature ≤ 53.5 °F (Figure 1A,B). Likewise, when we categorized the AAT according to quantiles, the same findings were observed, where patients living at an AAT > 62.69 °F had longer OS and DSS (Figure 1C,D). The univariate Cox regression showed that, with each 5 °F incremental increase in the AAT, there was a 2% improvement in OS (HR 0.98 [95% CI 0.97–0.99], $p < 0.001$) and 2.6% improvement in DSS (HR 0.974 [95% CI 0.96–0.98], $p < 0.001$). In the adjusted model, a 5 °F incremental increase in the AAT was an independent predictor of OS [HR 0.96 (95% CI 0.95–0.97), $p < 0.001$] and DSS [HR 0.96 (95% CI 0.95–0.97), $p < 0.001$]. The Cox regression model adjusted for covariates showed that living at an AAT > 53.5 °F was an independent predictor of OS (HR 0.89 [95% CI 0.86–0.92], $p < 0.001$) and DSS (HR 0.87 [95% CI 0.84–0.90], $p < 0.001$), Table 2.

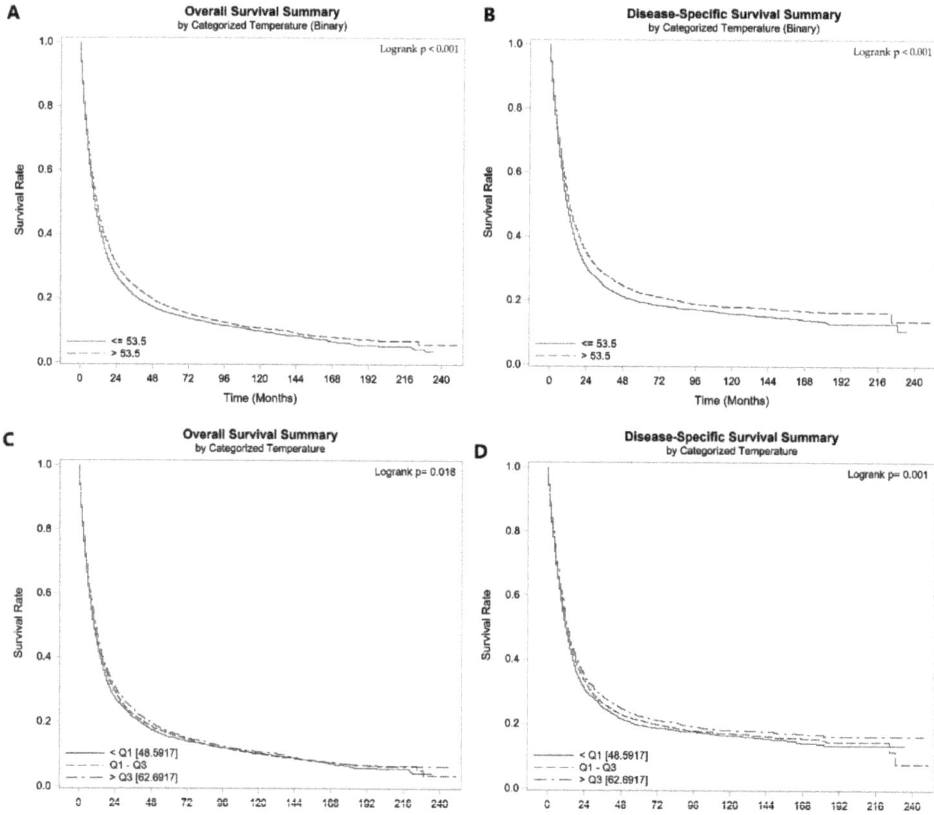


**Figure 1.** Patients with esophageal cancer: Kaplan–Meier Curve of (**A**) OS of patients living at ATT ≤ 53.5 and >53.5, (**B**) DSS of patients living at ATT ≤ 53.5 and >53.5, (**C**) OS of patients living at different quartiles of ATT, (**D**) DSS of patients living at different quartiles of ATT.

In the squamous subgroup, there were 4.1% and 4.2% improvements in OS and DSS, respectively ($p$ for adjusted HRs < 0.001) with each 5 °F increment in AAT. The multivariate regression showed that living at an AAT > 53.5 °F was an independent predictor of OS (HR 0.88 [95% CI 0.83–0.92], $p < 0.001$) and DSS (HR 0.87 [95% CI 0.82–0.92], $p < 0.001$), Table 2. The adenocarcinoma subgroup had similar results ($p < 0.001$), with living at an

AAT > 53.5 °F was an independent predictor of O (HR 0.90 [95% CI 0.86–0.94], $p < 0.001$) and DSS (HR 0.88 [95% CI 0.84–0.92], $p < 0.001$), Table 2.

**Table 2.** Multivariate analysis of AAT as a predictor of OS and DSS in the esophageal cancer cohort.

| AAT at Diagnosis | | | OS | | DSS | |
|---|---|---|---|---|---|---|
| | | | HR (95% CI) | *p*-Value | HR (95% CI) | *p*-Value |
| Overall population | Every 5-degree increment | | 0.964 (0.954–0.973) | <0.0001 | 0.959 (0.948–0.969) | <0.0001 |
| | Temperature at Diagnosis | <Q1 [48.59] | Ref. | | Ref. | |
| | | Q1–Q3 | 0.909 (0.873–0.945) | <0.0001 | 0.902 (0.865–0.942) | <0.0001 |
| | | >Q3 [62.69] | 0.873 (0.834–0.914) | <0.0001 | 0.854 (0.813–0.897) | <0.0001 |
| | Temperature at Diagnosis | ≤53.5 | Ref. | | Ref. | |
| | | >53.5 | 0.889 (0.860–0.918) | <0.0001 | 0.873 (0.843–0.904) | <0.0001 |
| Adenocarcinoma Subgroup | Every 5-degree increment | | 0.968 (0.955–0.980) | <0.0001 | 0.960 (0.947–0.974) | <0.0001 |
| | Temperature at Diagnosis | <Q1 [48.59] | Ref. | | Ref. | |
| | | Q1–Q3 | 0.924 (0.879–0.972) | 0.0023 | 0.917 (0.869–0.968) | 0.0018 |
| | | >Q3 [62.69] | 0.893 (0.842–0.947) | 0.0002 | 0.867 (0.814–0.924) | <0.0001 |
| | Temperature at Diagnosis | ≤53.5 | Ref. | | Ref. | |
| | | >53.5 | 0.902 (0.864–0.941) | <0.0001 | 0.879 (0.841–0.920) | <0.0001 |
| Squamous Subgroup | Every 5-degree increment | | 0.959 (0.944–0.975) | <0.0001 | 0.958 (0.941–0.975) | <0.0001 |
| | Temperature at Diagnosis | <Q1 [48.59] | Ref. | | Ref. | |
| | | Q1–Q3 | 0.903 (0.845–0.964) | 0.0023 | 0.897 (0.836–0.963) | 0.0026 |
| | | >Q3 [62.69] | 0.852 (0.791–0.918) | <0.0001 | 0.843 (0.778–0.913) | <0.0001 |
| | Temperature at Diagnosis | ≤53.5 | Ref. | | Ref. | |
| | | >53.5 | 0.877 (0.832–0.924) | <0.0001 | 0.871 (0.824–0.922) | <0.0001 |

Predictors: Temperature, Age (Continuous), Sex, Race, Stage, Histology, Grade, Primary Site, and Insurance Status.

B. Gastric cancer patients

1. Characteristics of the included patients

A total of 20,533 patients with GC patients from the SEER database were included in the analysis. The mean age of the study population was 68 years. 67% were male, 58% were non-Hispanic white, 56% were married, and 88% lived in urban areas. 66% were in the stomach, and 34% were at the esophagogastric junction. Within the stomach, cardia was the most common site (34%). Of all patients, 34% had grade I/II disease, and 53% had grade III/IV disease. Patients with stage I–IV cancer were included, with the majority (43%) with stage IV cancer. Patients living in warmer temperatures (>53.5 °F) had significantly older age ($p < 0.001$) and were more likely to be non-Hispanic white ($p < 0.001$) and had a higher grade ($p < 0.001$). Table 3.

**Table 3.** Characteristics of gastric cancer cohort according to temperature groups (n = 20,533 patients).

| | | ≤53.5 | >53.5 | Overall | *p*-Value |
|---|---|---|---|---|---|
| | N | 8025 (39.1) | 12,508 (60.9) | 20,533 (100%) | |
| Age | Mean/Std/N | 66.87/13.29/8025 | 68.51/13.31/12,508 | 67.87/13.33/20,533 | <0.001 |
| Sex | Male | 5399 (67.3%) | 8272 (66.1%) | 13,671 (66.6%) | 0.090 |
| | Female | 2626 (32.7%) | 4236 (33.9%) | 6862 (33.4%) | |
| Race | Non-Hispanic White | 4510 (56.2%) | 7366 (58.9%) | 11,876 (57.8%) | <0.001 |
| | Non-Hispanic Black | 1612 (20.1%) | 2221 (17.8%) | 3833 (18.7%) | |
| | Hispanic | 1041 (13.0%) | 1186 (9.5%) | 2227 (10.8%) | |
| | Other | 862 (10.7%) | 1735 (13.9%) | 2597 (12.6%) | |
| Marital Status | Married | 4517 (56.3%) | 6919 (55.3%) | 11,436 (55.7%) | 0.172 |
| | Single | 3508 (43.7%) | 5589 (44.7%) | 9097 (44.3%) | |
| Insurance Status | Insured | 3966 (49.4%) | 6144 (49.1%) | 10,110 (49.2%) | 0.844 |
| | Uninsured | 212 (2.6%) | 344 (2.8%) | 556 (2.7%) | |
| | Unknown | 3847 (47.9%) | 6020 (48.1%) | 9867 (48.1%) | |
| Primary Site | C160 Cardia, NOS | 2795 (34.8%) | 4212 (33.7%) | 7007 (34.1%) | 0.003 |
| | C161 Fundus of stomach | 309 (3.9%) | 446 (3.6%) | 755 (3.7%) | |
| | C162 Body of stomach | 605 (7.5%) | 979 (7.8%) | 1584 (7.7%) | |
| | C163 Gastric antrum | 1504 (18.7%) | 2487 (19.9%) | 3991 (19.4%) | |
| | C164 Pylorus | 252 (3.1%) | 325 (2.6%) | 577 (2.8%) | |
| | C165 Lesser curvature of the stomach, NOS | 585 (7.3%) | 1066 (8.5%) | 1651 (8.0%) | |
| | C166 Greater curvature of the stomach, NOS | 321 (4.0%) | 460 (3.7%) | 781 (3.8%) | |
| | C168 Overlapping lesion of the stomach | 516 (6.4%) | 769 (6.1%) | 1285 (6.3%) | |
| | C169 Stomach, NOS | 1138 (14.2%) | 1764 (14.1%) | 2902 (14.1%) | |
| Site | Stomach | 5198 (64.8%) | 8264 (66.1%) | 13,462 (65.6%) | 0.056 |
| | Esophagus GE Junction | 2827 (35.2%) | 4244 (33.9%) | 7071 (34.4%) | |
| Stage | Localized | 2136 (26.6%) | 3472 (27.8%) | 5608 (27.3%) | 0.003 |
| | Regional | 2537 (31.6%) | 4112 (32.9%) | 6649 (32.4%) | |
| | Distant | 3352 (41.8%) | 4924 (39.4%) | 8276 (40.3%) | |
| Grade | I/II | 2682 (33.4%) | 4327 (34.6%) | 7009 (34.1%) | <0.001 |
| | III/IV | 4160 (51.8%) | 6644 (53.1%) | 10,804 (52.6%) | |
| | Unknown | 1183 (14.7%) | 1537 (12.3%) | 2720 (13.2%) | |

2. Impact of AAT at Diagnosis on survival outcomes

The median OS and DSS of GC patients were 11.0 (95% CI 11.0, 12.0) and 13.0 (95% CI 13.0, 14.0) months, respectively. Patients living at an AAT > 53.5 °F had significantly longer OS (13.0 [95% CI 12.0, 13.0] versus 10.0 [95% CI not defined] months; $p < 0.001$) and DSS (15.0 [95% CI 14.0, 16.0] versus 11.0 (95% CI 11.0, 12.0) months; $p < 0.001$) than patients living at a temperature ≤ 53.5 °F (Figure 2A,B). Likewise, when we categorized the AAT according to quantiles, the same findings were observed, where patients living at an AAT > 62.57 °F had longer OS and DSS (Figure 2C,D).

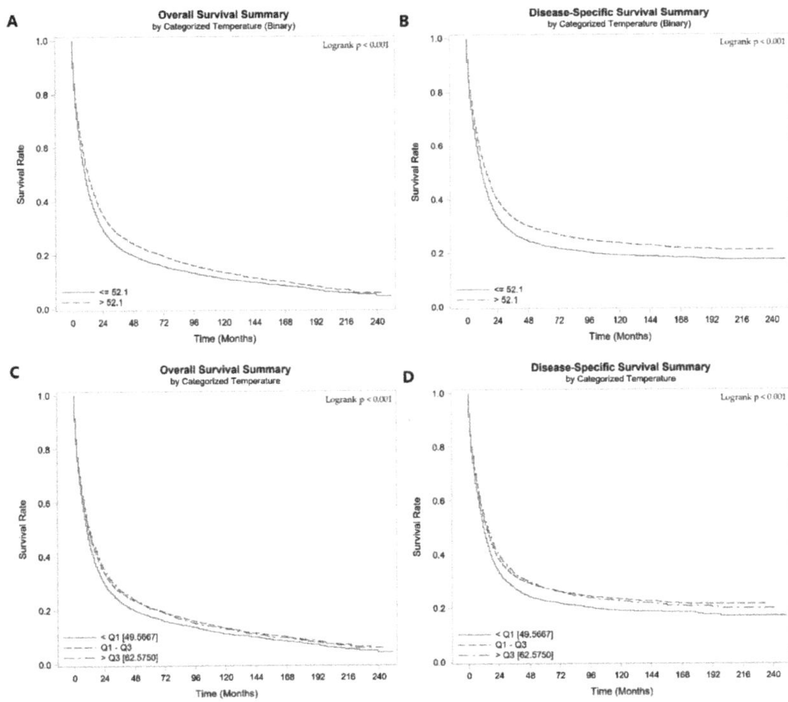

**Figure 2.** Patients with gastric cancer: Kaplan–Meier Curve of (**A**) OS of patients living at ATT ≤ 53.5 and >53.5, (**B**) DSS of patients living at ATT ≤ 53.5 and >53.5, (**C**) OS of patients living at different quartiles of ATT, (**D**) DSS of patients living at different quartiles of ATT.

The multivariate Cox regression showed that a 5 °F incremental increase in the AAT was an independent predictor of OS (HR 0.96 [95% CI 0.95–0.97], $p < 0.001$) and DSS (HR 0.96 [95% CI 0.95–0.97], $p < 0.001$). There were a 12.5% improvement in OS (HR 0.88 [95% CI 0.85–0.90], $p < 0.001$) and a 14.2% improvement in DSS (HR 0.86 [95% CI 0.83–0.89], $p < 0.001$) in patients living at an AAT > 53.5 °F, Table 4.

**Table 4.** Multivariate analysis of AAT as a predictor of OS and DSS in the gastric cancer cohort.

| Temperature at Diagnosis | | OS | | DSS | |
|---|---|---|---|---|---|
| | | **Hazard Ratio (95% CI)** | ***p*-Value** | **Hazard Ratio (95% CI)** | ***p*-Value** |
| Every 5-degree increment | | 0.961 (0.952–0.971) | <0.0001 | 0.955 (0.945–0.965) | <0.0001 |
| AAT at Diagnosis (Categorical) | <Q1 [49.5667] | Ref. | | Ref. | |
| | Q1–Q3 | 0.904 (0.871–0.938) | <0.0001 | 0.886 (0.851–0.923) | <0.0001 |
| | >Q3 [62.5750] | 0.869 (0.833–0.907) | <0.0001 | 0.855 (0.816–0.895) | <0.0001 |
| The temperature at Diagnosis (Categorical—Binary) | ≤53.5 | Ref. | | Ref. | |
| | >53.5 | 0.875 (0.848–0.903) | <0.0001 | 0.858 (0.829–0.887) | <0.0001 |

Predictors: Temperature, Age (Continuous), Sex, Race, Stage, Histology, Grade, Primary Site, and Insurance Status.

## 4. Discussion

Recent reports have revealed higher cancer incidence and less favorable oncological outcomes in countries with colder climates [26,27]. Interestingly, animal studies at our institution have demonstrated a pro-tumorigenic and metastatic response to sub-thermoneutral temperature in cancer models [23]. In the present population-based study, we demonstrated that higher AAT is associated with more favorable survival outcomes and significantly prolongs the OS and DSS of GEC patients. The results indicated that EC and GC patients had 3.4% and 4% improvements in OS with every 5 °F incremental increase in AAT, respectively. Likewise, EC and GC patients had 4% improvements in DSS with every 5 °F incremental increase in AAT.

The present study's findings agree with a growing body of evidence suggesting a positive correlation between environmental temperature and survival outcomes of cancer patients. In a recent analysis of 6479 breast cancer patients, Gandhi et al. observed a trend towards worse DSS and OS with a high thermogenesis score, which indicates chronic cold stress [31]. The prognostic value of environmental temperature was also evident in Sharma et al., in which countries with the coldest temperatures had the highest cancer-related mortality rates [28]. Our recent population-based study found that, for every 5 °F incremental increase, there was a 2% improvement in OS in patients with breast cancer [29]. Interestingly, Wang et al. studied the association between latitude and GC clinical outcomes using the Chinese Cancer Genome Atlas database. After adjusting for confounding factors, samples at low latitudes, usually associated with higher temperatures, had a significantly better clinical response and OS than samples at high latitudes [32].

Despite the growing interest in the impact of cold stress or environmental temperatures on the survival of cancer patients, limited data is available to explain the mechanistic pathways that form the basis of the association between cold stress and worse survival. The current literature suggests a significant influence of cold stress on tumor genetics and microenvironment. Past studies have indicated that cold stress induces tumorigenesis by increasing the frequency of somatic mutations [33]. In Wang et al., tumor mutation burden was lower and DNA repair activities were higher in GC samples of patients living at lower latitudes than in patients living at higher latitudes [32]. Cold stress may also alter the tumor microenvironment and host immune response, favoring tumor spread and metastasis. It was found that GC samples from high-latitude regions had a high burden of immune cell infiltration [32]. The cold stress-induced impaired antitumor immune responses were also evident in MacDonald et al., in which sub thermoneutral temperature suppressed functional $CD8^+$ T and led to the overexpression of suppressors of antitumor immune responses [19]. In cases with high thermogenesis scores, a typical pro-tumorigenesis/metastatic microenvironment was noted, including upregulated glucocorticoid receptor (GR) signaling pathway, anti-apoptotic activities, lower interferon-gamma (IFN-$\gamma$), cytolytic activity, and chemokines-mediated cytotoxic T lymphocytes (CTLs) responses [31,34]. Cold stress was also found to activate programmed death receptor-1 (PD-1), which suppresses cytotoxic T cells and helps tumor cells to evade the immune response [35]. According to Wang et al., patients living at high latitudes had higher expression of the PD-L1 gene, further supporting the potential role of cold stress in impairing antitumor immune responses [32].

Other possible explanations for the negative correlation between temperature and survival in cancer patients include the induction of higher angiogenesis and tumor invasiveness mediated by the adrenergic signaling pathway [31,36,37].

As mentioned above, our results align with previous epidemiological studies showing a significant association between environmental temperatures and the survival of cancer patients. When coupled with experimental evidence demonstrating pro-angiogenic and pro-metastatic responses to sub-thermoneutral housing temperature in cancer models [21], the results of the present study suggest the need to adjust for housing temperature during the evaluation of novel therapies. Kokolus et al. showed that lower housing temperatures (20–26 °C; 68–79 °F) significantly trigger the immunosuppressive microenvironment through overexpression of immunosuppressive cells and suppression of antitumor immune response [23]. On the other hand, tumor bearing mice housed at thermoneutral temperature (30–31 °C; 86–88 °F) had higher antigen specific $CD8^+$ T-cells, as well as a reduction in tumor growth rate and metastasis. Housing temperatures may explain the variation in response to immunotherapy in cancer models. Environmental temperature can also be considered a potential confounder in clinical immunotherapy trials. This becomes more relevant in GEC patients due to the ongoing efforts to introduce effective novel immunotherapies for advanced cases.

The results of the present study give rise to the question of whether patients with GEC who live in colder climates could benefit from adjuvant therapies targeting neuronal thermoreceptive pathways. For example, cold stress-induced neuroendocrine activation was found to induce breast cancer spread and metastasis via the β-adrenergic signaling pathway, an effect that was reversed after administrating a non-selective β-blocker [38]. These findings led to early clinical trials investigating add-on non-selective β-blockers in metastatic melanoma and breast cancer, which showed promising antitumor activity and reduced levels of metastatic biomarkers [39,40]. Our team at Roswell Park is using propranolol, a non-selective beta blocker, in two different clinical trials in esophageal cancer to potentially improve antitumor immunity and clinical outcomes (NCT05651594, PI: Mukherjee and NCT04682158, PI: Singh).

Our study is one of the rare population-based reports that evaluated the association between environmental temperatures and the survival of cancer patients. The study retrieved the data of a large cohort of GEC patients from the SEER database, which covers 35% of the US population. In addition, the AAT was based on county-specific data to account for potential variations in the environmental temperatures within the same region. However, we acknowledge the existence of methodological limitations. Firstly, our study is based on a retrospective collection of real-world data from routine clinical practice, which can introduce misclassification and ascertainment biases. The standardization of outcome reporting and definitions was not feasible. The available data limited expanding our adjusted multivariate analysis and accounting for additional confounding factors, such as patients' response to environmental temperature, tumor markers, chemotherapeutic regimens, or other treatment-specific factors that can impact the survival of GEC patients. Similarly, some other factors such as diet, incidence of *Helicobacter pylori* infection could not be accounted for in the analysis due to unavailability of such data in the SEER database. Healthcare delivery is also impacted by logistic limitations in colder weather. For example, travelling to high-volume and comprehensive cancer centers may be limited in cold weather which may impact the overall outcomes. Compared to individuals living in temperate regions, individuals who live in low-average temperature areas have differences in temperature-dependent host factors, such as their home environment, basic lifestyle, clothing, food, and beverage choices. The composition of their gut microbiome may also be altered [41,42]. Consequently, it may affect their ability to limit tumor development and growth. Due to the unavailability of data regarding the treatment received and its appropriateness, or the environmental temperature-dependent host factors in the SEER database, we could not incorporate these factors into our analysis. We acknowledge the role of such factors in altering survival outcomes. In addition, it was not possible to account for the residency change, in which patients might have been exposed to variable AAT.

In conclusion, the present study suggests a positive impact of higher environmental temperatures on the survival outcomes of patients with GEC. Patients with GEC living in warmer temperatures had a significantly longer OS and DSS, regardless of the pathologic subtype. Despite the methodological limitations implicated in a SEER database analysis, our findings, combined with the previously published animal experiments from our group, highlight the need to consider housing temperatures during the assessment of cancer models and environmental temperature as a potential confounder during the evaluation of the outcomes of GEC patients. In addition, novel therapies targeting neural thermoreceptive pathways may have a role in GEC patients. Future mechanistic studies are warranted to better understand the association between environmental temperature and cancer survival and study the impact of this association on treatment options.

**Author Contributions:** Conceptualization, S.G. and S.M.; Methodology, K.A. and A.G. (Anthony George); Software, K.A. and A.G. (Anthony George); Validation, S.M. and A.M.R.; Formal analysis,

K.A. and A.G. (Anthony George); Investigation, K.G., B.S. and A.G. (Ashish Gupta); Resources, A.G. (Ashish Gupta) and B.S.; Data curation, B.S. and A.G. (Ashish Gupta); Writing—Original draft preparation, K.G., B.S. and S.M.; Writing—Review and editing, S.M., A.S. and E.R.; Visualization, K.G., A.M.R. and S.M.; Supervision, E.R. and S.M.; Project administration, B.S. and S.M.; Funding acquisition, S.M. All authors have read and agreed to the published version of the manuscript.

**Funding:** This research received no external funding.

**Institutional Review Board Statement:** Not applicable.

**Informed Consent Statement:** Not applicable.

**Data Availability Statement:** Data are contained within the article.

**Conflicts of Interest:** The authors declare no conflict of interest.

## References


1. Sung, H.; Ferlay, J.; Siegel, R.L.; Laversanne, M.; Soerjomataram, I.; Jemal, A.; Bray, F. Global Cancer Statistics 2020: GLOBOCAN Estimates of Incidence and Mortality Worldwide for 36 Cancers in 185 Countries. *CA Cancer J. Clin.* **2021**, *71*, 209–249. [CrossRef] [PubMed]
2. Siegel, R.L.; Miller, K.D.; Fuchs, H.E.; Jemal, A. Cancer statistics, 2022. *CA Cancer J. Clin.* **2022**, *72*, 7–33. [CrossRef] [PubMed]
3. Stomach (Gastric) Cancer Survival Rates. Available online: https://www.cancer.org/cancer/stomach-cancer/detection-diagnosis-staging/survival-rates.html (accessed on 24 December 2022).
4. Survival Rates for Esophageal Cancer | Esophageal Cancer Outlook. Available online: https://www.cancer.org/cancer/esophagus-cancer/detection-diagnosis-staging/survival-rates.html (accessed on 24 December 2022).
5. Jim, M.A.; Pinheiro, P.S.; Carreira, H.; Espey, D.K.; Wiggins, C.L.; Weir, H.K. Stomach Cancer Survival in the United States by Race and Stage (2001–2009): Findings from the CONCORD-2 Study. *Cancer* **2017**, *123* (Suppl. 24), 4994. [CrossRef] [PubMed]
6. Napier, K.J.; Scheerer, M.; Misra, S. Esophageal cancer: A Review of epidemiology, pathogenesis, staging workup and treatment modalities. *World J. Gastrointest. Oncol.* **2014**, *6*, 112–120. [CrossRef] [PubMed]
7. Kwon, S.; Kim, J.; Kim, T.; Jeong, W.; Park, E.C. Association between gastric cancer and the risk of depression among South Korean adults. *BMC Psychiatry* **2022**, *22*, 207. [CrossRef]
8. Smyth, E.C.; Lagergren, J.; Fitzgerald, R.C.; Lordick, F.; Shah, M.A.; Lagergren, P.; Cunningham, D. Oesophageal Cancer. *Nat. Rev. Dis. Prim.* **2017**, *3*, 17048. [CrossRef]
9. Wroblewski, L.E.; Peek, R.M.; Wilson, K.T. *Helicobacter pylori* and Gastric Cancer: Factors That Modulate Disease Risk. *Clin. Microbiol. Rev.* **2010**, *23*, 713. [CrossRef]
10. Bae, J.M.; Kim, E.H. Epstein-Barr Virus and Gastric Cancer Risk: A Meta-analysis With Meta-regression of Case-control Studies. *J. Prev. Med. Public Health* **2016**, *49*, 97. [CrossRef]
11. Park, J.-M.; Ryu, W.-S.; Kim, J.-H.; Park, S.-S.; Kim, S.-J.; Kim, C.-S.; Mok, Y.-J. Prognostic Factors for Advanced Gastric Cancer: Stage-stratified Analysis of Patients who Underwent Curative Resection. *Cancer Res. Treat.* **2006**, *38*, 13. [CrossRef]
12. Jiang, N.; Ge, X.-L.; Zhang, Z.-Y.; Liu, J.; Wang, P.-P.; Sun, X.-C.; Yang, M. Prognostic factors for patients with esophageal cancer receiving definitive radiotherapy alone: A retrospective analysis. *Cancer Manag. Res.* **2021**, *13*, 3229–3234. [CrossRef]
13. Kulig, P.; Nowakowski, P.; Sierzęga, M.; Pach, R.; Majewska, O.; Markiewicz, A.; Kołodziejczyk, P.; Kulig, J.; Richter, P. Analysis of Prognostic Factors Affecting Short-term and Long-term Outcomes of Gastric Cancer Resection. *Anticancer Res.* **2021**, *41*, 3523–3534. [CrossRef] [PubMed]
14. Huang, F.L.; Yu, S.J. Esophageal cancer: Risk factors, genetic association, and treatment. *Asian J. Surg.* **2018**, *41*, 210–215. [CrossRef] [PubMed]
15. Chitti, B.; Pham, A.; Marcott, S.; Wang, X.; Potters, L.; Wernicke, A.G.; Parashar, B. Temporal Changes in Esophageal Cancer Mortality by Geographic Region: A Population-based Analysis. *Cureus* **2018**, *10*, e3596. [CrossRef] [PubMed]
16. Rana, N.; Gosain, R.; Lemini, R.; Wang, C.; Gabriel, E.; Mohammed, T.; Siromoni, B.; Mukherjee, S. Socio-Demographic Disparities in Gastric Adenocarcinoma: A Population-Based Study. *Cancers* **2020**, *12*, 157. [CrossRef] [PubMed]
17. Liu, Y.; Tian, S.; Ning, B.; Huang, T.; Li, Y.; Wei, Y. Stress and cancer: The mechanisms of immune dysregulation and management. *Front. Immunol.* **2022**, *13*, 1032294. [CrossRef] [PubMed]
18. Eng, J.W.-L.; Reed, C.B.; Kokolus, K.M.; Pitoniak, R.; Utley, A.; Bucsek, M.J.; Ma, W.W.; Repasky, E.A.; Hylander, B.L. Housing temperature-induced stress drives therapeutic resistance in murine tumour models through β2-adrenergic receptor activation. *Nat. Commun.* **2015**, *6*, 6426. [CrossRef]
19. MacDonald, C.; Ministero, S.; Pandey, M.; Robinson, D.; Hong, E.F.; Hylander, B.; McCarthy, P.; Gordon, C.; Repasky, E.; Mohammadpour, H. Comparing thermal stress reduction strategies that influence MDSC accumulation in tumor bearing mice. *Cell Immunol.* **2021**, *361*, 104285. [CrossRef]
20. Vialard, F.; Olivier, M. Thermoneutrality and Immunity: How Does Cold Stress. Affect. Disease? *Front. Immunol.* **2020**, *11*, 3031. [CrossRef]

21. Messmer, M.N.; Kokolus, K.M.; Eng, J.W.L.; Abrams, S.I.; Repasky, E.A. Mild cold-stress depresses immune responses: Implications for cancer models involving laboratory mice. *Bioessays* **2014**, *36*, 884. [CrossRef]
22. Eckerling, A.; Ricon-Becker, I.; Sorski, L.; Sandbank, E.; Ben-Eliyahu, S. Stress and cancer: Mechanisms, significance and future directions. *Nat. Rev. Cancer* **2021**, *21*, 767–785. [CrossRef]
23. Kokolus, K.M.; Capitano, M.L.; Lee, C.T.; Eng, J.W.; Waight, J.D.; Hylander, B.L.; Sexton, S.; Hong, C.C.; Gordon, C.J.; Abrams, S.I.; et al. Baseline tumor growth and immune control in laboratory mice are significantly influenced by subthermoneutral housing temperature. *Proc. Natl. Acad. Sci. USA* **2013**, *110*, 20176–20181. [CrossRef] [PubMed]
24. Mohammadpour, H.; MacDonald, C.R.; McCarthy, P.L.; Abrams, S.I.; Repasky, E.A. β2-adrenergic receptor signaling regulates metabolic pathways critical to myeloid-derived suppressor cell function within the TME. *Cell Rep.* **2021**, *37*, 109883. [CrossRef] [PubMed]
25. Voskarides, K. The "cancer–cold" hypothesis and possible extensions for the Nordic populations. *Scand. J. Public Health* **2019**, *47*, 477–481. [CrossRef] [PubMed]
26. Shah, V.; Rieger, R.H.; Pan, L.X. Precipitation and Climate Zone Explains the Geographical Disparity in the Invasive Cancer Incidence Rates in the United States. *Environ. Eng. Sci.* **2022**, *36*, 1452–1458. [CrossRef]
27. Sharma, A.; Sharma, T.; Panwar, M.S.; Sharma, D.; Bundel, R.; Hamilton, R.T.; A Radosevich, J.; Mandal, C.C. Colder environments are associated with a greater cancer incidence in the female population of the United States. *Tumour Biol.* **2017**, *39*, 1010428317724784. [CrossRef]
28. Sharma, A.; Verma, H.K.; Joshi, S.; Panwar, M.S.; Mandal, C.C. A link between cold environment and cancer. *Tumour Biol.* **2015**, *36*, 5953–5964. [CrossRef] [PubMed]
29. Gupta, A.; Attwood, K.; Gupta, K.; Gandhi, A.; Edge, S.; Takabe, K.; Gandhi, S. CLO22-051: Influence of Environmental Temperature on Pathological Complete Response and Overall Survival in Breast Cancer: A National Cancer Database Population-Based Study. *J. Natl. Compr. Cancer Netw.* **2022**, *20*, CLO22-051. [CrossRef]
30. NCEI. National Centers for Environmental Information (NCEI). Monthly Climate Tables. 2019. Available online: https://www.ncei.noaa.gov/ (accessed on 28 June 2022).
31. Gandhi, S.; Oshi, M.; Murthy, V.; Repasky, E.A.; Takabe, K. Enhanced thermogenesis in triple-negative breast cancer is associated with pro-tumor immune microenvironment. *Cancers* **2021**, *13*, 2559. [CrossRef]
32. Wang, L.; Cai, M.; Song, Y.; Bai, J.; Sun, W.; Yu, J.; Du, S.; Lu, J.; Fu, S. Multidimensional difference analysis in gastric cancer patients between high and low latitude. *Front. Genet.* **2022**, *13*, 944492. [CrossRef]
33. Saini, R.; Singh, A.K.; Dhanapal, S.; Saeed, T.H.; Hyde, G.J.; Baskar, R. Brief temperature stress during reproductive stages alters meiotic recombination and somatic mutation rates in the progeny of Arabidopsis. *BMC Plant Biol.* **2017**, *17*, 103. [CrossRef]
34. Kach, J.; Conzen, S.D.; Szmulewitz, R.Z. Glucocorticoid receptor signaling in breast and prostate cancers: Emergence as a therapeutic target. *Sci. Transl. Med.* **2015**, *7*, 305ps19. [CrossRef] [PubMed]
35. Bucsek, M.J.; Qiao, G.; MacDonald, C.R.; Giridharan, T.; Evans, L.; Niedzwecki, B.; Liu, H.; Kokolus, K.M.; Eng, J.W.-L.; Messmer, M.N.; et al. β-Adrenergic signaling in mice housed at standard temperatures suppresses an effector phenotype in CD8+ T cells and undermines checkpoint inhibitor therapy. *Cancer Res.* **2017**, *77*, 5639–5651. [CrossRef]
36. Chang, A.; Le, C.P.; Walker, A.K.; Creed, S.J.; Pon, C.K.; Albold, S.; Carroll, D.; Halls, M.L.; Lane, J.R.; Riedel, B.; et al. β2-Adrenoceptors on tumor cells play a critical role in stress-enhanced metastasis in a mouse model of breast cancer. *Brain Behav. Immun.* **2016**, *57*, 106–115. [CrossRef] [PubMed]
37. Lim, S.; Honek, J.; Xue, Y.; Seki, T.; Cao, Z.; Andersson, P.; Yang, X.; Hosaka, K.; Cao, Y. Cold-induced activation of brown adipose tissue and adipose angiogenesis in mice. *Nat. Protoc.* **2012**, *7*, 606–615. [CrossRef] [PubMed]
38. Sloan, E.K.; Priceman, S.J.; Cox, B.F.; Yu, S.; Pimentel, M.A.; Tangkanangnukul, V.; Arevalo, J.M.G.; Morizono, K.; Karanikolas, B.D.W.; Wu, L.; et al. Sympathetic nervous system induces a metastatic switch in primary breast cancer. *Cancer Res.* **2010**, *70*, 7042. [CrossRef] [PubMed]
39. Gandhi, S.; Pandey, M.R.; Attwood, K.; Ji, W.; Witkiewicz, A.K.; Knudsen, E.S.; Allen, C.; Tario, J.D.; Wallace, P.K.; Cedeno, C.D.; et al. Phase I Clinical Trial of Combination Propranolol and Pembrolizumab in Locally Advanced and Metastatic Melanoma: Safety, Tolerability, and Preliminary Evidence of Antitumor Activity. *Clin. Cancer Res.* **2021**, *27*, 87–95. [CrossRef]
40. Hiller, J.G.; Cole, S.W.; Crone, E.M.; Byrne, D.J.; Shackleford, D.M.; Pang, J.M.B.; Henderson, M.A.; Nightingale, S.S.; Ho, K.M.; Myles, P.S.; et al. Preoperative β-Blockade with Propranolol Reduces Biomarkers of Metastasis in Breast Cancer: A Phase II Randomized Trial. *Clin. Cancer Res.* **2020**, *26*, 1803–1811. [CrossRef]
41. Li, J.; Bates, K.A.; Hoang, K.L.; Hector, T.E.; Knowles, S.C.L.; King, K.C. Experimental temperatures shape host microbiome diversity and composition. *Glob. Change Biol.* **2023**, *29*, 41–56. [CrossRef]
42. Sepulveda, J.; Moeller, A.H. The Effects of Temperature on Animal Gut Microbiomes. *Front. Microbiol.* **2020**, *11*, 384. [CrossRef]

*cancers*

MDPI

*Article*

# National Burden and Trends for 29 Groups of Cancer in Mexico from 1990 to 2019: A Secondary Analysis of the Global Burden of Disease Study 2019

**Saul A. Beltran-Ontiveros [1], Jose A. Contreras-Gutierrez [1], Erik Lizarraga-Verdugo [1], Erick P. Gutierrez-Grijalva [2], Kenia Lopez-Lopez [3], Emilio H. Lora-Fierro [1], Miguel A. Trujillo-Rojas [4], Jose M. Moreno-Ortiz [4], Diana L. Cardoso-Angulo [1], Emir Leal-Leon [5], Jose R. Zatarain-Lopez [1], Hector M. Cuen-Diaz [1], Marisol Montoya-Moreno [1], Brisceyda Arce-Bojorquez [1], Juan L. Rochin-Teran [1], Daniel E. Cuen-Lazcano [1], Victor A. Contreras-Rodriguez [6], Ricardo Lascurain [7], Liliana Carmona-Aparicio [8], Elvia Coballase-Urrutia [8], Francisco Gallardo-Vera [9] and Daniel Diaz [10,*]**

1 Centro de Investigación y Docencia en Salud, Universidad Autónoma de Sinaloa, Culiacán Rosales 80030, Sinaloa, Mexico; saul.beltran@uas.edu.mx (S.A.B.-O.); eriklizarraga@uas.edu.mx (E.L.-V.); diana.cardoso@uas.edu.mx (D.L.C.-A.); marisol.montoya@uas.edu.mx (M.M.-M.); brisceyda.arce@uas.edu.mx (B.A.-B.)
2 Cátedras CONACYT, Centro de Investigación en Alimentación y Desarrollo, A.C., Culiacán Rosales 80110, Sinaloa, Mexico; erick.gutierrez@ciad.mx
3 Laboratorio de Biomedicina Molecular, Facultad de Ciencias Químico Biológicas, Universidad Autónoma de Sinaloa, Culiacán Rosales 80019, Sinaloa, Mexico; kenia.lopez@uas.edu.mx
4 Instituto de Genética Humana "Dr. Enrique Corona Rivera", Centro Universitario de Ciencias de la Salud, Universidad de Guadalajara, Guadalajara 44340, Jalisco, Mexico; migueltrojas@alumnos.udg.mx (M.A.T.-R.); miguel.moreno@academicos.udg.mx (J.M.M.-O.)
5 Laboratorio de Genética y Biología Molecular, Facultad de Ciencias Químico Biológicas, Universidad Autónoma de Sinaloa, Culiacán Rosales 80019, Sinaloa, Mexico; emir.leal@uas.edu.mx
6 Unidad Académica de Criminalística, Criminología y Ciencias Forenses, Universidad Autónoma de Sinaloa, Culiacán Rosales 80040, Sinaloa, Mexico; victorcontreras@uas.edu.mx
7 Unidad de Vinculación Científica, Facultad de Medicina, Universidad Nacional Autónoma de México en el Instituto Nacional de Medicina Genómica, Tlalpan 14610, Ciudad de México, Mexico; rlascurain@facmed.unam.mx
8 Laboratorio de Neurociencias II, Instituto Nacional de Pediatría, Coyoacán 04530, Ciudad de México, Mexico; c_apariccio@ciencias.unam.mx (L.C.-A.); ecoballaseu@pediatria.gob.mx (E.C.-U.)
9 Laboratorio de Biología Molecular y Bioseguridad Nivel III, Centro Médico Naval, Coyoacán 04470, Ciudad de México, Mexico; jfgallardo@ciencias.unam.mx
10 Facultad de Ciencias, Universidad Nacional Autónoma de México, Coyoacán 04510, Ciudad de México, Mexico
* Correspondence: ddiaz@ciencias.unam.mx

**Simple Summary:** Cancer is a significant contributor to morbidity and mortality worldwide. The purpose of this study was to analyze the cancer burden and trends of 29 groups of malignant neoplasms in Mexico by sex and age from 1990 to 2019. In 2019, there were 222.1 thousand incident cases and 105.6 thousand deaths due to cancer in the general population. The number of new cases and deaths from the 29 cancer groups increased between 10% and 436% from 1990 to 2019, with different patterns by sex and age. Breast, cervical, and colorectal cancers were the leading causes of death among women, while prostate, lung, and colorectal cancers were the leading causes of death among men. In Mexico, malignant neoplasms were the third leading cause of death in 2019, causing significant health loss. The existence of gender disparities emphasizes the need for cancer-specific targeted prevention, diagnosis, and treatment.

**Abstract:** The global burden of cancer is on the rise, with varying national patterns. To gain a better understanding and control of cancer, it is essential to provide national estimates. Therefore, we present a comparative description of cancer incidence and mortality rates in Mexico from 1990 to 2019, by age and sex for 29 different cancer groups. Based on public data from the Global Burden of Disease Study 2019, we evaluated the national burden of cancer by analyzing counts and crude and age-standardized rates per 100,000 people with 95% uncertainty intervals for 2019 and trends using the annual percentage change from 1990 to 2019. In 2019, cancer resulted in 222,060 incident cases and 105,591 deaths. In 2019, the highest incidence of cancer was observed in non-melanoma skin cancer, prostate cancer, and breast cancer. Additionally, 53% of deaths were attributed to six cancer groups (lung, colorectal, stomach, prostate, breast, and pancreatic). From 1990 to 2019, there was an increasing trend in incidence and mortality rates, which varied by 10–436% among cancer groups. Furthermore, there were cancer-specific sex differences in crude and age-standardized rates. The results show an increase in the national cancer burden with sex-specific patterns of change. These findings can guide national efforts to reduce health loss due to cancer.

**Keywords:** burden of disease; cancer epidemiology; cancer mortality; malignant neoplasm; public health

## 1. Introduction

Cancer is a significant cause of morbidity and mortality worldwide [1]. In 2019, it was the second leading cause of death, with an estimated 23.6 million new cases (17.2 million when excluding non-melanoma skin cancer) and 10.0 million deaths [2]. The incidence and mortality rates of cancer have been increasing, with an expected rise to 28.4 million cases by 2040, a 47% increase from 2020 [3]. If exposure to behavioral and environmental risk factors contributing to the cancer burden continues to increase, the global burden of cancer may worsen [4].

The United Nations and the World Health Organization have recognized the need to reduce the burden of cancer and develop strategies for national-level cancer control planning and implementation through the Sustainable Development Goals. However, there are regional and national differences in cancer morbidity and mortality associated with varying levels of exposure to population risk factors due to socioeconomic changes [5]. Therefore, understanding the local cancer epidemiology is crucial for informing cancer control efforts, including prioritizing resource allocation, implementing public health policies, and improving health system planning [6]. Previous studies in Mexico have described the specific burden of certain cancer groups at both national and state levels [7–12]. Furthermore, various studies have evaluated the national burden of cancer, encompassing multiple groups of malignant neoplasms from 1970 to 2015 [13–16]. However, due to the changing pattern and increasing trend of cancer burden, it is crucial to provide timely, reliable, and accurate estimates of the national burden of cancer.

The objective of this study is to compare the incidence and mortality rates of 29 types of cancer in Mexico in 2019 by sex and age, with trends from 1990 to 2019. The data used in this study were from the Global Burden of Disease Study 2019 (GBD 2019), which is a comprehensive global effort to systematically assess the major causes of health loss at the global, regional, and national levels [17]. The presented results provide updated information for a better understanding of the current context of evolution and trends of the national burden of cancer in Mexico. This information can be used to implement concrete public health actions to promote cancer control, diagnosis, and treatment programs.

## 2. Methods

### 2.1. GBD Study Overview

This observational study is a secondary analysis of results published in the Global Burden of Disease Study 2019 (GBD 2019). The GBD 2019 is produced by the Institute of Health Metrics and Evaluation (IHME), which includes a vast network of global collaborators, institutions, and partnerships involved in health policy and practice. This annual iteration was published in a series of four Capstone Papers [17–20], which describe in detail the trends in fertility, demography, and health loss due to 369 diseases and injuries and their corresponding 87 risk factors from 1990 to 2019. The estimates produced by the GBD

2019 represent the most comprehensive assessment of global health, providing timely and reliable results for 204 countries and territories by sex and age group. This study was produced and supervised by members of the GBD Collaborative Network from Mexico and adheres to GBD protocol.

### 2.2. Estimation of the Burden of Cancer in Mexico and Reporting Standards

The GBD 2019 report incorporates both fatal and non-fatal outcomes and provides a comprehensive hierarchical list of causes with four levels. Among the 22 groups at Level 2, 'neoplasms' (both benign and malignant) are included. At Level 3, there are 29 malignant neoplasms (cancers) and one group of benign neoplasms. The source for this information is https://vizhub.healthdata.org/gbd-compare/, accessed on 31 October 2023.

A detailed description of the approach, modeling framework, and steps taken by the GBD to generate the specific burden for neoplasms (total, benign, and malignant) is provided elsewhere [17]. Previous GBD studies have reported the methodology used to estimate the global, national, and regional burden of the 29 cancer groups, including case definition, data input sources, data processing, and statistical analysis [2,6]. The specific analytical flowchart used to produce cancer estimates is available online at https://ghdx.healthdata.org/gbd-2019/code/cod-2 (accessed on 2 November 2023).

This secondary analysis utilized publicly available data from the Global Health Data Exchange (GHDx), an online repository of the Institute for Health Metrics and Evaluation (IHME) (https://ghdx.healthdata.org, accessed on 11 August 2023). The GHDx provides GBD results for use in scientific publications, health policy, dissemination, and reporting. The results for Mexico were downloaded as CSV files from the GHDx online query tool (https://vizhub.healthdata.org/gbd-results/, accessed on 11 August 2023). To depict the cancer burden in Mexico between 1990 and 2019, we utilized crude counts of incidence and deaths caused by 29 groups of malignant neoplasms. Furthermore, we obtained crude and age-standardized rates per 100,000 individuals at the national level for each year, sex, and 5-year age groups. To compare the trends in these measures, we also downloaded the annual percentage change from 1990 to 2019.

Tables and figures were utilized to provide a comparative description of the burden of 29 cancer groups in Mexico for 2019, along with trends from 1990 to 2019. The data are presented as point estimates with 95% uncertainty intervals (95% UI), which were generated by the GBD 2019.

## 3. Results

### 3.1. National Burden of Disease Due to 29 Malignant Neoplasms during 2019

In Mexico, the 29 groups of malignant neoplasms mapped by the GBD caused an estimated 222,060 new cases in 2019. According to their national incidence (thousand new cases, 95% CI), non-melanoma skin cancer (41.3, 34.3 to 48.7), prostate cancer (27.1, 20.6 to 36.0), breast cancer (24.4, 19.9 to 29.9), colorectal cancer (17.5, 15.0 to 20.1), cervical cancer (12.2, 9.6 to 16.5), and stomach cancer (11.3, 9.8 to 13.0) were the top six ranked cancer groups in 2019 and contributed 60.2% of the total cases due to malignant neoplasm. In contrast, with incidence estimates ranging from 213 to 439 new cases, mesothelioma, other pharynx cancer, and nasopharyngeal cancer had the lowest incidence in Mexico during 2019 (Figure 1a and Table 1). The age-standardized incidence rate of these 29 malignant neoplasms varied substantially between 0.18 and 35.66 cases per 100,000 people. According to Supplementary Table S1, non-melanoma skin cancer and nasopharyngeal cancer had the highest and lowest rates, respectively.

In 2019, there were an estimated 105,591 deaths attributed to 29 types of cancer in Mexico. Of these malignant neoplasms, 52.9% were caused by six types of cancer: lung (11,002 deaths, 10.4% of the total), colorectal (10,518, 9.9%), stomach (10,095, 9.6%), prostate (9257, 8.8%), breast (8097, 7.7%), and pancreatic (6853, 6.5%). In 2019, the fewest cancer deaths were attributed to mesothelioma, other pharynx cancer, and nasopharyngeal cancer (range: 174–353 deaths; see Table 1 and Figure 1c). The highest age-standardized death rates per 100,000 people were observed for lung, colorectal, stomach, and prostate cancer (range: 8.78 to 9.74; see Supplementary Table S1).

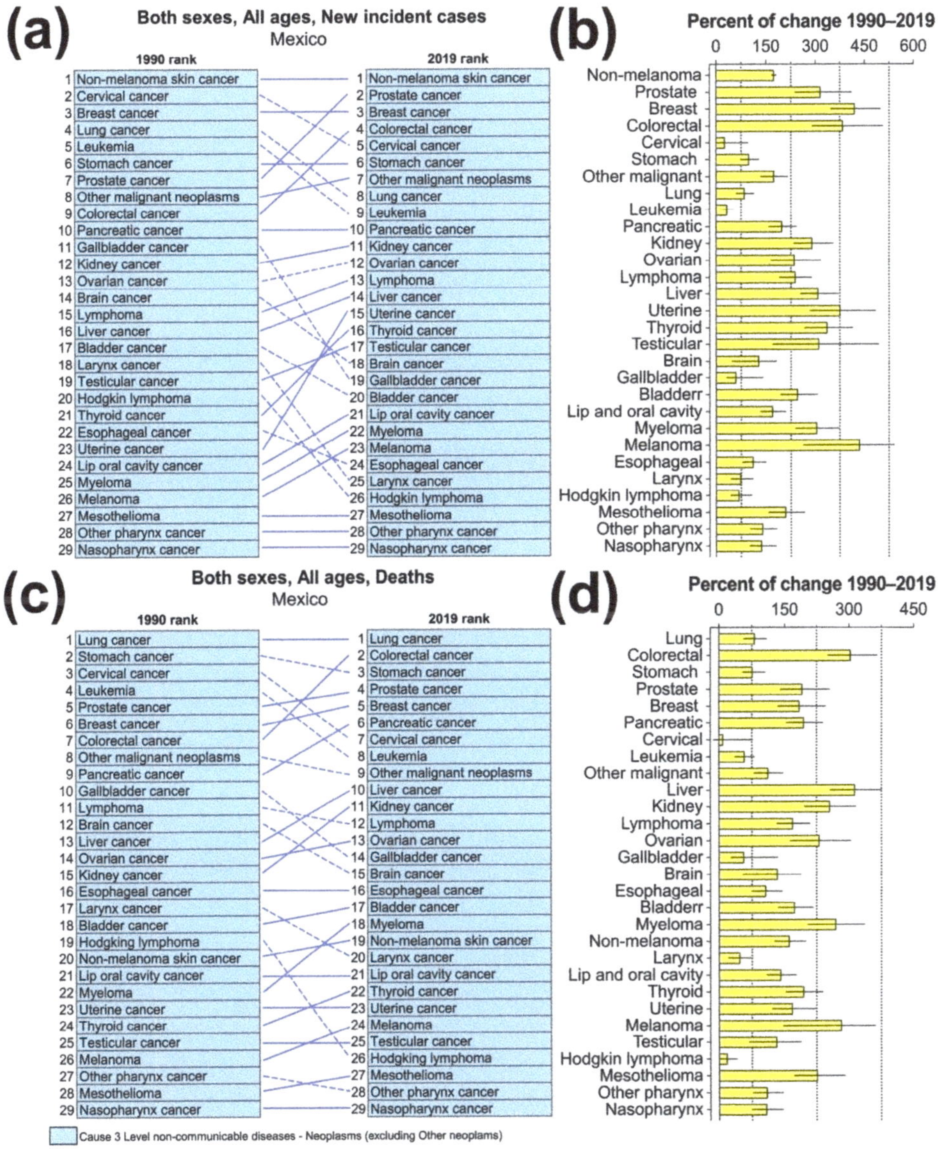


**Figure 1.** National ranking with percentage of annual change from 1990 to 2019 in the number of cases (**a**,**b**) and deaths (**c**,**d**) by cancer group.

**Table 1.** Total and sex-specific incidence and mortality by cancer group in Mexico in 2019.

| Group of Cancer | Incidence (Counts, 95% UI) | | | Deaths (Counts, 95% UI) | | |
|---|---|---|---|---|---|---|
| | Total | Female | Male | Total | Female | Male |
| Bladder cancer | 3071 (2633 to 3597) | 1009 (835 to 1224) | 2062 (1672 to 2529) | 1665 (1417 to 1929) | 571 (473 to 689) | 1094 (896 to 1321) |
| Brain and central nervous system cancer | 3473 (2515 to 4098) | 1547 (958 to 1954) | 1925 (1355 to 2369) | 2777 (2034 to 3274) | 1219 (754 to 1540) | 1558 (1099 to 1928) |
| Breast cancer | 24,442 (19,918 to 29,949) | 24,312 (19,777 to 29,810) | 130 (104 to 161) | 8097 (6718 to 9852) | 8024 (6649 to 9777) | 73 (60 to 90) |
| Cervical cancer | 12,195 (9656 to 16,527) | 12,195 (9656 to 16,527) | - | 6104 (4904 to 8120) | 6104 (4904 to 8120) | - |
| Colon and rectum cancer | 17,470 (15,042 to 20,060) | 8044 (6598 to 9771) | 9426 (7750 to 11,611) | 10,518 (9036 to 12,022) | 4917 (4101 to 5914) | 5601 (4599 to 6802) |
| Esophageal cancer | 1668 (1417 to 1962) | 443 (367 to 533) | 1226 (990 to 1495) | 1720 (1456 to 2008) | 453 (375 to 544) | 1267 (1018 to 1541) |
| Gallbladder and biliary tract cancer | 3109 (2591 to 4180) | 2139 (1706 to 3137) | 970 (761 to 1226) | 2910 (2415 to 3865) | 2005 (1588 to 2960) | 905 (697 to 1150) |
| Hodgkin lymphoma | 1383 (1147 to 1769) | 572 (431 to 862) | 811 (639 to 1053) | 632 (520 to 806) | 252 (186 to 366) | 381 (301 to 483) |
| Kidney cancer | 6321 (5374 to 7371) | 2451 (2032 to 2966) | 3870 (3069 to 4794) | 3461 (2918 to 4045) | 1278 (1057 to 1541) | 2182 (1704 to 2730) |
| Larynx cancer | 1493 (1241 to 1789) | 216 (174 to 297) | 1277 (1033 to 1562) | 1118 (926 to 1333) | 162 (131 to 223) | 957 (775 to 1159) |
| Leukemia | 7787 (6810 to 8825) | 3677 (3103 to 4338) | 4111 (3469 to 4853) | 5249 (4603 to 5958) | 2431 (2049 to 2867) | 2818 (2351 to 3372) |
| Lip and oral cavity cancer | 1913 (1648 to 2195) | 793 (654 to 955) | 1121 (908 to 1366) | 1109 (958 to 1264) | 439 (366 to 529) | 670 (552 to 813) |
| Liver cancer | 3973 (3436 to 4550) | 1943 (1611 to 2345) | 2030 (1661 to 2472) | 4183 (3606 to 4792) | 2054 (1705 to 2475) | 2128 (1731 to 2586) |
| Malignant skin melanoma | 1725 (1296 to 2243) | 846 (516 to 1111) | 879 (543 to 1281) | 874 (618 to 1158) | 382 (224 to 500) | 492 (305 to 736) |
| Mesothelioma | 439 (364 to 517) | 146 (87 to 186) | 294 (237 to 362) | 353 (294 to 415) | 115 (69 to 146) | 238 (193 to 289) |
| Multiple myeloma | 1873 (1512 to 2206) | 892 (692 to 1100) | 981 (687 to 1252) | 1444 (1152 to 1714) | 664 (529 to 820) | 780 (550 to 1001) |
| Nasopharynx cancer | 213 (181 to 251) | 62 (51 to 75) | 151 (121 to 188) | 174 (146 to 204) | 45 (37 to 55) | 129 (103 to 158) |
| Non-Hodgkin lymphoma | 5069 (4363 to 5862) | 2202 (1809 to 2702) | 2867 (2335 to 3487) | 3399 (2944 to 3876) | 1521 (1262 to 1841) | 1878 (1526 to 2290) |
| Non-melanoma skin cancer | 41,320 (34,279 to 48,728) | 21,263 (17,507 to 25,200) | 20,057 (16,717 to 23,577) | 1286 (1093 to 1478) | 583 (482 to 695) | 703 (567 to 851) |
| Other malignant neoplasms | 10,938 (9495 to 12,555) | 5625 (4695 to 6724) | 5313 (4325 to 6389) | 5161 (4415 to 5949) | 2437 (1997 to 2937) | 2724 (2195 to 3313) |
| Other pharynx cancer | 332 (280 to 392) | 89 (73 to 107) | 243 (194 to 300) | 280 (235 to 327) | 68 (57 to 82) | 212 (168 to 258) |
| Ovarian cancer | 5341 (4256 to 6599) | 5341 (4256 to 6599) | - | 3340 (2688 to 4120) | 3340 (2688 to 4120) | - |
| Pancreatic cancer | 6674 (5744 to 7683) | 3463 (2848 to 4191) | 3212 (2579 to 3941) | 6853 (5866 to 7853) | 3583 (2973 to 4308) | 3270 (2649 to 3966) |
| Prostate cancer | 27,097 (20,602 to 36,017) | - | 27,097 (20,602 to 36,017) | 9256 (7077 to 12,679) | - | 9256 (7077 to 12,679) |
| Stomach cancer | 11,272 (9786 to 13,049) | 5298 (4393 to 6401) | 5973 (4926 to 7343) | 10,095 (8688 to 11,605) | 4656 (3860 to 5612 | 5439 (4465 to 6589) |
| Testicular cancer | 3495 (2050 to 4892) | - | 3495 (2050 to 4892) | 662 (520 to 854) | - | 662 (520 to 854) |
| Thyroid cancer | 3534 (2967 to 4174) | 2589 (2094 to 3163) | 945 (755 to 1168) | 944 (811 to 1089) | 636 (521 to 768) | 309 (244 to 381) |
| Tracheal, bronchus, and lung cancer | 10,890 (9400 to 12,582) | 3961 (3271 to 4801) | 6930 (5682 to 8476) | 11,002 (9425 to 12,698) | 3827 (3121 to 4659) | 7176 (5881 to 8671) |
| Uterine cancer | 3550 (2870 to 4333) | 3550 (2870 to 4333) | - | 923 (760 to 1121) | 923 (760 to 1121) | - |

### 3.2. National Trends in Crude Incidence and Mortality Due to 29 Malignant Neoplasms from 1990 to 2019

Figure 1a shows that seven cancer groups maintained their incidence ranking at the national level between 1990 and 2019, including non-melanoma skin cancer, breast cancer, stomach cancer, and pancreatic cancer in the top 10. Furthermore, among the 13 cancer groups that increased their ranking, prostate, colorectal, uterine, and thyroid cancer showed the most significant advancement. In contrast, the greatest declines were observed in cases of laryngeal cancer and Hodgkin lymphoma, gallbladder cancer, and brain cancer. Despite the different patterns of change observed, all 29 groups of cancer showed a positive percentage of annual change from 1990 to 2019, albeit variable (Figure 1b). The incidence increases ranged from 27% (−1 to 97) for cervical cancer to 436% (264 to 541) for melanoma (Supplementary Table S2). Several cancer types experienced significant increases, including colorectal, prostate, uterine, thyroid, breast, testicular, and liver cancer, with increases ranging from 310% to 421%.

The national ranking of cancer-related deaths revealed that six cancer types (lung, esophageal, lip, oral cavity, uterine, testicular, and nasopharynx) maintained their positions from 1990 to 2019, while 13 cancer types moved up in rank (Figure 1c). Colorectal cancer experienced the highest increase, moving from the seventh to the second position. However, 10 cancer groups experienced a decrease in rank, with Hodgkin lymphoma, cervical cancer, leukemia, and brain cancer showing the largest decreases. It is worth noting that all 29 cancer groups had a positive percentage annual change in mortality from 1990 to 2019 (refer to Figure 1d). Liver cancer, colorectal cancer, melanoma, myeloma, kidney cancer, and ovarian cancer had the six highest increases in the numbers of deaths they caused, with values ranging from 232% to 314% (Supplementary Table S2).

### 3.3. National Cancer-Specific Trends from 1990 to 2019 in Age-Standardized Incidence and Mortality Rates

From 1990 to 2019, the age-standardized incidence and mortality rates (per 100,000 people) of 29 cancer groups in Mexico showed a contrasting pattern of change. Supplementary Table S3 shows that 17 out of 29 malignant neoplasms had an increasing trend in age-standardized incidence rate during this period. Testicular cancer (190.7%), melanoma (116.8%), and colorectal cancer (89.2%) showed the largest increases, as shown in Supplementary Figure S1. In contrast, the age-standardized incidence rates per 100,000 for cervical cancer decreased by 47.9%, gallbladder cancer by 42.7%, laryngeal cancer by 37.6%, and lung cancer by 32.8%.

Over the period, 16 out of 29 cancer groups had a decrease in their age-standardized death rates, but with wide variability in their time series (Figure 2). According to Supplementary Table S3, there were significant decreases in the incidence of cervical cancer, laryngeal cancer, gallbladder cancer, Hodgkin lymphoma, stomach cancer, and lung cancer (ranging from −35.5% to −58.3%). However, liver cancer (52.1%), melanoma (44.3%), and colorectal cancer (41.7%) showed substantial increases. To aid in interpreting the intricate patterns of results, Supplementary Figure S2 summarizes the percentage of change in age-standardized rates, ordered from the cancer with the largest increase to the cancer with the largest decrease. The figure illustrates that the percentage change varied by measure and cancer group.

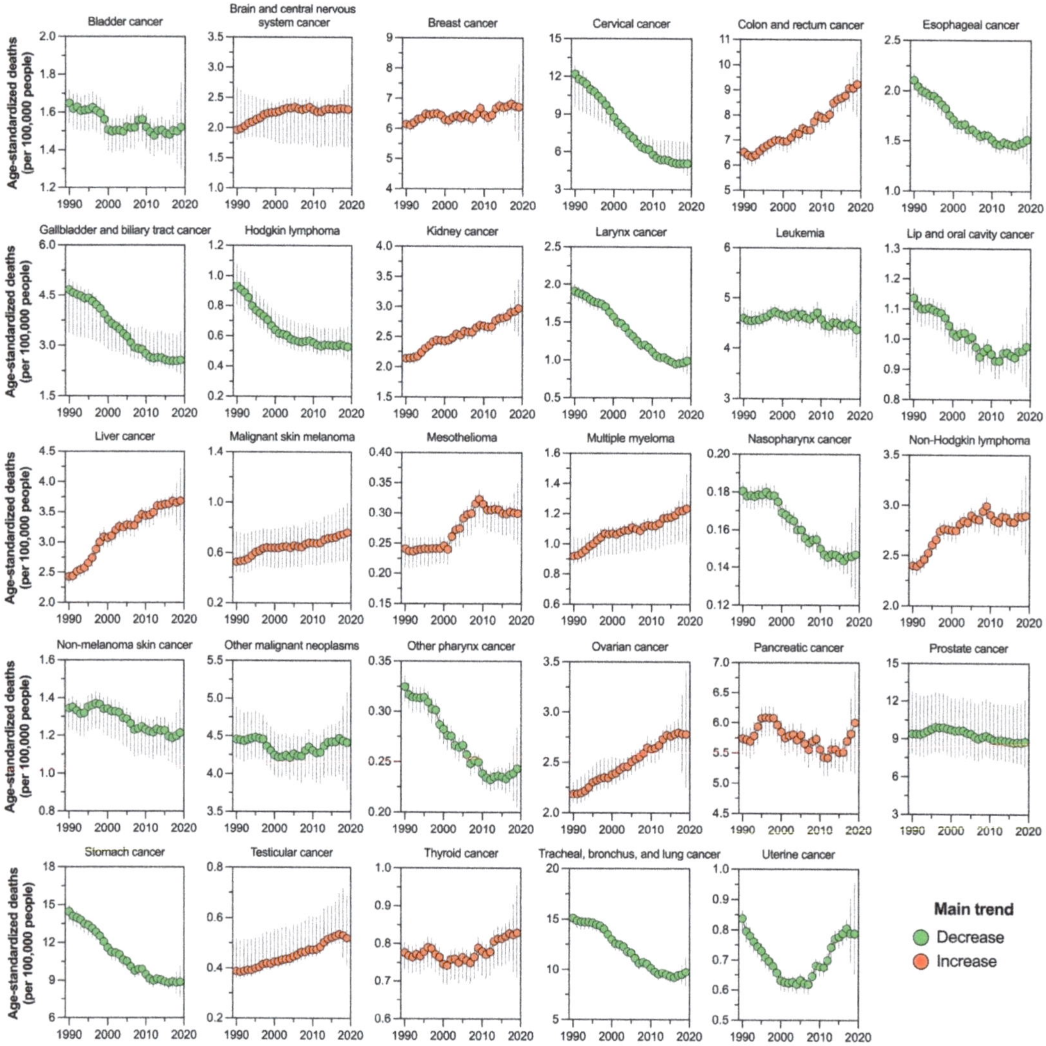


**Figure 2.** Cancer-specific trends from 1990 to 2019 of the age-standardized death rates (per 100,000) in Mexico.

### *3.4. National Burden of 29 Cancer Groups by Sex and Age Group in 2109*

In 2019, the burden of disease due to cancer in Mexico exhibited a distinct age-specific distribution by sex. The crude incidence was lower in the early age groups (1–24 years) for both sexes. However, in women, there was a rapid increase in cancer incidence starting at 35–39 years of age. The highest number of cases was concentrated between 40 and 84 years of age, with a peak of 14,853 new cases in the 60–64 age group. In contrast, the number of incident cases among men increased gradually and occurred at older ages, starting at 45–49 years and peaking at 70–74 years with 12,291 new cases (Figure 3a). A similar pattern was found for mortality, with the highest number of deaths occurring in the 70–74 age group for women (5999 deaths) and in the 75–79 age group for men (7146 deaths) due to cancer (Figure 3b).

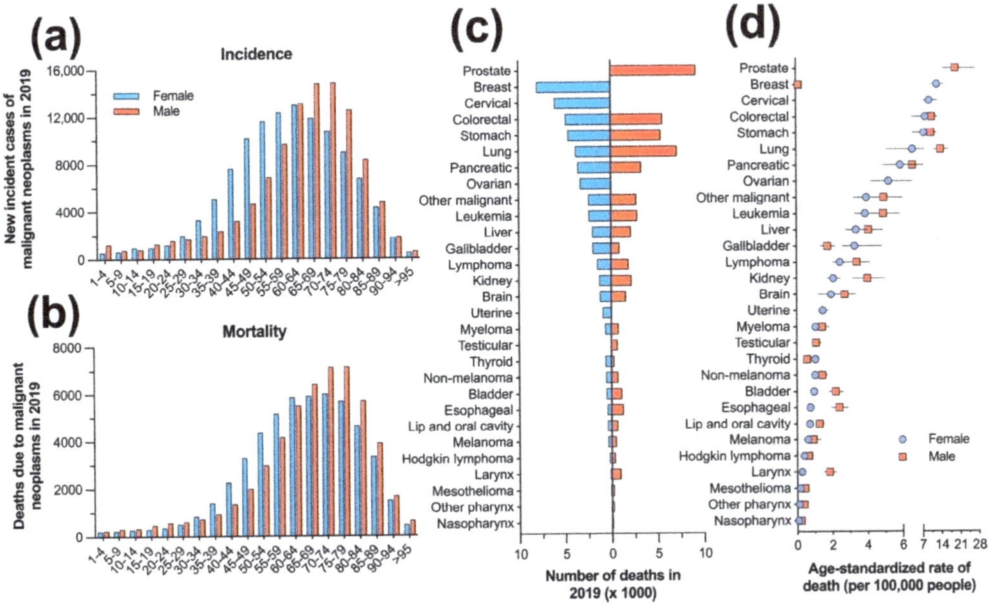


**Figure 3.** Sex- and age-specific distribution of the incident cases (**a**) and deaths (**b**) due to malignant neoplasms in Mexico during 2019, cancer-specific death counts (**c**), and age-standardized rate of death per 100,000 people by sex (**d**).

To analyze sex differences among the 29 cancer groups, we compared the crude counts and age-standardized rates per 100,000 people (Table 1 and Supplementary Table S1). Breast cancer (24,312 cases), non-melanoma (21,263 cases), and cervical cancer (12,195 cases) were the most common types of cancer in women, while prostate cancer, melanoma, and colorectal cancer (with a range of 9426 to 27,097 cases, Supplementary Figure S3a) were the most common in men. Prostate cancer was the leading cause of incident cases in men, with an age-standardized rate of 52.3 (40.0 to 70.1) per 100,000 people. In women, breast cancer was the leading cause with an estimated rate of 36.81 (30.02 to 45.01) cases per 100,000 people, while men had a negligible rate of 0.23 (0.19 to 0.29 cases) (Supplementary Figure S3b).

Breast cancer caused an estimated 8024 deaths among women in Mexico in 2019, followed by cervical cancer and colorectal cancer in second and third place with 6104 and 4917 deaths, respectively. Among men, prostate cancer was the leading cause of death from malignant neoplasms with 9256 deaths, followed by lung and colorectal cancers with 7176 and 5601 deaths, respectively (refer to Figure 3c). The age-standardized death rate varied significantly by cancer group in both sexes. Prostate cancer had the highest death rate among men, with 19.4 (14.8 to 26.7) deaths per 100,000 people. Among women, breast cancer had the highest death rate, with 12.5 (10.3 to 15.2) deaths per 100,000 people. The death rates for other neoplasms varied from 0.07 to 9.53 and 0.1 to 13.8 deaths per 100,000 people in women and men, respectively (Figure 3d).

Finally, based on the incidence (Supplementary Figure S4) and mortality (Figure 4) rates per 100,000 people, there was a contrasting pattern of age-specific burden between sexes that varied by cancer type in Mexico in 2019. Overall, except for brain cancer, leukemia, Hodgkin lymphoma, and testicular cancer, most malignant neoplasms tended to have the highest burden in older ages. Several cancer groups, including bladder, brain, esophageal, Hodgkin lymphoma, kidney, larynx, lip and oral cavity, mesothelioma, nasopharynx, other pharynx, and lung cancer, had higher rates in men than in women.

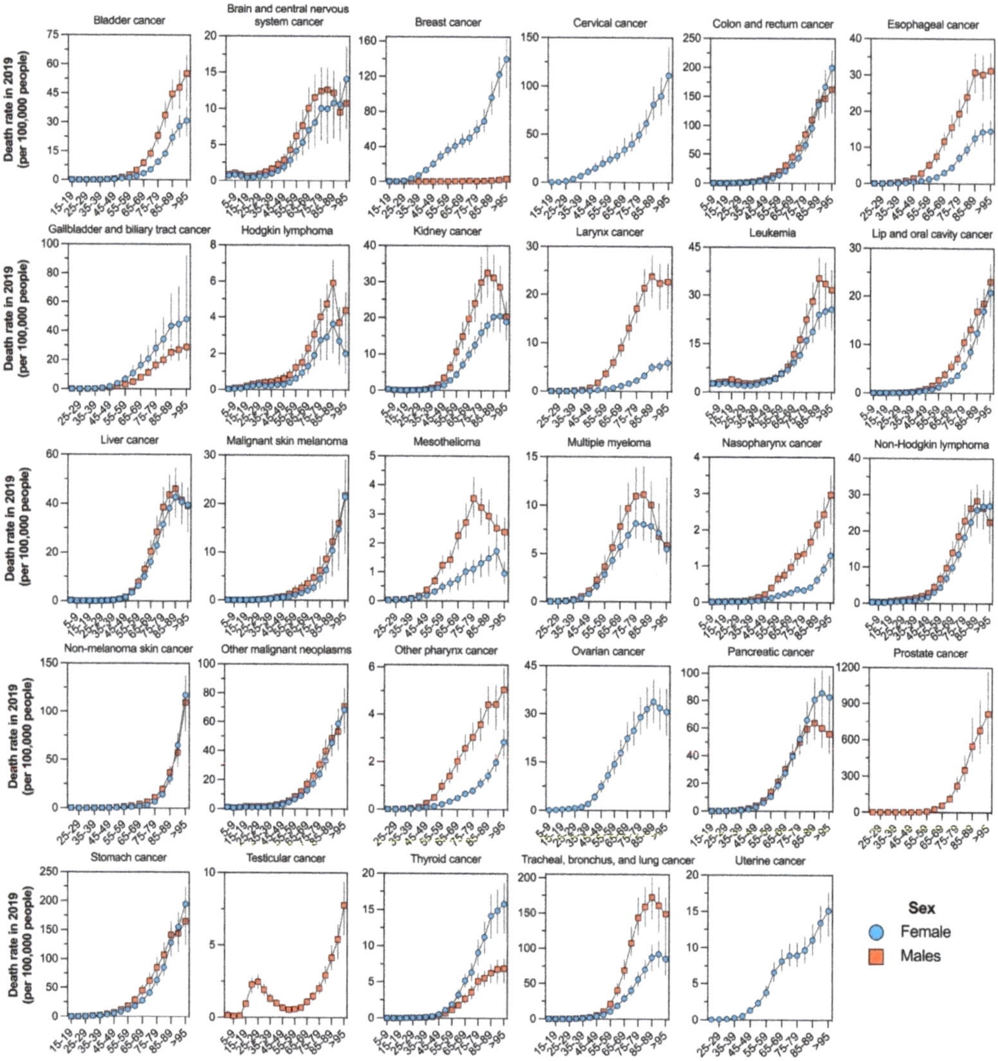


**Figure 4.** Age-specific rate of death (per 100,000 people) by sex for each group of cancers in Mexico during 2019.

## 4. Discussion

Although neoplasms (benign and malignant) moved from the second to the third leading cause of death in Mexico between 1990 and 2019, mortality rates caused by this group of diseases increased by 126.05% during this period. This increase was driven by the 29 groups of malignant neoplasms reported in this study (source: https://vizhub.healthdata.org/gbd-compare/, accessed on 10 August 2023). Our study found that lung cancer remained the leading cause of mortality from 1990 to 2019. Colorectal cancer moved up from seventh to second place, followed by stomach cancer, which dropped from second to third. Prostate cancer, breast cancer, and pancreatic cancer completed the list of the six most common causes of cancer death in Mexico in 2019. This pattern differs partially from a previous study that identified lung cancer, stomach cancer, liver cancer, prostate cancer, breast cancer, and cervical cancer as the top six causes of cancer-related deaths between

2000 and 2013 [15]. These findings may indicate a shift in the mortality pattern of cancer over the past two decades.

Other studies based on national databases from Mexico [7] have confirmed the rise in colorectal cancer mortality, which has also been documented globally [21]. The rise in colorectal cancer mortality is linked to a trend of higher incidence, even in early onset cases (<50 years of age) [22]. However, the absence of national screening strategies in Mexico may worsen this trend due to the detection of a large number of new cases at advanced stages, leading to higher mortality rates. Our results indicate that in 2019, the top six ranked cancer groups in Mexico were non-melanoma skin cancer, prostate cancer, breast cancer, colorectal cancer, cervical cancer, and stomach cancer among the 29 groups of malignant neoplasms in terms of incidence. The rise in cancer morbidity and mortality may be linked to various behavioral and environmental risk factors, including smoking, alcohol consumption, diet, radiation exposure, certain infections, and hormonal imbalances [23]. In Mexico, the prevalence of risk factors such as alcohol and tobacco consumption is high [15]. Therefore, further studies are necessary to determine the association between cancer mortality and risk factors.

Cancer affecting non-reproductive tissues has a higher incidence and mortality rate in males, resulting in roughly double the mortality rate compared to females [24]. Previous studies have shown that female cancer patients tend to have better survival rates than males [25]. However, in the Mexican population, overall mortality was slightly higher in females. The incidence of cancer in males is understudied despite the well-known disparity. This may be due to researchers assuming that known causes explain the disparity. According to GBD 2017 estimates, non-melanoma skin cancer was the most prevalent form of cancer among women globally, followed by breast cancer. In males, non-melanoma skin cancer had the most significant impact, followed by tracheal, bronchus, lung, and prostate cancer [6]. Our results showed that in comparison to this global trend, breast cancer has become the most prevalent cancer among females in Mexico, surpassing non-melanoma skin cancer. Cervical cancer, colorectal cancer, and ovarian cancer followed in frequency. Among males, prostate cancer has overtaken non-melanoma skin cancer, followed by colorectal, tracheal, bronchus, and lung cancer. The reasons for this differential pattern in Mexico remain unclear. However, the reasons for the differences in cancer rates and outcomes between sexes are not fully understood. Biological sex significantly influences organismal development and physiology, affecting processes such as cell signaling, metabolism, and immune responses [26,27]. The higher incidence of gallstones among women is likely the reason for the excess risk of gallbladder and biliary tract cancer in females [28]. Similarly, factors such as smoking and occupational exposures can be attributed to the higher portion of the male excess in urinary bladder cancer [29]. Additionally, the incidence of thyroid cases is more than double in women than that in men, a disparity that has been documented in other countries. Although the biological causes of this difference are not yet conclusive, it is speculated that non-biological factors may play a role. For instance, there is a possibility that women have more opportunities for incidental detection in clinical settings [30].

As anticipated, both sexes exhibited a higher incidence and mortality at older ages. Aging has been shown to accelerate cancer mortality, which may be influenced by various factors such as comorbidities, less intense detection, and lower likelihood of undergoing aggressive treatment [31]. In recent decades, Latin America has experienced a significant increase in life expectancy, resulting in a growing population of older adults. The rise in incidence and mortality rates in Mexico since 1990 can be partially attributed to this aging population. As a result, more individuals are expected to be diagnosed with cancer and experience cancer-related fatalities. A previous study demonstrated that advanced age may influence oncologists to avoid intensive cancer therapy, even in cases where patients are highly functional and have no comorbidities [32]. As a result, this group may have a worse prognosis and be undertreated, contributing to the mortality rate. Although our study did not categorize age groups, our results are consistent with global trends. The age-specific distribution showed that cancer incidence among children and teenagers was notably lower compared to older populations [33]. Furthermore, certain types of cancer disproportionately affect specific age groups. Leukemia is the primary contributor to cancer incidence among young individuals in the child and teenage age range [34]. A previous study in Mexico found that leukemia and other malignant neoplasms accounted for almost 70% of the cancer burden in younger age groups [14]. The present study shows a significant change in the prevalence of leukemia over time, with a decline in its ranking from fifth in 1990 to ninth in 2019. The changing landscape of cancer epidemiology suggests possible alterations in risk factors, diagnostic capabilities, or treatment modalities over time [35].

Lung cancer is the primary cause of death among respiratory system cancers, but its incidence in Mexico has decreased since 1990. Tobacco smoke is a significant contributing factor in the development of lung cancer, and it is widely recognized. Approximately 90% of lung cancer cases in men and 78% in women are estimated to be caused by tobacco smoke [36]. Tobacco consumption in Mexico has declined over the past few decades, especially among males [8]. Mexican healthcare systems aim to effectively address this issue by implementing advertising campaigns and initiatives to raise public awareness, particularly regarding lung cancer.

Colorectal cancer has a higher incidence among gastrointestinal tract cancers, and this incidence has increased nationally in recent years. This trend is consistent with the global trend, as the global incidence of colorectal cancer has more than doubled from 1990 to 2019 [21]. Other low- and middle-income countries, like Mexico, are also experiencing an increase in incident cases of colorectal cancer. In developed countries, there has been a trend of either decrease or stabilization [37]. It is possible that these trends are influenced by an increase in the prevalence of risk factors associated with diet and lifestyle [4]. Obesity and physical inactivity are two factors strongly associated with colorectal cancer [38] and are increasing nationally. Currently, 17% of the population is physically inactive and over 70% are overweight or obese [39]. These factors are modifiable, indicating potential for prevention. Given that this this cancer has one of the highest incidence and mortality rates, it should be a priority in the country's public policies design. This should focus on improving access to screening tests and early detection, which would help to reduce the number of cases and deaths.

Prostate cancer is one of the most significant tumors of the genitourinary system and has the second-highest incidence rate. The incidence of this ailment is increasing. However, Mexico has a relatively low incidence rate compared to other Latin American and Caribbean countries, ranking higher only than Argentina, Honduras, Ecuador, and Bolivia [40]. Testicular cancer is another type of cancer that affects the genitourinary system and is relevant in Mexico. The national incidence of this cancer differs from that observed in the rest of the world. However, there is a lack of studies on the epidemiology and risk factors of this cancer type in Mexico. Therefore, more research is necessary to implement public policies that could reduce the burden of this disease. Although the global incidence rate has increased, the mortality rate has improved. Unfortunately, Mexico has one of the highest mortality rates [41].

Breast and cervical cancer are the most frequently diagnosed gynecological cancers. Breast cancer has consistently ranked as the third most prevalent malignant neoplasm over the past three decades. In 2019, it represented 7.67% of total deaths, ranking fifth, with a slight increase over the period. The increase in obesity prevalence in Mexico can be attributed to various factors, including changes in diet, physical activity, reproductive choices, and detection at a more advanced stage [42,43]. Studies have found that obesity is a significant risk factor for developing this neoplasia regardless of socioeconomic level, region, or locality [44]. Breast cancer disproportionately affects lower-income populations, but it can impact women of all ages and income levels [12]. In 2002, the Ministry of Health extended and expanded official health regulations and legislation concerning the management of breast cancer through an official technical directive. Mexico has seen a significant decrease in cervical cancer incidence in recent years due to successful campaigns aimed at combating human papillomavirus (HPV). This is because most cervical cancer cases are caused by chronic infection by oncogenic subtypes of HPV. In 2012, Mexico launched a vaccination program for girls aged 11 years to reduce the overall burden of cervical cancer and other diseases caused by HPV [45]. Around 80% of 11-year-old girls in Mexico were covered by vaccination programs. However, vaccination coverage has drastically decreased in recent years, from 11.22% in 2020 to 0.45% in 2021. This decline is mainly due to health efforts being focused on managing the COVID-19 pandemic [11].

Reducing cancer in Mexico is crucial due to disparities in the public healthcare system. The system is primarily composed of employment-based social security systems, and medical services for oncological diagnosis and prognosis are inadequate due to limited infrastructure. Mexico has only 212 radiotherapy units, 358 nuclear medicine units, and 2582 imaging units for the entire population [46]. Therefore, the Mexican government should allocate more resources to improve medical coverage. To achieve more accurate rates, new diagnostic tools and improved registration systems are necessary. National and local governments require additional resources for healthcare and epidemiological surveillance of cancer. Additionally, medical public campaigns for primary healthcare are lacking to increase awareness of the risk factors associated with cancer groups that affect the Mexican population and to prevent an increase in preventable cancer cases. The accurate diagnosis and registration of all cancer cases, including oncological characteristics such as cancer type, staging, and follow-up, are necessary for reliable data. It is important to note that people from rural communities are often excluded from these statistical surveys due to the lack of universal healthcare. The Mexican Congress has established a national cancer registry. However, since its establishment in 2017, it has only included the registration of childhood cancer cases. Therefore, it needs to be expanded to cover the entire population.

This observational study is based on a secondary analysis of data generated by the GBD for Mexico. Therefore, some of the estimates presented here should be interpreted with caution due to the following limitations. The challenges in cancer data collection include (1) insufficient cancer-specific data categorized by year, age, and sex; (2) limited availability of diverse data sources, such as nationally representative studies; (3) varying levels of completeness and time lags in high-quality data; (4) a reduced number of studies on cancer risk factors; and (5) high variability in the data, which may lead to an underestimation of the number of people affected by cancer.

## 5. Conclusions

Cancer remains a significant public health issue in Mexico, marked by rising incidence and mortality rates. While these statistical trends do not directly apply to an individual patient, they play a crucial role in aiding governments, policymakers, health professionals, and researchers in comprehending the impact of cancer on the population. These trends enable them to develop strategies to reduce the cancer burden and to manage and treat cancer. The increasing burden of cancer in Mexico emphasizes the necessity for sustained efforts to address underlying risk factors and enhance access to screening, treatment, and patient care. With appropriate strategies and investments, it is feasible to mitigate the impact of cancer on the health of the Mexican population and improve outcomes.

**Supplementary Materials:** The following supporting information can be downloaded at https://www.mdpi.com/article/10.3390/cancers16010149/s1, Figure S1. Cancer-specific trends and annual percentage change from 1990 to 2019 of the age-standardized incidence rate (per 100,000 people) in Mexico; Figure S2. Cancer-specific annual percentage changes from 1990 to 2019 of age-standardized incidence (a) and mortality (b) rates per 100,000 population in Mexico; Figure S3. Cancer-specific incidence rates (a) and age-standardized mortality rates (per 100,000 people) by sex (b) in Mexico in 2019.; Figure S4. Age-specific incidence rate (per 100,000 people) by sex for each cancer group in Mexico during 2019; Table S1. Total and sex-specific and age-standardized incidence and mortality rates (per 100,000 people) by cancer group in Mexico during 2019; Table S2. Percentage change from 1990 to 2019 in crude incidence and mortality due to 29 malignant neoplasms in Mexico; Table S3. Percentage change from 1990 to 2019 of age-standardized incidence and mortality rates (per 100,000 population) due to 29 malignant neoplasms in Mexico.

**Author Contributions:** Conceptualization, supervision, and project administration, S.A.B.-O. and D.D.; methodology, data curation, and visualization D.D.; software and formal analysis, D.D.; investigation, E.L.-V., E.P.G.-G. and K.L.-L.; writing—original draft preparation, S.A.B.-O., E.L.-V., K.L.-L. and D.D.; writing—review and editing, J.A.C.-G., M.A.T.-R., J.M.M.-O., D.L.C.-A., E.L.-L., J.R.Z.-L., E.H.L.-F., J.L.R.-T., H.M.C.-D., M.M.-M., B.A.-B., D.E.C.-L., V.A.C.-R., R.L., L.C.-A., E.C.-U. and F.G.-V. All authors have read and agreed to the published version of the manuscript.

**Funding:** This research received no external funding.

**Institutional Review Board Statement:** Not applicable.

**Informed Consent Statement:** Not applicable.

**Data Availability Statement:** All data used are available at https://ghdx.healthdata.org (accessed on: 31 October 2023).

**Conflicts of Interest:** The authors declare no conflict of interest.

## References

1. Bray, F.; Ferlay, J.; Soerjomataram, I.; Siegel, R.L.; Torre, L.A.; Jemal, A. Global cancer statistics 2018: GLOBOCAN estimates of incidence and mortality worldwide for 36 cancers in 185 countries. *CA Cancer J. Clin.* **2018**, *68*, 394–424. [CrossRef] [PubMed]
2. Kocarnik, J.M.; Compton, K.; Dean, F.E.; Fu, W.; Gaw, B.L.; Harvey, J.D.; Henrikson, H.J.; Lu, D.; Pennini, A.; Xu, R.; et al. Cancer Incidence, Mortality, Years of Life Lost, Years Lived with Disability, and Disability-Adjusted Life Years for 29 Cancer Groups From 2010 to 2019: A Systematic Analysis for the Global Burden of Disease Study 2019. *JAMA Oncol.* **2022**, *8*, 420–444. [CrossRef] [PubMed]
3. Sung, H.; Ferlay, J.; Siegel, R.L.; Laversanne, M.; Soerjomataram, I.; Jemal, A.; Bray, F. Global Cancer Statistics 2020: GLOBOCAN Estimates of Incidence and Mortality Worldwide for 36 Cancers in 185 Countries. *CA Cancer J. Clin.* **2021**, *71*, 209–249. [CrossRef] [PubMed]
4. Tran, K.B.; Lang, J.J.; Compton, K.; Xu, R.; Acheson, A.R.; Henrikson, H.J.; Kocarnik, J.M.; Penberthy, L.; Aali, A.; Abbas, Q. The global burden of cancer attributable to risk factors, 2010–2019: A systematic analysis for the Global Burden of Disease Study 2019. *Lancet* **2022**, *400*, 563–591. [CrossRef]
5. Lin, L.; Li, Z.; Yan, L.; Liu, Y.; Yang, H.; Li, H. Global, regional, and national cancer incidence and death for 29 cancer groups in 2019 and trends analysis of the global cancer burden, 1990–2019. *J. Hematol. Oncol.* **2021**, *14*, 197. [CrossRef]
6. Fitzmaurice, C.; Abate, D.; Abbasi, N.; Abbastabar, H.; Abd-Allah, F.; Abdel-Rahman, O.; Abdelalim, A.; Abdoli, A.; Abdollahpour, I.; Abdulle, A.S.M.; et al. Global, Regional, and National Cancer Incidence, Mortality, Years of Life Lost, Years Lived with Disability, and Disability-Adjusted Life-Years for 29 Cancer Groups, 1990 to 2017: A Systematic Analysis for the Global Burden of Disease Study. *JAMA Oncol.* **2019**, *5*, 1749–1768. [CrossRef]
7. Espinosa-Tamez, P.; Suazo-Zepeda, E.; Sánchez-Blas, H.; Meneses-Medina, M.; Huitzil-Meléndez, F.D.; Van Loon, K.; Potter, M.B.; Lajous, M. National and state-level colorectal cancer mortality trends in Mexico, 1998–2018. *Salud Pública México* **2022**, *64*, 5–13. [CrossRef]
8. Torres-Dominguez, J.A.; Betancourt, A.M.; Mejia, L.S.P.; Noveron, N.R. Lung cancer mortality trends in Mexico, 1998–2018: The impact of the General Law on Tobacco Control. *Rev. Bras. Epidemiol.* **2022**, *25*, e220003. [CrossRef]
9. Beltran-Ontiveros, S.A.; Fernandez-Galindo, M.A.; Moreno-Ortiz, J.M.; Contreras-Gutierrez, J.A.; Maduena-Molina, J.; Arambula-Meraz, E.; Leal-Leon, E.; Becerril-Camacho, D.M.; Picos-Cardenas, V.J.; Angulo-Rojo, C.; et al. Incidence, Mortality, and Trends of Prostate Cancer in Mexico from 2000 to 2019: Results from the Global Burden of Disease Study 2019. *Cancers* **2022**, *14*, 3184. [CrossRef]
10. Torres-Sánchez, L.E.; Espinoza-Giacinto, R.; Rojas-Martínez, R.; Escamilla-Nuñez, C.; Vázquez-Salas, R.A.; Campuzano, J.C.; Lazcano-Ponce, E. Comportamiento de la mortalidad por cáncer de próstata en México de acuerdo al índice de marginación estatal, de 1980 a 2013. *Salud Pública México* **2016**, *58*, 179–186. [CrossRef]
11. Munoz-Bello, J.O.; Carrillo-Garcia, A.; Lizano, M. Epidemiology and Molecular Biology of HPV Variants in Cervical Cancer: The State of the Art in Mexico. *Int. J. Mol. Sci.* **2022**, *23*, 8566. [CrossRef] [PubMed]
12. Knaul, F.M.; Nigenda, G.; Lozano, R.; Arreola-Ornelas, H.; Langer, A.; Frenk, J. Breast cancer in Mexico: A pressing priority. *Reprod. Health Matters* **2008**, *16*, 113–123. [CrossRef] [PubMed]
13. Malvezzi, M.; Bosetti, C.; Chatenoud, L.; Rodriguez, T.; Levi, F.; Negri, E.; La Vecchia, C. Trends in cancer mortality in Mexico, 1970–1999. *Ann. Oncol.* **2004**, *15*, 1712–1718. [CrossRef] [PubMed]
14. Gomez-Dantes, H.; Lamadrid-Figueroa, H.; Cahuana-Hurtado, L.; Silverman-Retana, O.; Montero, P.; Gonzalez-Robledo, M.C.; Fitzmaurice, C.; Pain, A.; Allen, C.; Dicker, D.J.; et al. The burden of cancer in Mexico, 1990–2013. *Salud Pública México* **2016**, *58*, 118–131. [CrossRef] [PubMed]
15. Mohar-Betancourt, A.; Reynoso-Noveron, N.; Armas-Texta, D.; Gutierrez-Delgado, C.; Torres-Dominguez, J.A. Cancer Trends in Mexico: Essential Data for the Creation and Follow-Up of Public Policies. *J. Glob. Oncol.* **2017**, *3*, 740–748. [CrossRef] [PubMed]

16. Aldaco-Sarvide, F.; Pérez-Pérez, P.; Cervantes-Sánchez, M.G.; Torrecillas-Torres, L.; Erazo-Valle-Solís, A.A.; Cabrera-Galeana, P.; Motola-Kuba, D.; Anaya, P.; Rivera, S.; Cárdenas-Cárdenas, E. Mortality from cancer in Mexico: 2015 update. *Gac. Mex. Oncol.* **2022**, *17*, 28–34. [CrossRef]
17. Vos, T.; Lim, S.S.; Abbafati, C.; Abbas, K.M.; Abbasi, M.; Abbasifard, M.; Abbasi-Kangevari, M.; Abbastabar, H.; Abd-Allah, F.; Abdelalim, A.; et al. Global burden of 369 diseases and injuries in 204 countries and territories, 1990–2019: A systematic analysis for the Global Burden of Disease Study 2019. *Lancet* **2020**, *396*, 1204–1222. [CrossRef] [PubMed]
18. Murray, C.J.; Aravkin, A.Y.; Zheng, P.; Abbafati, C.; Abbas, K.M.; Abbasi-Kangevari, M.; Abd-Allah, F.; Abdelalim, A.; Abdollahi, M.; Abdollahpour, I. Global burden of 87 risk factors in 204 countries and territories, 1990–2019: A systematic analysis for the Global Burden of Disease Study 2019. *Lancet* **2020**, *396*, 1223–1249. [CrossRef]
19. Vollset, S.E.; Goren, E.; Yuan, C.W.; Cao, J.; Smith, A.E.; Hsiao, T.; Bisignano, C.; Azhar, G.S.; Castro, E.; Chalek, J.; et al. Fertility, mortality, migration, and population scenarios for 195 countries and territories from 2017 to 2100: A forecasting analysis for the Global Burden of Disease Study. *Lancet* **2020**, *396*, 1285–1306. [CrossRef]
20. Wang, H.; Abbas, K.M.; Abbasifard, M.; Abbasi-Kangevari, M.; Abbastabar, H.; Abd-Allah, F.; Abdelalim, A.; Abolhassani, H.; Abreu, L.G.; Abrigo, M.R. Global age-sex-specific fertility, mortality, healthy life expectancy (HALE), and population estimates in 204 countries and territories, 1950–2019: A comprehensive demographic analysis for the Global Burden of Disease Study 2019. *Lancet* **2020**, *396*, 1160–1203. [CrossRef]
21. Sharma, R.; Abbasi-Kangevari, M.; Abd-Rabu, R.; Abidi, H.; Abu-Gharbieh, E.; Acuna, J.M.; Adhikari, S.; Advani, S.M.; Afzal, M.S.; Meybodi, M.A. Global, regional, and national burden of colorectal cancer and its risk factors, 1990–2019: A systematic analysis for the Global Burden of Disease Study 2019. *Lancet Gastroenterol. Hepatol.* **2022**, *7*, 627–647. [CrossRef] [PubMed]
22. Gu, W.J.; Pei, J.P.; Lyu, J.; Akimoto, N.; Haruki, K.; Ogino, S.; Zhang, C.D. The Burden of Early-Onset Colorectal Cancer and Its Risk Factors from 1990 to 2019: A Systematic Analysis for the Global Burden of Disease Study 2019. *Cancers* **2022**, *14*, 3502. [CrossRef]
23. Yildirim-Kahriman, S. Non-intrinsic cancer risk factors. *Exp. Oncol.* **2021**, *43*, 290–297. [CrossRef] [PubMed]
24. Haupt, S.; Caramia, F.; Klein, S.L.; Rubin, J.B.; Haupt, Y. Sex disparities matter in cancer development and therapy. *Nat. Rev. Cancer* **2021**, *21*, 393–407. [CrossRef] [PubMed]
25. Afshar, N.; English, D.R.; Thursfield, V.; Mitchell, P.L.; Te Marvelde, L.; Farrugia, H.; Giles, G.G.; Milne, R.L. Differences in cancer survival by sex: A population-based study using cancer registry data. *Cancer Causes Control* **2018**, *29*, 1059–1069. [CrossRef] [PubMed]
26. Dong, M.; Cioffi, G.; Wang, J.; Waite, K.A.; Ostrom, Q.T.; Kruchko, C.; Lathia, J.D.; Rubin, J.B.; Berens, M.E.; Connor, J.; et al. Sex Differences in Cancer Incidence and Survival: A Pan-Cancer Analysis. *Cancer Epidemiol. Biomark. Prev.* **2020**, *29*, 1389–1397. [CrossRef] [PubMed]
27. Kim, H.I.; Lim, H.; Moon, A. Sex Differences in Cancer: Epidemiology, Genetics and Therapy. *Biomol. Ther.* **2018**, *26*, 335–342. [CrossRef] [PubMed]
28. Rawla, P.; Sunkara, T.; Thandra, K.C.; Barsouk, A. Epidemiology of gallbladder cancer. *Clin. Exp. Hepatol.* **2019**, *5*, 93–102. [CrossRef]
29. Henley, S.J.; Thomas, C.C.; Sharapova, S.R.; Momin, B.; Massetti, G.M.; Winn, D.M.; Armour, B.S.; Richardson, L.C. Vital Signs: Disparities in Tobacco-Related Cancer Incidence and Mortality—United States, 2004–2013. *MMWR Morb. Mortal. Wkly. Rep.* **2016**, *65*, 1212–1218. [CrossRef]
30. Kitahara, C.M.; Schneider, A.B. Epidemiology of Thyroid Cancer. *Cancer Epidemiol. Biomark. Prev.* **2022**, *31*, 1284–1297. [CrossRef]
31. Hashim, D.; Carioli, G.; Malvezzi, M.; Bertuccio, P.; Waxman, S.; Negri, E.; La Vecchia, C.; Boffetta, P. Cancer mortality in the oldest old: A global overview. *Aging* **2020**, *12*, 16744–16758. [CrossRef] [PubMed]
32. Foster, J.A.; Salinas, G.D.; Mansell, D.; Williamson, J.C.; Casebeer, L.L. How does older age influence oncologists' cancer management? *Oncologist* **2010**, *15*, 584–592. [CrossRef] [PubMed]
33. Bhakta, N.; Force, L.M.; Allemani, C.; Atun, R.; Bray, F.; Coleman, M.P.; Steliarova-Foucher, E.; Frazier, A.L.; Robison, L.L.; Rodriguez-Galindo, C.; et al. Childhood cancer burden: A review of global estimates. *Lancet Oncol.* **2019**, *20*, e42–e53. [CrossRef] [PubMed]
34. Miller, K.D.; Fidler-Benaoudia, M.; Keegan, T.H.; Hipp, H.S.; Jemal, A.; Siegel, R.L. Cancer statistics for adolescents and young adults, 2020. *CA Cancer J. Clin.* **2020**, *70*, 443–459. [CrossRef] [PubMed]
35. Ruiz-Arguelles, G.J. Advances in the diagnosis and treatment of acute and chronic leukemia in Mexico. *Salud Pública México* **2016**, *58*, 291–295. [CrossRef]
36. Zhang, Y.; Luo, G.; Etxeberria, J.; Hao, Y. Global Patterns and Trends in Lung Cancer Incidence: A Population-Based Study. *J. Thorac. Oncol.* **2021**, *16*, 933–944. [CrossRef]
37. Arnold, M.; Sierra, M.S.; Laversanne, M.; Soerjomataram, I.; Jemal, A.; Bray, F. Global patterns and trends in colorectal cancer incidence and mortality. *Gut* **2017**, *66*, 683–691. [CrossRef]
38. Mandic, M.; Li, H.; Safizadeh, F.; Niedermaier, T.; Hoffmeister, M.; Brenner, H. Is the association of overweight and obesity with colorectal cancer underestimated? An umbrella review of systematic reviews and meta-analyses. *Eur. J. Epidemiol.* **2023**, *38*, 135–144. [CrossRef]
39. Medina, C.; Jauregui, A.; Hernandez, C.; Shamah, T.; Barquera, S. Physical inactivity and sitting time prevalence and trends in Mexican adults. Results from three national surveys. *PLoS ONE* **2021**, *16*, e0253137. [CrossRef]

40. Pineros, M.; Laversanne, M.; Barrios, E.; Cancela, M.C.; de Vries, E.; Pardo, C.; Bray, F. An updated profile of the cancer burden, patterns and trends in Latin America and the Caribbean. *Lancet Reg. Health Am.* **2022**, *13*, 100294. [CrossRef]
41. Znaor, A.; Skakkebaek, N.E.; Rajpert-De Meyts, E.; Kulis, T.; Laversanne, M.; Gurney, J.; Sarfati, D.; McGlynn, K.A.; Bray, F. Global patterns in testicular cancer incidence and mortality in 2020. *Int. J. Cancer* **2022**, *151*, 692–698. [CrossRef] [PubMed]
42. Avgerinos, K.I.; Spyrou, N.; Mantzoros, C.S.; Dalamaga, M. Obesity and cancer risk: Emerging biological mechanisms and perspectives. *Metabolism* **2019**, *92*, 121–135. [CrossRef] [PubMed]
43. Sharma, R. Breast cancer incidence, mortality and mortality-to-incidence ratio (MIR) are associated with human development, 1990–2016: Evidence from Global Burden of Disease Study 2016. *Breast Cancer* **2019**, *26*, 428–445. [CrossRef] [PubMed]
44. Barquera, S.; Hernández-Barrera, L.; Trejo-Valdivia, B.; Shamah, T.; Campos-Nonato, I.; Rivera-Dommarco, J. Obesity in Mexico, prevalence and trends in adults. Ensanut 2018–2019. *Salud Pública México* **2020**, *62*, 682–692. [CrossRef]
45. Restrepo, F.D.l.H.; Guzman, N.A.; Gomez, A.D.l.H.; Ruiz, C. Policies and processes for human papillomavirus vaccination in Latin America and the Caribbean. *Rev. Panam. Salud Pública* **2018**, *41*, e124. [CrossRef]
46. Brau-Figueroa, H.; Palafox-Parrilla, A.; Parrilla-Taylor, P.; Mohar, A. Infraestructura oncológica en el Sistema de Salud Mexicano. *Salud Pública México* **2022**, *64*, 105–106. [CrossRef]

cancers

MDPI

*Review*

# Novel Insights in Venous Thromboembolism Risk Assessment Methods in Ambulatory Cancer Patients: From the Guidelines to Clinical Practice

Anca Drăgan [1,*] and Adrian Ştefan Drăgan [2]

1 Department of Cardiovascular Anaesthesiology and Intensive Care, Emergency Institute for Cardiovascular Diseases "Prof. Dr. C C Iliescu", 258 Fundeni Road, 022328 Bucharest, Romania
2 Faculty of General Medicine, Carol Davila University of Medicine and Pharmacy, 8 Eroii Sanitari Blvd, 050474 Bucharest, Romania; dragan.adrian.stefan24@gmail.com
* Correspondence: anca.dragan1978.14@gmail.com; Tel.: +40-760587855

**Simple Summary:** Cancer patients are at greater risk of developing venous thromboembolism compared to the general population, which can lead to a decreased quality of life, a worsened prognosis, and increased treatment costs. Guidelines provide clear strategies for preventing thrombosis in hospitalized cancer patients and those undergoing surgery. For ambulatory cancer patients, thromboprophylaxis is recommended only for those who are at high risk. However, this can be challenging in clinical practice. The current guidelines do not provide sufficient information on this problem. Imaging and biomarker screening techniques are underutilized in practice. Although new risk scores, nomograms, and strategies have been developed using biomarkers and clinical and genetic features, many of these methods have not yet been validated. Machine learning algorithms have already been studied with promising results. This review presents the current knowledge on venous thromboembolism risk assessment in ambulatory cancer patient settings.

**Abstract:** Many cancer patients will experience venous thromboembolism (VTE) at some stage, with the highest rate in the initial period following diagnosis. Novel cancer therapies may further enhance the risk. VTE in a cancer setting is associated with poor prognostic, a decreased quality of life, and high healthcare costs. If thromboprophylaxis in hospitalized cancer patients and perioperative settings is widely accepted in clinical practice and supported by the guidelines, it is not the same situation in ambulatory cancer patient settings. The guidelines do not recommend primary thromboprophylaxis, except in high-risk cases. However, nowadays, risk stratification is still challenging, although many tools have been developed. The Khrorana score remains the most used method, but it has many limits. This narrative review aims to present the current relevant knowledge of VTE risk assessment in ambulatory cancer patients, starting from the guideline recommendations and continuing with the specific risk assessment methods and machine learning models approaches. Biomarkers, genetic, and clinical features were tested alone or in groups. Old and new models used in VTE risk assessment are exposed, underlining their clinical utility. Imaging and biomolecular approaches to VTE screening of outpatients with cancer are also presented, which could help clinical decisions.

**Keywords:** venous thromboembolism risk; ambulatory cancer; risk assessment

## 1. Introduction

Cancer patients often present with a prothrombotic state due to the abnormalities in each component of Virchow's triad, thus contributing to thrombosis. Researchers estimated that VTE would occur in 4–20% of cancer patients at some stage, with the highest risk immediately following cancer diagnosis [1]. In the last period, the VTE incidence in oncologic patients has increased in the context of the higher performance of imaging techniques and the development of new cancer treatments that improved survival [2].

After cancer diagnosis, the 12-month cumulative VTE incidence was 3%, a percentage nine times higher when compared to the general population [2].

However, despite improved cancer treatment, VTE in cancer patients is strongly associated with a poor prognosis. The cumulative mortality in VTE cancer patients was 27.7% after one month, 48.7% after three months, 68.2% at one year, and 84.1% after five years, which is much higher than the cumulative mortality in cancer patients without VTE (7.5%, 17%, 38.5%, and 84.1%, respectively) [3]. Pulmonary embolism (PE) was associated with a poorer prognosis than venous thrombosis [3]. The one-year mortality of the PE cancer patients was 73% in Sørensen et al.'s study, as compared to 39.3% in the non-cancer cohort [3].

Khorana et al. reported that 17.1% of the patients recently diagnosed with cancer and with VTE events would develop recurrent episodes of VTE during a nine-month follow-up period [4]. The total costs related to the healthcare of the patients with VTE recurrence were very high, suggesting the necessity of reducing VTE risk in cancer patients [4].

Thromboprophylaxis in hospitalized cancer patients and perioperative settings is widely accepted in clinical practice and supported by the guidelines. However, most cancer patients would develop VTE in the outpatient setting. Primary thromboprophylaxis is not routinely recommended, except for high-risk cancer patients. Selecting an ambulatory cancer patient who would benefit from thromboprophylaxis is still challenging because of the specific bleeding risk. The Khrorana score is mainly the recommended tool in this setting, but many limits of this old score have been reported. Novel approaches have been proposed. Clinical features, routine hematologic and coagulation lab testing, new biomarkers, and genetic data, separately or grouped, were introduced in the novel risk scores, nomograms, or machine learning algorithms to accurately assess the VTE risk in ambulatory cancer patients in general and specific tumors. This narrative review aims to present the current relevant knowledge in this setting starting from the guideline recommendations and continuing with the specific risk assessment methods to help clinicians in their decision regarding primary thromboprophylaxis in ambulatory cancer patients (Figure 1). The future directions provided by the recent research papers are also presented.

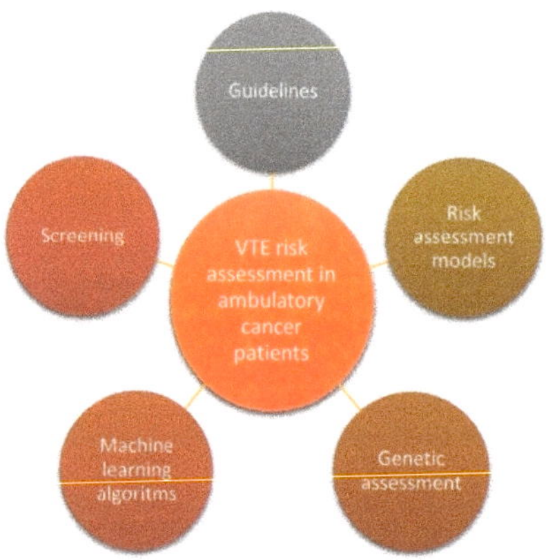


**Figure 1.** The current relevant knowledge in VTE risk assessment in ambulatory cancer patients. Abbreviations: VTE—venous thromboembolism.

## 2. Guideline Recommendations

The European Society for Medical Oncology (ESMO) 2010 practical guidelines proposed the Khrorana model to identify ambulatory cancer patients who are clinically at high risk for VTE [5]. The new 2023 ESMO guideline suggested the use of the same Khrorana model, but also the Vienna-CATS and COMPASS-CAT methods [6].

The same guideline strongly recommended ultrasound diagnosis and computer tomography (CT) pulmonary angiogram if deep venous thrombosis (DVT) or pulmonary embolism (PE), respectively, were suspected in cancer patients [6]. The D-dimer levels and the clinical prediction rules have not been recommended in this setting [6].

The new 2023 American Society of Clinical Oncology (ASCO) guideline considers only the Khrorana score in stratifying the risk in this setting [7]. The American Society of Hematology (ASH) 2021 guidelines provided strong and conditional recommendations for not using thromboprophylaxis on low and intermediate-risk ambulatory oncologic patients receiving cancer chemotherapy, respectively [8]. A validated risk assessment tool (i.e., Khorana score) together with clinical judgment and experience were recommended for patient classification [8]. The hereditary thrombophilia tests were suggested by the 2023 update in ambulatory cancer patients receiving systemic therapy with VTE family history determined to be at low or intermediate risk for VTE [9].

The European Society of Cardiology (ESC) 2022 cardio-oncology guideline recommended the baseline clinical and biomarkers assessment of the patient diagnosed with cancer [10]. Multidisciplinary monitoring during the specific treatments was also proposed [10,11]. The ESC 2022 cardio-oncology guideline emphasized the high incidence of VTE among cancer patients and recommended imaging screening in patients with clinically suspected VTE [10]. Lower-extremity venous ultrasonography is the method that has to be used in DVT diagnosis, as well as contrast-enhanced CT [10]. After detailing the patient-, cancer-, and treatment-related risk factors, the guideline proposed the TBIP method in the anticoagulation decision. It represents an acronym for thromboembolic risk, bleeding risk, drug–drug interactions, and patient preferences [10].

The ESC guideline recommended that the VTE risk assessment in ambulatory patients be individually determined and only found the Khorana and COMPASS-CAT scores useful in this setting [10]. Khrorana risk assessment was also recommended by the American College of Cardiology in ambulatory oncologic patients [12].

Table 1 summarizes the relevant guideline recommendations on VTE risk assessment in ambulatory oncologic patients.

**Table 1.** The relevant guideline recommendations on VTE risk assessment in ambulatory oncologic patients.

| Guideline | Reference | Main Findings | Recommendation |
|---|---|---|---|
| ESMO 2023 | [6] | • Ultrasound diagnosis in suspected DVT and diagnosis by CTPA in suspected PE, without using clinical prediction rules and D-dimer level | Class I, Level of evidence A |
| | | • Apixaban, rivaroxaban or LMWH may be considered for primary thromboprophylaxis for a maximum of 6 months in high-thrombosis-risk ambulatory cancer patients starting systemic anticancer treatment. | Class I, Level of evidence B |
| | | • Primary thromboprophylaxis is suggested when a VTE risk is estimated to be >8–10% at 6 months. | Class II, Level of evidence C |
| | | • Cancer patients should be offered a CAT risk assessment and have an opportunity to discuss their particular risks. | Class III, Level of evidence B |
| | | • Khrorana score (cut-off 2), COMPASS-CAT, and Vienna-CATS should be used for risk stratification | Class III, Level of evidence C |
| | | • LMWH given at a higher dose for a maximum of 3 months may be considered for ambulatory pancreatic cancer patients on first-line systemic anticancer treatment,. | Class II, Level of evidence C |

**Table 1.** *Cont.*

| Guideline | Reference | Main Findings | Recommendation |
|---|---|---|---|
| ASCO 2023 | [7] | • Routine pharmacologic thromboprophylaxis should not be offered to all outpatients with cancer | Evidence-based<br>Intermediate-High quality<br>Strong recommendation |
| | | • High-risk outpatients with cancer (Khorana score ≥ 2 before starting a new systemic chemotherapy regimen) may be offered thromboprophylaxis with apixaban, rivaroxaban, or LMWH provided there are no significant risk factors for bleeding and no drug interactions. Such therapy should be accompanied by a discussion with the patient about the relative benefits and harms, drug cost, and duration of prophylaxis in this setting | Evidence-based<br>Evidence quality:<br>Intermediate to High for apixaban and rivaroxaban,<br>Intermediate for LMWH<br>Moderate recommendation |
| | | • Patients with multiple myeloma receiving thalidomide- or lenalidomide-based regimens with chemotherapy and/or dexamethasone should be offered pharmacologic thromboprophylaxis with either aspirin or LMWH for lower-risk patients and LMWH for higher-risk patients | Evidence-based<br>Intermediate evidence quality<br>Strong recommendation |
| ESC 2022 | [10] | • The venous ultrasonography or contrast-enhanced CT were recommended as screening when clinical signs of DVT were present | |
| | | • The CT pulmonary angiography was recommended as screening when clinical signs of PE are present | |
| | | • TBIP assessment | Class I |
| | | • VTE risk should be individually determined (Khorana score or COMPASS-CAT) | - |
| | | • For ambulatory patients with cancer at high risk of thrombosis receiving systemic therapy, primary thromboprophylaxis with a NOAC (apixaban or rivaroxaban) or LMWH may be considered, provided there are no significant contraindications. | Class IIb, Level of evidence B |
| | | • The patients at high risk of thrombosis receiving systemic therapy are those with locally advanced/metastatic pancreas or lung cancer or Khorana score ≥ 2 | |
| | | • A discussion with the patient about the relative benefits and harms, cancer prognosis, drug cost, and duration of treatment is recommended prior to prophylactic anticoagulation for the primary prevention of VTE | Class I, Level of evidence C |
| ASH 2021 | [8] | • For low-risk thrombosis patients receiving systemic therapy, no thromboprophylaxis is recommended over parenteral thromboprophylaxis | Strong recommendation, moderate certainty in the evidence of effects |
| | | • For intermediate-risk thrombosis patients receiving systemic therapy, no prophylaxis is suggested over parenteral prophylaxis | Conditional recommendation, moderate certainty in the evidence of effects |
| | | • For high-risk thrombosis patients receiving systemic therapy thromboprophylaxis (LMWH or DOAC) are suggested over no thromboprophylaxis<br>• Classification of patients as being low-, intermediate-, or high-risk for VTE should be based on a validated risk assessment tool (i.e., Khorana score) complemented by clinical judgment and experience. | Conditional recommendation, moderate certainty in the evidence of effects |

Abbreviations: ASCO, American Society of Clinical Oncology; ASH American Society of Hematology; COMPASS-CAT, Comparison of Methods for Thromboembolic Risk Assessment with Clinical Perceptions and Awareness in real-life patients-Cancer-Associated Thrombosis; CAT, cancer-associated thrombosis; CT, Computed tomography; CTPA, CT pulmonary angiogram; ESC, European Society of Cardiology; DOAC, direct oral anticoagulants; DVT, deep venous thrombosis; ESMO, European Society for Medical Oncology; LMWH, low molecular weight heparin; PE, pulmonary embolism; TBIP, thromboembolic risk, bleeding risk, drug–drug interactions, patient preferences; Vienna-CATS, Vienna Cancer and Thrombosis Study; VTE, venous thromboembolism.

## 3. VTE Screening in Ambulatory High-Risk Oncologic Patients

Cancer and thrombosis are strongly related. VTE can be the first clinical sign of undiagnosed cancer, especially when the event is unprovoked [13], while cancer represents a risk factor in VTE occurrence. In this last setting, guidelines issued recommendations for hospitalized and surgical cancer patients and high-risk outpatients. Gainsbury et al. found a 10.1% prevalence of preoperative deep venous thrombosis (DVT) in asymptomatic patients undergoing major oncologic surgery and suggested the preoperative screening with lower extremity venous duplex ultrasound (US) in this setting [14]. Increasing age, recent diagnosis of sepsis, and a history of prior VTE were significantly associated with preoperative DVT [14].

Detecting VTE high-risk outpatients with cancer is still challenging. VTE screening may be an answer in this setting. In total, 6.6% of venous thrombosis was found by Heidrich et al. in all tumor patients [15]. The same authors reported a much higher incidence of 33% when using an imaging prospective approach [15]. Loftus et al. researched the role of venous US screening in incidentally detecting VTE in high-risk patients with cancer in a multicenter trial. The studied 117 patients were asymptomatic, had a Khorana score $\geq 3$, and were starting new systemic chemotherapy [16]. The lower-limb venous US and a contrast-enhanced CT baseline screening discovered 9% incidental VTE (6% DVT, 1% pulmonary embolism, 1% DVT and pulmonary embolism) [16]. The patients were screened further every four weeks for a 12-week period with venous US and at 12 weeks with contrast-enhanced CT [16]. Researchers proposed the lower-limb venous US screening in addition to the oncologic surveillance CT in high-risk ambulatory cancer patients setting with a Khorana score $\geq 3$ [16].

This approach could help in early VTE detection in latent stages, preventing VTE progression and thus decreasing morbidity and costs [16]. Kourlaba et al. also reported US screening of high-risk cancer patients as a cost-effective strategy compared to clinical surveillance, even when all patients with a positive first US underwent a second US [17]. Kunapareddy et al. proposed an electronic alert to identify high-risk patients and suggest US screening for early detection [18]. Holmes et al. reported the success of a multidisciplinary program related to Venous Thromboembolism Prevention in the Ambulatory Cancer Clinic (VTEPACC) [19]. The high-risk patients identified by Khorana and Protecht scores ($\geq$3 points) were offered a hematology consultation to consider VTE prophylaxis, further referring the results of the consultation to the oncologist [19].

VTE risk was predicted by baseline D-dimer levels [20,21]. Niimi et al. recently reported the optimal D-dimer cut-off value of 4.0 μg/mL for predicting DVT in patients with malignancy [22]. Its association with risk assessment scores performed better in VTE prediction [21,22]. D-dimer was reported in another study as part of the thromboembolism risk assessment when added to fibrinogen level [23]. Oi et al. found that high D-dimer levels at VTE diagnosis were associated with an increased risk for short-term and long-term mortality and with long-term recurrent VTE, especially in patients with active cancer [24]. During a median follow-up of 30 months, D-dimer positively correlated with the reoccurrence of VTE ($p$ = 0.0299) and mortality in cancer patients with VTE ($p$ < 0.0001) and without VTE ($p$ = 0.0008) [25]. D-dimer level positively correlated in Koch et al.'s study with VTE reoccurrence and mortality during a 30-month period [25]. The relationship with mortality was reported both in cancer patients who presented VTE and in cancer patients without VTE [25].

Another VTE risk factor is the soluble P-selectin (sP-selectin). A cut-off level of 53.1 ng/mL could predict VTE in cancer patients with no difference between tumor sites [26]. Zhang et al. recommended sP-selectin level for early identification of cancer-associated VTE and monitoring [27].

Khorana et al. recently studied the biomarkers distribution in patients with and without VTE diagnosed with cancer [28]. In the two groups, there were reported baseline lower levels of stromal cell-derived factor-1, thyroid-stimulating hormone, and monocyte chemotactic protein 4 and higher levels of growth hormone and interleukin-1 receptor type

1 [28]. ST2, IL-8, and C-reactive protein were significantly different between survivors and those who died [28].

Table 2 presents the relevant studies presenting modalities and importance of VTE screening among ambulatory cancer patients.

**Table 2.** The relevant studies presenting modalities and importance of VTE screening among ambulatory cancer patients.

| Screening Modality | Authors (Year) [Ref] | No. Patients | VTE Detected (%) | Type of Tumors | Main Findings |
|---|---|---|---|---|---|
| Lower limb venous duplex US | Gainsbury et al. (2018) [14] | 346 | 10.1 | Solid cancer | High-risk cancer patients may benefit from screening lower extremity venous duplex US before surgery. |
| Lower limb duplex US and/or venography | Heidrich et al. (2009) [15] | 97 | 33 | Various types | Regular screening for thrombosis is indicated even in asymptomatic tumor patients |
| Lower limb duplex US and contrast-enhanced chest CT | Loftus et al. (2022) [16] | 117 | 58 | Solid cancers | Suggested to add US screening to routine oncologic surveillance CT in high-risk ambulatory cancer patients (Khorana score $\geq$ 3) |
| Lower limb venous US | Kourlaba et al. (2017) [17] | 907 | - | various | Screening high-risk cancer patients via US to detect asymptomatic DVT is a cost-effective strategy over clinical surveillance |
| Automated alert Lower limb venous US | Kunapareddy et al. (2019) [18] | 194 | 12.5 | various | An automated alert may help in early detection of DVT in high-risk cancer patients |
| VTEPACC model | Holmes et al. (2020) [19] | 918 | 23.2 | various | VTEPACC involves a multidisciplinary approach |
| D-dimer F 1 + 2 | Ay et al. (2009) [20] | 821 | 7.6 | various | The cumulative probability of developing VTE after 6 months was highest in patients with both elevated D-dimer and elevated F 1 + 2 |
| Baseline D-dimer | Schorling et al. (2020) [21] | 100 | 11.2 | Solid cancers | VTE risk was well predicted by baseline D-dimer levels. |
| D-dimer | Niim et al. (2023 [22] | 208 | 28.4 | various | The optimal D-dimer cut-off value for the DVT diagnosis in cancer patients was 4.0 µg/mL. |
| D-dimer | Oi et al. (2020) [24] | 2852 | | various | Elevated levels at diagnosis were associated with an increased risk for short-term and long-term mortality. |
| D-dimer | Koch et al. (2023) [25] | 526 | 39.73 | various | Levels above the 10-fold upper reference limit contain diagnostic and prognostic information |
| sP-selectin | Ay et al. (2008) [26] | 687 | 6.4 | various | Higher levels independently predict VTE in cancer patients |
| sP-selectin | Zhang (2023) [27] | 1882 | 24.17 | various | Metaanalysis. Role in early identification and monitoring A higher level in Asian cancer patients |
| Various biomarkers | Khorana (2022) [28] | 124 | 50 | various | SDF-1 and TSH were the strongest predictors of VTE |

Abbreviations: CT, computed tomography; DVT, deep venous thrombosis; F 1 + 2, prothrombin fragment 1 + 2; SDF-1, stromal cell-derived factor1; VTE, venous thromboembolism; VTEPACC, Venous Thromboembolism Prevention in the Ambulatory Cancer Clinic; TSH, thyroid-stimulating hormone; US, ultrasonography.

microRNAs (miRNAs) represent a promising class of biomarkers in VTE prediction in cancer, but until now, only a few small-sample-size studies, lacking external validation, have investigated their role in this setting [29]. The long non-coding RNAs (lncRNAs) may have a role as well in VTE pathogenesis [30]. Ten lncRNAs were implicated in VTE pathogenesis, but future research is needed in this setting [30].

Genetic assessment may help VTE risk stratify and prognostic in the cancer population. Thrombogenesis-related genetic polymorphisms are already studied in this setting and are integrated in specific risk scores alone, or together with clinical features. However, more prospective studies are required before clinical application.

## 4. VTE Risk Assessment Using Scores

Because the CAT risk factors are multifactorial, risk scores have been developed to find oncologic outpatients who need anticoagulation treatment. The Khorana score was the first proposed [31]. The type of cancer, some components of the complete blood count, and body mass index were assessed. A value $\geq 2$ was retained by the guidelines as describing high-risk patients [6,7,32], although a value of more than 3 was initially proposed [31]. Khorana et al. validated the method in a cohort with 34.6% breast cancer patients and 18.9% lung cancer patients [31]. The rest of Khorana et al.'s cohort had colon, ovarian, gastric, and pancreatic cancers, lymphomas, and other tumor types [31]. Mulder et al.'s meta-analysis reported the Khorana score as a tool for selecting high-risk VTE in oncologic patients [33], and Akasaka-Kihara et al. validated it in the Japanese cancer population [34]. Ramos-Esquivel et al. recently found the Khorana score to perform an accurate categorization of VTE risk in ambulatory Hispanic patients who were newly diagnosed with solid tumors and were receiving systemic chemotherapy [35]. El-Sayed et al. reported a calculated VTE occurrence probability of 87.5% when using the Khorana score at cut-off levels $\geq 3$ in patients with hematological malignancy [36]. However, many researchers found the universal use of the Khorana score in primary thromboprophylaxis risk assessment inappropriate. Ha et al. (2023) only partially validated the Khorana score in the Korean population [37]. Khorana could stratify the 6-month VTE risk only in selected cancer populations [33,38–40]. Verzeroli et al. (2023) recently found that the Khorana score was not able to discriminate between low and high VTE risk in newly diagnosticated metastatic cancer (non-small cell lung, gastric, colorectal, and breast cancers) for whom systemic chemotherapy was indicated [41]. This score was unable to stratify VTE risk in lung cancer [39,42,43], endometrial [40], MM [44], myeloid leukemia [45], hepatocellular carcinoma [46], uterine [47], or lymphoid malignancies [48]. Although this risk score was suboptimal in VTE risk prediction, other studies found it more useful in mortality prediction [41,43] or when a value $\geq 2$ was tested [49,50] in the VTE setting.

Ay et al. [51] proposed a new VTE risk assessment method in patients by adding two biomarkers, D-dimer and sP-selectin, to the Khorana score. Higher D-dimer (cut-off 1.44 μg/mL) and sP-selectin (cut-off 53.1 ng/mL) levels were reported previously by the authors to be associated with VTE [20,26] in a Vienna Cancer and Thrombosis Study (Vienna CATS). In a multinational, prospective cohort study, the Vienna CATS method discriminated better than the Khorana score between low- and high-risk VTE patients [52]. The eligible patients were those with advanced cancer who underwent chemotherapy or had started chemotherapy in the previous three months [52]. In hematological malignancy, the calculated probability of VTE occurrence was the same when using Vienna CATS or Khorana score at cut-off values of $\geq 3$ [36]. A value more than or equal to 3 of the Vienna CATS risk score was significantly associated with VTE complications in Japanese patients with advanced cancer who were receiving chemotherapy [53].

Verso et al. proposed another risk score, the PROTECHT score, that added gemcitabine and platinum-based chemotherapy to Khorana score variables [54]. Moik did not sustain the use of these variables in prediction models [55]. The gemcitabine therapy has not been associated with an increased VTE risk, while platinum-based treatment had only limited predictive value beyond tumor site category and D-dimer levels [55]. However, in van Es et al.'s study, the PROTECHT score performed better discrimination than the Khorana score in the VTE risk assessment [52]. Ramos-Esquivel et al. also found PROTECHT (cut-off 3) among the scores that could categorize the VTE risk in newly diagnosed solid tumors in the Hispanic population [56]. Other studies reported this score as suboptimal in VTE risk assessment [49,50], proposing a 2-value threshold to improve the results [49].

Another risk score proposed in this setting was CONKO [57]. From the Khorana score variables, BMI was replaced by WHO performance status [57]. In Qin et al.'s (2023) study,

Khorana, Vienna CATS, PROTECHT, and CONKO risk scores moderately assessed the VTE risk in hospitalized metastatic colorectal cancer inpatients [58], but the prediction was enhanced when KRAS and BRAF mutations were added to the scores [58]. In ambulatory oncologic patients, the VTE risk stratification by CONKO was suboptimal [49,52], although in the Hispanic population the results were more encouraging [56]. HYPERSCAN study reported that CONKO scores significantly stratified patients for VTE risk, while the KRS and the PROTECHT failed in ambulatory lung cancer patients [59]. In this setting, future research is awaited. Yan et al.'s systematic review regarding VTE risk assessment models for use in ambulatory patients with lung cancer is expected to be published soon [60].

Papinger et al. proposed a modified Vienna CATS, the CATS/MICA score, that integrated the tumor site category and D-dimer level to predict the VTE risk in ambulatory patients with solid cancers [61]. The new Vienna CATS and the CONKO scores significantly stratified patients for VTE risk in lung cancer [59]. Verzeroli et al. reported that a modified Vienna CATS score > 60 points was an independent risk factor for mortality in outpatients with metastatic cancer during chemotherapy [41].

Gerotziafas et al. proposed the COMPASS-CAT model, another VTE risk assessment method in a breast, colorectal, lung, or ovarian cancer cohort [62]. COMPASS-CAT takes into account several aspects referring to the time the cancer was diagnosed, the stage of the disease, previous VTE occurrences, platelet count, the presence of central venous catheter and the cardiovascular risk factors, the specific anti-hormonal treatment or with anthracycline, and recent hospitalization in acute medical setting [62]. The model presented in Gerotziafas et al.'s study had a good sensitivity of 88% but a lower specificity of 52% [62]. There was a strong association between catheter-related thrombosis and high Khorana, PROTECHT, and COMPASS-CAT scores [63]. COMPASS-CAT better identified more patients in high-risk group in non-small cell lung cancer [42]. Rupa-Matysek et al. reported that the COMPASS-CAT model was the most accurate predictor of VTE in lung cancer patients, compared to Khorana, PROTECHT, and CONKO scores [64]. In a large retrospective external validation study, the COMPASS-CAT model had good negative predictive value, with moderate discrimination and poor calibration power [65]. Pestana et al. (2023) reported a high VTE risk when evaluated by the COMPASS-CAT model (score $\geq 7$) in breast cancer patients [66] and proposed the combination of this model with IL-10 levels to improve the method [66].

Cella et al. proposed a new assessment tool, the ONKOTEV score, an easy-to-use and cost-effective model based on clinical information, avoiding highly selective biochemical parameters. The ONKOTEV score offers one point for a Khorana score > 2, previous venous thromboembolism, metastatic disease, and vascular/lymphatic macroscopic compression [67]. In their prospective study, the area under the curve of ONKOTEV over the Khorana score was reported at 3 months (71.9% vs. 57.9%, $p = 0.001$), 6 months (75.4% vs. 58.6%, $p < 0.001$), and 12 months (69.8% vs. 58.3%, $p = 0.014$) [67]. Cella et al. (2023) validated this model in the ONKOTEV-2, a multicenter prognostic study on ambulatory patients with solid tumors undergoing active treatments [68]. The most represented tumors were breast (18.1%), gastroesophageal adenocarcinoma (16.5%), colon (12.7%), lung (11.1%), rectum (10.8%), and pancreatic cancers (7.5%) [68]. Di Nisio et al. reported that the performance of the Khorana, PROTECHT, CONKO, and ONKOTEV scores improved at the threshold of 2 points, compared to 3 points [49]. The scores' accuracy decreased over time, suggesting the need for periodic re-evaluation [49]. An ONKOTEV score $\geq 2$ was associated with a higher VTE occurrence in patients with pancreatic cancer, including ambulatory ones [69]. ONKOTEV score performed better than PROTECHT, COMPASS-CAT, CONKO, Khorana, and the CATS/MICA score in VTE risk assessment in hospitalized medical patients with primary lung cancer [70]. An ONKOTEV score $\geq 2$ was also a predictor of survival and thromboembolic events in cholangiocarcinoma [71].

Table 3 summarizes the relevant studies related to the scores used in VTE risk assessment in ambulatory cancer patients.

**Table 3.** The relevant studies related to the main risk scores used for selecting high-risk outpatients with cancer who would benefit from primary thromboprophylaxis.

| Score | Authors (Year) [Reference] | Study Population | | | | | | | Observation |
|---|---|---|---|---|---|---|---|---|---|
| | | No. | Type of Cancer | Age | Male (%) | Ethnicity/ Race | Metastasis (%) | VTE (%) | |
| Khorana | Khorana et al. (2008) [31] | 2801 | breast, lung, ovarian sarcoma colon lymphomas | | 32.7 | US | 36.9 | 2.2 | • Validation in an independent cohort (1365 patients).<br>• Cut-off KRS = 3 |
| | Austin et al. (2019) [40] | 87 | pancreatic | 66.2 | - | UK | 86.2 | 26.8 | • Retrospective<br>• KRS was associated with VTE in endometrial cancer only |
| | | 154 | endometrial | 67.5 | | | 27.3 | 5.7 | |
| | | 205 | colorectal | 64 | | | 16.6 | 9.8 | |
| | | 193 | ovarian | 60.2 | | | 67.9 | 10.2 | |
| | | 91 | cervical | 48.9 | | | 0 | 0 | |
| | Mulder et al. (2019) [33] | 34,555 | various | - | - | various | - | 6.9% | • Meta-analysis<br>• At cut-off 2, KRS helps to select high-risk patients, but with limitations in lung and hematologic cancers |
| | Di Nisio et al. (2019) [49] | 770 | various types | - | - | Multinational | 70 | - | • KRS performance improved when using the threshold of 2 points |
| | van Es et al. (2020) [39] | 3293 | solid cancers | 61 | 59 | various | 68 | - | • Meta-analysis<br>• KRS did not stratify the VTE risk in lung cancer patients |
| | Akasaka-Kihara et al. (2021) [34] | 27,687 | various | 67 | 52.3 | Japanese | 23.5 | 5.26 | • External validation of KRS<br>• Cut-off KRS = 2<br>• Cut-off for BMI = 25 |
| | Guman et al. (2021) [50] | 2729 | advanced solid tumors | 63 | 51 | Dutch | - | 5.9 | • Retrospective multicentre study<br>• Poor overall discrimination of KRS, PROTECHT, 5-SNP |
| | Ramos-Esquivel et al. (2022) [35] | 708 | solid tumors | 59.04 | 37.4 | Hispanic | - | 4.23 | • Support KRS use in Hispanic patients |
| | Overvad et al. (2022) [38] | 40,218 | various | 65 | 44.6 | Danish | - | 2.5 | • KRS did not stratify the risk of VTE in all cancer types. |
| | Verzeroli et al. (2023) [41] | 1286 | NSCL, colorectal, gastric, breast | 65 | 55 | Caucasian | 100 | 9.7 | • KRS did not discriminate between low and high VTE<br>• At cut-off levels $\geq$ 3, independently predicted mortality |
| | El-Sayed et al. (2023) [36] | 81 | hematology | 42.6 | 49.4 | Egyptian | 2.7 | 9.8 | • At cut-off levels $\geq$ 3, the calculated VTE probability was 87.5% |
| | Ha et al. (2023) [37] | 11,714 | various | 59 | 40.5 | East Asian | - | 1.77 | • Partially validated KRS in Korean cancer patients |

**Table 3.** *Cont.*

| Score | Authors (Year) [Reference] | Study Population | | | | | | | Observation |
|---|---|---|---|---|---|---|---|---|---|
| | | No. | Type of Cancer | Age | Male (%) | Ethnicity/ Race | Metastasis (%) | VTE (%) | |
| PROTECHT | van Es et al. (2017) [52] | 876 | solid advanced cancers | 64 | 59 | Dutch Italian French Mexican | 66 | 6.1 | • Multinational prospective study<br>• Vienna CATS and PROTECHT predicted better than KRS the VTE occurrence. |
| | Di Nisio et al. (2019) [49] | 770 | various types | - | - | Multinational | 70 | - | • PROTECHT performance improved when using the threshold of 2 points |
| | Guman et al. (2021) [50] | 2729 | advanced solid tumors | 63 | 51 | Dutch | - | 5.9 | • Retrospective multicenter study<br>• Poor overall discrimination of KRS, PROTECHT, 5-SNP |
| | Ramos-Esquivel et al. (2023) [56] | 708 | solid tumours | - | - | Hispanic | - | 4.45 | • Poor overall discriminatory performance for predicting all patients at VTE risk. |
| ONKOTEV | Cella et al. (2017) [67] | 843 | various types | 59 | 33.6 | Italian, Germany | 55.2 | 8.6 | • Prospective<br>• ONKOTEV score was proposed |
| | Godinho et al. (2020) [69] | 165 | pancreatic | 73 | 54.5 | Portuguese | 55.8 | 30.9 | • Retrospective<br>• ONKOTEV score ≥ 2 stratifies VTE risk in pancreatic cancer |
| | Cella et al. (2023) [68] | 425 | various types | 61 | 43.1 | Italian, Germany, UK | 68 | 2.6 | • External validation ONKOTEV |
| COMPASS-CAT | Gerotziafas et al. (2016) [61] | 1023 | breast colorectal lung ovarian | 55 | 18.9 | Multinational | 39.6 | 8.5 | • COMPASS-CAT proposal |
| | Spyropoulos et al. (2020) [65] | 3814 | breast lung colorectal ovarian | 64 | 21 | US | 18.8 | 5.85 | • External validation of COMPASS-CAT |
| | Abdel-Razeq et al. (2023) [42] | 508 | NSCLC | 58.4 | 79.7 | Jordanian | 65.6 | 15 | • retrospective<br>• COMPASS-CAT better identified high-risk VTE patients compared to KRS |
| Vienna CATS | Ay et al. (2010) [51] | 819 | various types | 62 | 55.44% | Austrian | 37.1 | 7.4 | • Proposed to add D-dimer and sP-selectin to KRS assessment |
| | van Es et al. (2017) [52] | 876 | solid advanced cancers | 64 | 59 | Dutch Italian French Mexican | 66 | 6.1 | • Multinational, prospective study.<br>• Vienna CATS and PROTECHT predicted better than KRS the VTE occurrence. |
| | Harada et al. (2023) [53] | 190 | solid cancers | 69 | 73 | Japanese | 100 | 8.94 | • single-center, prospective study<br>• unresectable cancer patients<br>• levels ≥ 3 were significantly associated with VTE occurrence |

**Table 3.** *Cont.*

| Score | Authors (Year) [Reference] | Study Population | | | | | | | Observation |
|---|---|---|---|---|---|---|---|---|---|
| | | No. | Type of Cancer | Age | Male (%) | Ethnicity/ Race | Metastasis (%) | VTE (%) | |
| Vienna CATS | El-Sayed et al. (2023) [36] | 81 | hematology | 42.6 | 49.4 | Egyptian | 2.7 | 9.8 | • Prospective study<br>• At cut-off levels $\geq$ 3, the VTE occurrence calculated probability was 87.5% |
| CATS/ MICA | Pabinger et al. (2018) [61] | 1423 CATS<br>832 MICA | solid cancers | 62.9 CATS<br>63.7 MICA | 54.2 CATS<br>57.3 MICA | Austrian Dutch Franch Italian Mexican | 61.7 | 6.3 | • The data from the CATS cohort (1423) were used to select variables.<br>• The score was externally validated in the MICA cohort (832). |
| | Verzeroli et al. (2023) [41] | 1286 | NSCL, colorectal, gastric, breast | 65 | 55 | Caucasian | 100 | 9.7 | • The cut-off 60 assessed better than KRS the VTE risk<br>• The levels $\geq$ 60, independently predicted mortality |

The missing values were either unavailable or non-applicable. Abbreviations: CATS, Vienna Cancer and Thrombosis Study cohort; COMPASS-CAT, COMPASS-CAT, Comparison of Methods for Thromboembolic Risk Assessment with Clinical Perceptions and Awareness in real-life patients-Cancer-Associated Thrombosis; MICA, Multinational Cohort Study to Identify Cancer Patients at High Risk of Venous Thromboembolism; KRS, Khorana score; No. number; NSCL, non-small cell lung; Vienna-CATS, Vienna Cancer and Thrombosis Study; VTE, venous thromboembolism; UK, United Kingdom; US, United States.

Zhang et al. studied the systemic immune-inflammation index (SII) and the prognosis nutritional index (PNI) in VTE prediction in gastrointestinal cancer patients [72]. The SII was an auxiliary diagnostic test for patients with venous thrombosis in general, with an AUC of 0.861 (95% CI: 0.820–0.902; $p < 0.001$), a sensitivity of 78.1%, and a specificity of 73.1% for an SII > 755.54 [73]. SII (cut-off 504.80) paired with PNI (cut-off 45.57) were part of the two nomograms proposed to predict VTE risk in gastrointestinal cancer [72]. Model A (age, tumor location, therapy, PNI, SII) and Model B (age, tumor location, therapy, PNI, SII and D dimer) presented an AUC of 0.806 (95% CI: 0.782–0.830) and 0.832 (95% CI: 0.810–0.855), respectively, as compared to Khorana score's 0.592 (95% CI: 0.562–0.621) [72]. Zhang et al. also tested SII in lung cancer patients and developed a new nomogram model (the inflammatory marker, coagulation indicator, and tumor features) to perform an accurate prediction of VTE [74]. The SII cut-off was 851.51, and the new nomogram presented an AUC of 0.708, compared to the Khorana score's 0.600 [74].

Li et al.' new nomogram contains common data from the electronic health record, some demographic data (Asian/Pacific islander), the original Khorana score, but with cancer subtypes that were revised, and cancer and patient risk factors such as hormonal/target therapy, advanced cancer, previous VTE occurrence, recent hospitalization, and history of immobility [75].

Approximately 50% of cancer patients receiving modern systemic therapy were stratified into a high-risk group (a 6-month VTE risk of 8–10%) and the other half into a low-risk group (a 6-month VTE risk of 3%) [75]. This novel tool appeared generalizable in variate age, sex, and race/ethnicity subgroups but needs further validation [75].

In the ambulatory cancer population, there is no universal method for the VTE risk assessment. Thus, new specific risk scores have been developed. In newly diagnosed NSCLC outpatients who undergo chemotherapy, Thrombo-NSCLC (FVIII and sP-selectin values) predicted VTE significantly better than the Khorana score [76]. Gomez-Rosas et al. recently proposed a new risk tool, the Hypercan score, to stratify lung cancer patients for VTE and mortality risk [59]. This score contains information regarding ECOG performance and D dimer and stratifies the patients into low- and high-risk groups [59]. Using the Hypercan score, the cumulative incidence of VTE was 6% in the low- and 25% in the high-risk group [59]. Li et al. proposed and validated a new nomogram for VTE risk prediction in patients recently diagnosed with lung cancer [77]. Some clinical and therapeutic features and genetic parameters were incorporated into the new assessment system: overweight, adenocarcinoma, stage III-IV, central venous catheters, D-dimer levels $\geq$ 2.06 mg/L, prothrombin time $\geq$ 11.45 s, fibrinogen levels $\geq$ 3.33 g/L, triglyceride $\geq$ 1.37 mmol/L, ROS1 rearrangement, chemotherapy history and radiotherapy history [77]. In lymphoma patients, the ThroLy score was proposed. It was designed for both hospitalized and outpatient settings and included data referring to tumor spread (mediastinal involvement, extranodal localization), frailty (reduced mobility, BMI > 30 kg/m$^2$), the presence of previous arterial or venous thromboembolic events, anemia (hemoglobin level < 100 g/L), neutropenia [78]. ThroLy not only predicted VTE in Hodgkin lymphoma, but also survival [79]. It has been studied in diffuse large B-cell lymphoma settings as well [80]. A simplified model was proposed (high-risk with a score $\geq$ 3 and low-risk score < 3) [80]. Others did not find this score an accurate model for predicting VTE events in patients at higher risk of VTE [81]. An adapted TiC-Onco risk score to lymphoma settings was proposed by Bastos-Oreiro et al. [82] with promising results. The TiC-LYMPHO score incorporated the same genetic variables included in the TiC-ONCO score and some of the clinical variables associated with VTE in the studied population (the type of lymphoma according to the WHO classification, mediastinal involvement, Ann Arbor stage, bed rest for >3 days, and a family or personal history of VTE) [82]. López Sacerio et al. (2023) found five predictive factors—hypercholesterolemia, tumoral activity, use of thrombogenic drugs, diabetes mellitus, and immobilization—that were integrated into a predictor model of VTE in patients with hospitalized hematologic malignancies [83].

The IMPEDE VTE score (immunomodulatory agent; body mass index ≥ 25 kg/m$^2$; pelvic, hip or femur fracture; erythropoietin stimulating agent; dexamethasone/doxorubicin; Asian ethnicity/race; VTE history; tunneled line/central venous catheter; existing thromboprophylaxis) was developed and validated by Sanfilippo et al. (2019) as a VTE risk prediction score in multiple myeloma (MM) [84]. Recently, Sanfilippo et al. (2023) reported that adding D-dimer to the IMPEDE VTE score could improve VTE prediction among MM patients [85].

The PICOS score (primary tumors with high thrombogenicity, immobilization, chemotherapy, obesity, and steroid) was proposed by Wolpert et al. as a helpful tool for the identification of patients with brain metastasis at high risk for VTE [86].

Kubo et al. found that the D-dimer combined with the Glasgow prognostic score accurately predicted VTE in stage IIIC and IVA of ovarian cancer (AUC: 0.846; $p < 0.001$) [87]. D-dimer could significantly predict VTE in all gynecologic cancer patients. Optimal reported D-dimer cut-off values were 3.1, 3.2, and 3.9 μg/mL in cervical, endometrial, and ovarian cancer patients, respectively [87].

## 5. Genetic-Based Risk Assessment Scores

Polygenic risk scores do not change during the cancer course. Thus, they could be potential predictors of cancer-associated VTE independent of cancer type. Both Factor V Leiden and ABO gene mutations were reported as independent predictors of VTE occurrence in moderate to high-risk outpatients with cancer undergoing chemotherapy [88].

Lindström et al. (2019) reported the results of a large genome-wide association study (GWAS) and the first transcriptome-wide association study (TWAS) on VTE risk. GWAS meta-analysis identified 34 independent genetic signals for VTE risk with 14 newly reported associations [89]. TWAS identified five additional genetic loci not previously associated with VTE (SPSB1, ERAP1, RP11-747H7.3, RP4-737E23.2, and replicated SH2B3) [89]. The researchers demonstrated that a genetic risk score based on 37 VTE-susceptibility variants can identify a subset of the population at high risk for developing VTE [89].

De Haan et al. designed a genetic score to select VTE high-risk patients [90]. This method contained data on 31 single-nucleotide polymorphisms (SNPs) associated with an increased risk [90]. The 5-SNP score (rs8176719, rs6025, rs1799963, rs2066865, and rs2036914) was created by adding one-by-one the SNPs with the highest odds ratios of VTE and similarly discriminated high-risk patients as 31 SNPs regarding both incidental and recurrent VTE events [91]. VTE risk increased with the number of prothrombotic risk alleles, independent of the cancer diagnosis [91]. The presence of both prothrombotic risk alleles and cancer represented a highly elevated VTE risk factor [91].

Other studies did not find the 5-SNP score to be superior to the Khorana score [50]. Jakobsen et al. reported an elevated discriminative effect of the 5-SNP score on VTE risk by combining it with the mean platelet volume, but the results were not focused on the cancer population [92].

The 5, 37, 297, extended 297, and 100 SNPs prospectively identified those cancer patients at high risk for VTE development in a population-based study [93]. The tumor type has not influenced the result [93]. The 36,150 patients of the UK Biobank cohort diagnosed with hematological or solid cancer were studied from the genetic point of view regarding VTE risk. In the 12 months post-cancer diagnosis, the germline genetic markers accurately selected the patients with an increased double risk for VTE occurrence. Guman et al. demonstrated that the tumor type and polygenic scores' performance were independent variables, as the latter remained consistent during the 12-month follow-up [93]. The VTE prediction was improved when the two variables were combined [93].

The TiC-Onco risk score integrated genetic (rs2232698, rs6025, rs5985, rs4524) and clinical risk factors. Muñoz et al. used it to identify patients with colorectal, esophagogastric, lung, or pancreatic cancer in the outpatient setting who are at high risk of VTE [94]. This method has to be followed at the moment cancer is suspected [94]. Its sensitivity was significantly higher than that of the Khorana, while the specificities of both scores were similar in the studied population [94]. TiC-LYMPHO, a modified TiC-Onco score, was proposed in lymphoma settings [82]. Neto et al. (2023) reported PROCR rs10747514 and RGS7 rs2502448 as valuable prognostic biomarkers regardless of VTE and significantly associated with the VTE risk in cervical cancer [95].

Recently, nine genetic variants (rs4524, rs6025, rs2232698, rs2227631, rs268, rs169713, rs11696364, rs5110, rs6003) were independently associated with VTE in outpatients with cancer [96]. Muñoz et al. developed and validated ONCOTHROMB, by combining this genetic profile with three clinical variables independently associated with VTE in outpatients with cancer. This score, with a higher AUC compared to the Khorana model (AUC, 0.781 vs. 0.580; $p < 0.001$) was recommended to be assessed at the moment cancer is suspected [96]. ONCOTHROMB presented a significantly higher sensitivity than Khorana (81.54% vs. 22.54%; $p < 0.001$), with a lower specificity (65.22% vs. 81.76%; $p < 0.0001$) [96].

## 6. Machine Learning Algorithms Tools

Artificial intelligence brings new methods to assess risk. Machine learning (ML) can develop many statistical algorithms that can learn from the pattern of the database. The highly flexible novel tools can discriminate better in a nonlinear setting [97,98]. The manual data analysis is eliminated when using ML algorithms, while a large volume of data can be reviewed, identifying more easily patterns and trends. The automatic and dynamic self-learning process leads to continuous improvement in decision making. ML may help save time and resources at the clinician level by reducing the data analysis time, optimizing medical decisions, and offering insights into other centers' experiences and databases. Thus, the clinician may have additional time to spend with patients to understand better their needs and disease. Of course, the input data must be correct and large enough to obtain accurate results. The parameters and ML algorithms must be continuously developed and optimized. Otherwise, the probability of high errors is high. The users must define the acceptable margins of the statistical error because the ML algorithms approach represents a probabilistic process. The ethical challenges in collecting and handling data represent another ML algorithm limitation. Clinicians must understand the advantages and the disadvantages of using the ML approach as they are the interface to the patients [99]. Clinical judgment still has its role in our era. The medical doctor is the one able to discriminate between clinical changes by integrating medical and social data. Still, the clinician is the one who can interpret the results of ML algorithms in the patient's context.

Machine learning algorithms can help assess the risk of venous thromboembolism (VTE) in ambulatory cancer patients. By accurately identifying high-risk VTE patients, healthcare professionals can provide them with the appropriate treatment. In Ferroni et al.'s (2017) study, a model based on multiple kernel learning (MKL) and random optimization (RO) was used to achieve this goal in chemotherapy-treated ambulatory cancer patients [100]. ML-RO-2 was the most accurate model compared to the Khorana score (positive likelihood ratio 1.68, negative likelihood ratio 0.24) [100]. ML-RO-2 presented an area under the precision–recall curve of 0.212, while the Khorana score' area was only 0.096 [100]. The strongest association was related to the blood lipids and body mass index/performance status, while the weaker was related to the tumor site/stage and drugs [100]. The second best-performing model was ML-RO-3 [100]. A study conducted by Ferroni et al. in 2017 validated the ML-RO-2 and ML-RO-3 approaches as a low-cost method for assessing VTE risk in oncologic patients [101]. The f-measure, a metric used in ML, calculated as a harmonic mean of $P$ (positive predictive value in ML) and $R$ (sensitivity in ML), measured the effectiveness of a classifier algorithm. ML-RO-2 and ML-RO-3 presented higher f-measures (0.213 and, respectively, 0.211) than the Khorana score (f-measure: 0.100) [101]. The study involved 608 patients, with a mean age of 63 years, with 58% of them having relapsing/metastatic solid cancers [101]. The incidence of deep venous thrombosis was 5.3%, while pulmonary embolism was diagnosed in 1.8% of cases [101]. Xu et al. (2023) developed and validated a new clinical prediction model for VTE in gastric cancer patients based on support vector machine (SVM), one of the ML algorithms [97]. The model's AUC, sensitivity, and specificity were 0.825, 0.710, and 0.802, respectively [97]. The top five predictors in the model were the clinical stage, the blood transfusion history, D-dimer, age, and fibrinogen degradation products [97].

Jin et al. reported that only linear discriminant analysis (AUC 0.773) and logistic regression (AUC 0.772) outperformed the Khorana score (AUC 0.642) in cancer-related VTE prediction [102]. The combination with D-dimer improved the models' performance [103]. The top five predictors of cancer-related VTE were D-dimer level, age, Charlson Comorbidity Index, length of stay, and previous VTE history [102].

Lei et al. recommended the random forest model as the best classifier for VTE prediction in lung cancer [103]. The model presented an AUC of 0.91 (95% CI: 0.893–0.926), a sensitivity of 0.714 (95% CI: 0.614–0.762), and a specificity of 0.965 (95% CI: 0.941–0.985) [103]. The five most relevant parameters were Karnofsky Performance Status, a history of VTE, recombinant human endostatin, EGFR-TKI, and platelet count [103].

Mantha et al. (Preprint) [104] conducted the first study of a deep-learning model that predicts the risk of cancer-associated VTE. The model was selected based on its C-index and potential usefulness in clinical practice [104]. The DeepHit model's most important predictors were plasma albumin, followed by the presence of metastatic disease [104]. Additionally, the use of systemic therapy, plasma electrolytes (sodium, potassium, chloride, and calcium), hemoglobin, glucose, and alkaline phosphatase were identified as VTE risk predictors [104]. Meng et al. found in hospitalized cancer patients that the extreme gradient boosting (XGBoost) model achieved the best performance in VTE prediction [105]. The five most significant features tested in the model were D-dimer level, diabetes, hypertension, pleural metastasis, and hematological malignancies [105]. Danilatou and colleagues demonstrated that the machine learning approach outperformed traditional scoring systems in predicting early and late mortality in critically ill patients with venous thromboembolism and cancer. In addition, they validated the model externally [106].

In the future, machine learning models have potential in clinical practice but require optimization with larger databases and multiple algorithms. It is crucial to adhere to the standardization of reporting provided by the Scientific and Standardization Committee (SSC) Subcommittee on Hemostasis & Malignancy of the International Society on Thrombosis and Hemostasis (ISTH). This involves the TRIPOD checklist (Transparent Reporting of a Multivariable Prediction Model for Individual Prognosis or Diagnosis), clearly defining predictors, defining the derivation population, and validating the model externally before implementing it [107].

This paper aims to present the current relevant knowledge in VTE risk assessment in ambulatory cancer patients, starting from the guideline recommendations and continuing with the specific risk assessment methods and machine learning models approaches. The main limitation of this review is its narrative character.

## 7. Conclusions and Future Directions

VTE risk assessment in ambulatory cancer patients is still challenging. High-risk cancer patients must be accurately discriminated against thromboprophylaxis, but the guidelines do not provide enough information. Many scores, nomograms, and models were developed, but none have optimally performed in this setting. Clinical features, biomarkers, and genetic patterns have been tested alone or grouped in cancer populations in general or specific cancer cohorts. The polygenic risk scores that do not change during the cancer course could be potential predictors of cancer-associated VTE independent of cancer type, but this idea needs further validation in prospective studies. Additionally, the expenses must be assessed better. The machine learning models might provide a potentially useful algorithm through learning and improving its performance based on the data they use. But, to apply these methods in clinical practice, they need to be optimized in larger databases.

**Author Contributions:** Conceptualization, A.D. and A.Ş.D.; methodology, A.D. and A.Ş.D.; validation, A.D. and A.Ş.D.; formal analysis A.D. and A.Ş.D.; investigation A.D. and A.Ş.D.; resources, A.D. and A.Ş.D.; data curation, A.D. and A.Ş.D.; writing—original draft preparation, A.D. and A.Ş.D.; writing—review and editing, A.D. and A.Ş.D.; visualization, A.D. and A.Ş.D.; supervision, A.D. and A.Ş.D.; project administration, A.D. and A.Ş.D.; funding acquisition, A.D. All authors have read and agreed to the published version of the manuscript.

**Funding:** This research received no external funding.

**Conflicts of Interest:** The authors declare no conflicts of interest.

## References

1. Abdol Razak, N.B.; Jones, G.; Bhandari, M.; Berndt, M.C.; Metharom, P. Cancer-Associated Thrombosis: An Overview of Mechanisms, Risk Factors, and Treatment. *Cancers* **2018**, *10*, 380. [CrossRef] [PubMed]
2. Mulder, F.I.; Horváth-Puhó, E.; van Es, N.; van Laarhoven, H.W.M.; Pedersen, L.; Moik, F.; Ay, C.; Büller, H.R.; Sørensen, H.T. Venous thromboembolism in cancer patients: A population-based cohort study. *Blood* **2021**, *137*, 1959–1969. [CrossRef] [PubMed]
3. Sørensen, H.T.; Pedersen, L.; van Es, N.; Büller, H.R.; Horváth-Puhó, E. Impact of venous thromboembolism on the mortality in patients with cancer: A population-based cohort study. *Lancet Reg. Health Eur.* **2023**, *34*, 100739. [CrossRef] [PubMed]
4. Khorana, A.A.; McCrae, K.R.; Milentijevic, D.; Laliberté, F.; Lejeune, D.; Crivera, C.; Lefebvre, P. Healthcare resource utilization and costs associated with venous thromboembolism recurrence in patients with cancer. *J. Med. Econ.* **2020**, *23*, 323–329. [CrossRef] [PubMed]
5. Falanga, A.; Marchetti, M. Cancer-associated thrombosis: Enhanced awareness and pathophysiologic complexity. *J. Thromb. Haemost.* **2023**, *21*, 1397–1408. [CrossRef] [PubMed]
6. Falanga, A.; Ay, C.; Di Nisio, M.; Gerotziafas, G.; Jara-Palomares, L.; Langer, F.; Lecumberri, R.; Mandala, M.; Maraveyas, A.; Pabinger, I.; et al. Venous thromboembolism in cancer patients: ESMO Clinical Practice Guideline. *Ann. Oncol.* **2023**, *34*, 452–467. [CrossRef] [PubMed]
7. Key, N.S.; Khorana, A.A.; Kuderer, N.M.; Bohlke, K.; Lee, A.Y.Y.; Arcelus, J.I.; Wong, S.L.; Balaban, E.P.; Flowers, C.R.; Gates, L.E.; et al. Venous Thromboembolism Prophylaxis and Treatment in Patients with Cancer: ASCO Guideline Update. *J. Clin. Oncol.* **2023**, *41*, 3063–3071. [CrossRef]
8. Lyman, G.H.; Carrier, M.; Ay, C.; Di Nisio, M.; Hicks, L.K.; Khorana, A.A.; Leavitt, A.D.; Lee, A.Y.Y.; Macbeth, F.; Morgan, R.L.; et al. American Society of Hematology 2021 guidelines for management of venous thromboembolism: Prevention and treatment in patients with cancer. *Blood Adv.* **2021**, *5*, 927–974. [CrossRef]
9. Middeldorp, S.; Nieuwlaat, R.; Baumann Kreuziger, L.; Coppens, M.; Houghton, D.E.; James, A.H.; Lang, E.; Moll, S.; Myers, T.; Bhatt, M.; et al. American Society of Hematology 2023 Guidelines for Management of Venous Thromboembolism: Thrombophilia Testing. *Blood Adv.* **2023**, *7*, 7101–7138. [CrossRef]
10. Lyon, A.R.; López-Fernández, T.; Couch, L.S.; Asteggiano, R.; Aznar, M.C.; Bergler-Klein, J.; Boriani, G.; Cardinale, D.; Cordoba, R.; Cosyns, B.; et al. 2022 ESC Guidelines on cardio-oncology developed in collaboration with the European Hematology Association (EHA), the European Society for Therapeutic Radiology and Oncology (ESTRO) and the International Cardio-Oncology Society (IC-OS). *Eur. Heart J.* **2022**, *43*, 4229–4361. [CrossRef]
11. Drăgan, A.; Sinescu, I. The Role of the Cardiac Biomarkers in the Renal Cell Carcinoma Multidisciplinary Management. *Diagnostics* **2023**, *13*, 1912. [CrossRef] [PubMed]
12. Mosarla, R.C.; Vaduganathan, M.; Qamar, A.; Moslehi, J.; Piazza, G.; Giugliano, R.P. Anticoagulation Strategies in Patients with Cancer: JACC Review Topic of the Week. *J. Am. Coll. Cardiol.* **2019**, *73*, 1336–1349. [CrossRef] [PubMed]
13. van Es, N.; Ay, C.; Jara-Palomares, L. Screening for Occult Cancer in Patients with Venous Thromboembolism: Past, Present, and Future. *Hamostaseologie* **2020**, *40*, 270–279. [CrossRef] [PubMed]
14. Gainsbury, M.L.; Erdrich, J.; Taubman, D.; Mirocha, J.; Manguso, N.; Amersi, F.; Silberman, A.W. Prevalence and Predictors of Preoperative Venous Thromboembolism in Asymptomatic Patients Undergoing Major Oncologic Surgery. *Ann. Surg. Oncol.* **2018**, *25*, 1640–1645. [CrossRef]
15. Heidrich, H.; Konau, E.; Hesse, P. Asymptomatic venous thrombosis in cancer patients—A problem often overlooked. Results of a retrospective and prospective study. *Vasa* **2009**, *38*, 160–166. [CrossRef]
16. Loftus, J.R.; Hu, Z.; Morin, B.R.; Hobbs, S.K.; Francis, C.W.; Khorana, A.A.; Rubens, D.J.; Kaproth-Joslin, K.A. Vascular Imaging in the Asymptomatic High-risk Cancer Population: A Role for Thrombosis Screening and Therapy Management. *J. Ultrasound Med.* **2022**, *41*, 225–236. [CrossRef]
17. Kourlaba, G.; Gourzoulidis, G.; Rasmussen, E.; Kontodimas, S.; Maniadakis, N. Cost Effectiveness of Ultrasound Screening, Cancer Patients, to Detect Asymptomatic Thrombosis. *Value Health* **2017**, *20*, A587. [CrossRef]
18. Kunapareddy, G.; Switzer, B.; Jain, P.; Conces, M.; Chen, Y.W.; Patel, B.; Patel, S.; Pinnamaneni, P.; Pohlman, B.; Angelini, D.E.; et al. Implementation of an electronic medical record tool for early detection of deep vein thrombosis in the ambulatory oncology setting. *Res. Pract. Thromb. Haemost.* **2019**, *3*, 226–233. [CrossRef]

19. Holmes, C.E.; Ades, S.; Gilchrist, S.; Douce, D.; Libby, K.; Rogala, B.; Parenteau, E.; Cushman, M.; Holm, A.K. Successful Model for Guideline Implementation to Prevent Cancer-Associated Thrombosis: Venous Thromboembolism Prevention in the Ambulatory Cancer Clinic. *JCO Oncol. Pract.* **2020**, *16*, e868–e874. [CrossRef]
20. Ay, C.; Vormittag, R.; Dunkler, D.; Simanek, R.; Chiriac, A.L.; Drach, J.; Quehenberger, P.; Wagner, O.; Zielinski, C.; Pabinger, I. D-dimer and prothrombin fragment 1 + 2 predict venous thromboembolism in patients with cancer: Results from the Vienna Cancer and Thrombosis Study. *J. Clin. Oncol.* **2009**, *27*, 4124–4129. [CrossRef]
21. Schorling, R.M.; Pfrepper, C.; Golombek, T.; Cella, C.A.; Muñoz-Unceta, N.; Siegemund, R.; Engel, C.; Petros, S.; Lordick, F.; Knödler, M. Evaluation of Biomarkers for the Prediction of Venous Thromboembolism in Ambulatory Cancer Patients. *Oncol. Res. Treat.* **2020**, *43*, 414–427. [CrossRef] [PubMed]
22. Niimi, K.; Nishida, K.; Lee, C.; Ikeda, S.; Kawai, Y.; Sugimoto, M.; Banno, H. Optimal D-Dimer Cutoff Values for Diagnosing Deep Vein Thrombosis in Patients with Comorbid Malignancies. *Ann. Vasc. Surg.* **2024**, *98*, 293–300. [CrossRef] [PubMed]
23. Alexander, M.; Harris, S.; Underhill, C.; Torres, J.; Sharma, S.; Lee, N.; Wong, H.; Eek, R.; Michael, M.; Tie, J.; et al. Risk-Directed Ambulatory Thromboprophylaxis in Lung and Gastrointestinal Cancers: The TARGET-TP Randomized Clinical Trial. *JAMA Oncol.* **2023**, *9*, 1536–1545. [CrossRef] [PubMed]
24. Oi, M.; Yamashita, Y.; Toyofuku, M.; Morimoto, T.; Motohashi, Y.; Tamura, T.; Kaitani, K.; Amano, H.; Takase, T.; Hiramori, S.; et al. D-dimer levels at diagnosis and long-term clinical outcomes in venous thromboembolism: From the COMMAND VTE Registry. *J. Thromb. Thrombolysis.* **2020**, *49*, 551–561. [CrossRef] [PubMed]
25. Koch, V.; Martin, S.S.; Gruber-Rouh, T.; Eichler, K.; Mahmoudi, S.; Leistner, D.M.; Scholtz, J.E.; Bernatz, S.; Puntmann, V.O.; Nagel, E.; et al. Cancer patients with venous thromboembolism: Diagnostic and prognostic value of elevated D-dimers. *Eur. J. Clin. Investig.* **2023**, *53*, e13914. [CrossRef] [PubMed]
26. Ay, C.; Simanek, R.; Vormittag, R.; Dunkler, D.; Alguel, G.; Koder, S.; Kornek, G.; Marosi, C.; Wagner, O.; Zielinski, C.; et al. High plasma levels of soluble P-selectin are predictive of venous thromboembolism in cancer patients: Results from the Vienna Cancer and Thrombosis Study (CATS). *Blood* **2008**, *112*, 2703–2708. [CrossRef] [PubMed]
27. Zhang, X.; Zhang, C.; Ma, Z.; Zhang, Y. Soluble P-selectin level in patients with cancer-associated venous and artery thromboembolism: A systematic review and meta-analysis. *Arch. Med. Sci.* **2023**, *19*, 274–282. [CrossRef] [PubMed]
28. Khorana, A.A.; Barnard, J.; Wun, T.; Vijapurkar, U.; Damaraju, C.V.; Moore, K.T.; Wildgoose, P.; McCrae, K.R. Biomarker signatures in cancer patients with and without venous thromboembolism events: A substudy of CASSINI. *Blood Adv.* **2022**, *6*, 1212–1221. [CrossRef]
29. Anijs, R.J.S.; Nguyen, Y.N.; Cannegieter, S.C.; Versteeg, H.H.; Buijs, J.T. MicroRNAs as prognostic biomarkers for (cancer-associated) venous thromboembolism. *J. Thromb. Haemost.* **2023**, *21*, 7–17. [CrossRef]
30. Marques, I.S.; Tavares, V.; Neto, B.V.; Mota, I.N.R.; Pereira, D.; Medeiros, R. Long Non-Coding RNAs in Venous Thromboembolism: Where Do We Stand? *Int. J. Mol. Sci.* **2023**, *24*, 12103. [CrossRef]
31. Khorana, A.A.; Kuderer, N.M.; Culakova, E.; Lyman, G.H.; Francis, C.W. Development and validation of a predictive model for chemotherapy-associated thrombosis. *Blood* **2008**, *111*, 4902–4907. [CrossRef] [PubMed]
32. Khorana, A.A.; DeSancho, M.T.; Liebman, H.; Rosovsky, R.; Connors, J.M.; Zwicker, J. Prediction and Prevention of Cancer-Associated Thromboembolism. *Oncologist* **2021**, *26*, e2–e7. [CrossRef] [PubMed]
33. Mulder, F.I.; Candeloro, M.; Kamphuisen, P.W.; Di Nisio, M.; Bossuyt, P.M.; Guman, N.; Smit, K.; Buller, H.R.; van Es, N.; CAT-prediction collaborators. The Khorana score for prediction of venous thromboembolism in cancer patients: A systematic review and meta-analysis. *Haematologica* **2019**, *104*, 1277–1287. [CrossRef] [PubMed]
34. Akasaka-Kihara, F.; Sueta, D.; Ishii, M.; Maki, Y.; Hirakawa, K.; Tabata, N.; Ito, M.; Yamanaga, K.; Fujisue, K.; Hoshiyama, T.; et al. Validation of the Khorana Venous Thromboembolism Risk Score in Japanese Cancer Patients. *JACC Asia* **2021**, *1*, 259–270. [CrossRef]
35. Ramos-Esquivel, A.; Marenco-Flores, A.; Hernández-Romero, G.; Umaña-Mora, C.; Céspedes-Calvo, A.; Mora-Hidalgo, R. Using the Khorana risk score to predict venous thromboembolism and overall survival in a cohort of Hispanic patients with solid malignancies. *Ecancermedicalscience* **2022**, *16*, 1470. [CrossRef] [PubMed]
36. El-Sayed, H.A.; Othman, M.; Azzam, H.; Bucciol, R.; Ebrahim, M.A.; El-Agdar, M.A.M.A.; Tera, Y.; Sakr, D.H.; Ghoneim, H.R.; Selim, T.E. Assessing the risk of venous thromboembolism in patients with haematological cancers using three prediction models. *J. Cancer Res. Clin. Oncol.* **2023**, *149*, 17771–17780. [CrossRef] [PubMed]
37. Ha, H.; Ko, Y.H.; Kim, K.; Hong, J.; Lee, G.W.; Jeong, S.H.; Bang, S.M.; Yoon, S.S. Application of the Khorana score for cancer-associated thrombosis prediction in patients of East Asian ethnicity undergoing ambulatory chemotherapy. *Thromb. J.* **2023**, *21*, 63. [CrossRef]
38. Overvad, T.F.; Ording, A.G.; Nielsen, P.B.; Skjøth, F.; Albertsen, I.E.; Noble, S.; Vistisen, A.K.; Gade, I.L.; Severinsen, M.T.; Piazza, G.; et al. Validation of the Khorana score for predicting venous thromboembolism in 40 218 patients with cancer initiating chemotherapy. *Blood Adv.* **2022**, *6*, 2967–2976. [CrossRef]
39. van Es, N.; Ventresca, M.; Di Nisio, M.; Zhou, Q.; Noble, S.; Crowther, M.; Briel, M.; Garcia, D.; Lyman, G.H.; Macbeth, F.; et al. IPDMA Heparin Use in Cancer Patients Research Group. The Khorana score for prediction of venous thromboembolism in cancer patients: An individual patient data meta-analysis. *J. Thromb. Haemost.* **2020**, *18*, 1940–1951. [CrossRef]
40. Austin, K.; George, J.; Robinson, E.J.; Scully, M.; Thomas, M.R. Retrospective Cohort Study of Venous Thromboembolism Rates in Ambulatory Cancer Patients: Association with Khorana Score and Other Risk Factors. *J. Hematol.* **2019**, *8*, 17–25. [CrossRef]

41. Verzeroli, C.; Giaccherini, C.; Russo, L.; Bolognini, S.; Gamba, S.; Tartari, C.J.; Schieppati, F.; Ticozzi, C.; Vignoli, A.; Masci, G.; et al. Utility of the Khorana and the new-Vienna CATS prediction scores in cancer patients of the HYPERCAN cohort. *J. Thromb. Haemost.* **2023**, *21*, 1869–1881. [CrossRef] [PubMed]
42. Abdel-Razeq, H.; Sharaf, B.; Al-Jaghbeer, M.J.; Abu-Fares, H.; Bater, R.; Shaer, M.A.; Abu-Jaish, H.; Laban, D.A.; Salamah, O.; Tamimi, F.; et al. COMPASS-CAT versus Khorana risk assessment model for predicting venous thromboembolic events in patients with non-small cell lung cancer on active treatment with chemotherapy and/or immunotherapy, the CK-RAM study. *J. Thromb. Thrombolysis* **2023**, *56*, 447–453. [CrossRef] [PubMed]
43. Mansfield, A.S.; Tafur, A.J.; Wang, C.E.; Kourelis, T.V.; Wysokinska, E.M.; Yang, P. Predictors of active cancer thromboembolic outcomes: Validation of the Khorana score among patients with lung cancer. *J. Thromb. Haemost.* **2016**, *14*, 1773–1778. [CrossRef] [PubMed]
44. Sanfilippo, K.M.; Carson, K.R.; Wang, T.F.; Luo, S.; Edwin, N.; Kuderer, N.; Keller, J.M.; Gage, B.F. Evaluation of the Khorana score for prediction of venous thromboembolism in patients with multiple myeloma. *Res. Pract. Thromb. Haemost.* **2022**, *6*, e12634. [CrossRef] [PubMed]
45. Mirza, A.S.; Yun, S.; Ali, N.A.; Shin, H.; O'Neil, J.L.; Elharake, M.; Schwartz, D.; Robinson, K.; Nowell, E.; Engle, G.; et al. Validation of the Khorana score in acute myeloid leukemia patients: A single-institution experience. *Thromb. J.* **2019**, *17*, 13. [CrossRef] [PubMed]
46. Wang, Y.; Attar, B.M.; Fuentes, H.E.; Yu, J.; Zhang, H.; Tafur, A.J. Performance of Khorana Risk Score for Prediction of Venous Thromboembolism in Patients with Hepatocellular Carcinoma. *Clin. Appl. Thromb. Hemost.* **2018**, *24*, 471–476. [CrossRef] [PubMed]
47. Piver, R.N.; Wagner, V.M.; Levine, M.D.; Backes, F.J.; Chambers, L.J.; Cohn, D.E.; Copeland, L.J.; Cosgrove, C.M.; Nagel, C.I.; O'Malley, D.M.; et al. Use of the Khorana score to predict venous thromboembolism in patients undergoing chemotherapy for uterine cancer. *Gynecol. Oncol. Rep.* **2023**, *46*, 101156. [CrossRef]
48. Rupa-Matysek, J.; Gil, L.; Kaźmierczak, M.; Barańska, M.; Komarnicki, M. Prediction of venous thromboembolism in newly diagnosed patients treated for lymphoid malignancies: Validation of the Khorana Risk Score. *Med. Oncol.* **2017**, *35*, 5. [CrossRef]
49. Di Nisio, M.; van Es, N.; Rotunno, L.; Anzoletti, N.; Falcone, L.; De Tursi, M.; Natoli, C.; Tinari, N.; Cavallo, I.; Valeriani, E.; et al. Long-term performance of risk scores for venous thromboembolism in ambulatory cancer patients. *J. Thromb. Thrombolysis* **2019**, *48*, 125–133. [CrossRef]
50. Guman, N.A.M.; van Geffen, R.J.; Mulder, F.I.; van Haaps, T.F.; Hovsepjan, V.; Labots, M.; Cirkel, G.A.; de Vos, F.Y.F.L.; Ten Tije, A.J.; Beerepoot, L.V.; et al. Evaluation of the Khorana, PROTECHT, and 5-SNP scores for prediction of venous thromboembolism in patients with cancer. *J. Thromb. Haemost.* **2021**, *19*, 2974–2983. [CrossRef]
51. Ay, C.; Dunkler, D.; Marosi, C.; Chiriac, A.L.; Vormittag, R.; Simanek, R.; Quehenberger, P.; Zielinski, C.; Pabinger, I. Prediction of venous thromboembolism in cancer patients. *Blood* **2010**, *116*, 5377–5382. [CrossRef] [PubMed]
52. van Es, N.; Di Nisio, M.; Cesarman, G.; Kleinjan, A.; Otten, H.M.; Mahé, I.; Wilts, I.T.; Twint, D.C.; Porreca, E.; Arrieta, O.; et al. Comparison of risk prediction scores for venous thromboembolism in cancer patients: A prospective cohort study. *Haematologica* **2017**, *102*, 1494–1501. [CrossRef] [PubMed]
53. Harada, Y.; Sato, A.; Nishioka, A.; Ogusu, S.; Matsumoto, M.; Sueoka, E.; Kawaguchi, A.; Kimura, S.; Sueoka-Aragane, N. Usefulness of blood biomarkers for predicting venous thromboembolism in Japanese patients with cancer. *Oncol. Lett.* **2023**, *25*, 180. [CrossRef] [PubMed]
54. Verso, M.; Agnelli, G.; Barni, S.; Gasparini, G.; LaBianca, R. A modified Khorana risk assessment score for venous thromboembolism in cancer patients receiving chemotherapy: The Protecht score. *Intern. Emerg. Med.* **2012**, *7*, 291–292. [CrossRef] [PubMed]
55. Moik, F.; van Es, N.; Posch, F.; Di Nisio, M.; Fuereder, T.; Preusser, M.; Pabinger, I.; Ay, C. Gemcitabine and Platinum-Based Agents for the Prediction of Cancer-Associated Venous Thromboembolism: Results from the Vienna Cancer and Thrombosis Study. *Cancers* **2020**, *12*, 2493. [CrossRef] [PubMed]
56. Ramos-Esquivel, A.; Marenco-Flores, A.; Hernández-Romero, G.; Céspedes-Calvo, A.; Mora-Hidalgo, R. Comparison among three predictive models for cancer-associated thromboembolism in a hispanic population. *J. Thromb. Thrombolysis* **2023**, *56*, 433–438. [CrossRef] [PubMed]
57. Pelzer, U.; Sinn, M.; Stieler, J.; Riess, H. Primary pharmacological prevention of thromboembolic events in ambulatory patients with advanced pancreatic cancer treated with chemotherapy? *Dtsch. Med. Wochenschr.* **2013**, *138*, 2084–2088.
58. Qin, L.; Liang, Z.; Xie, J.; Li, X. Estimating Venous Thromboembolism Risk in Metastatic Colorectal Cancer Inpatients: Validation of Existing Risk Scores and Development of New Risk Scores. *Clin. Appl. Thromb. Hemost.* **2023**, *29*, 10760296231196859. [CrossRef]
59. Gomez-Rosas, P.; Giaccherini, C.; Russo, L.; Verzeroli, C.; Gamba, S.; Tartari, C.J.; Bolognini, S.; Ticozzi, C.; Schieppati, F.; Barcella, L.; et al. A New Risk Prediction Model for Venous Thromboembolism and Death in Ambulatory Lung Cancer Patients. *Cancers* **2023**, *15*, 4588. [CrossRef]
60. Yan, A.R.; Samarawickrema, I.; Naunton, M.; Peterson, G.M.; Yip, D.; Mortazavi, R. Models for predicting venous thromboembolism in ambulatory patients with lung cancer: A systematic review protocol. *BMJ Open* **2021**, *11*, e055322. [CrossRef]
61. Pabinger, I.; van Es, N.; Heinze, G.; Posch, F.; Riedl, J.; Reitter, E.M.; Di Nisio, M.; Cesarman-Maus, G.; Kraaijpoel, N.; Zielinski, C.C.; et al. A clinical prediction model for cancer-associated venous thromboembolism: A development and validation study in two independent prospective cohorts. *Lancet Haematol.* **2018**, *5*, e289–e298. [CrossRef] [PubMed]

62. Gerotziafas, G.T.; Taher, A.; Abdel-Razeq, H.; AboElnazar, E.; Spyropoulos, A.C.; El Shemmari, S.; Larsen, A.K.; Elalamy, I.; COMPASS–CAT Working Group. A Predictive Score for Thrombosis Associated with Breast, Colorectal, Lung, or Ovarian Cancer: The Prospective COMPASS-Cancer-Associated Thrombosis Study. *Oncologist* **2017**, *22*, 1222–1231. [CrossRef] [PubMed]
63. Taglialatela, I.; Mariani, L.; Dotti, K.F.; Di Vico, L.; Pisanu, M.N.; Facchinetti, C.; De Braud, F.; Ferrari, L.A.M. Central venous catheters-related-thrombosis and risk factors in oncological patients: A retrospective evaluation of recent risk scores. *Tumori J.* **2023**, *109*, 363–369. [CrossRef] [PubMed]
64. Rupa-Matysek, J.; Lembicz, M.; Rogowska, E.K.; Gil, L.; Komarnicki, M.; Batura-Gabryel, H. Evaluation of risk factors and assessment models for predicting venous thromboembolism in lung cancer patients. *Med. Oncol.* **2018**, *35*, 63. [CrossRef] [PubMed]
65. Spyropoulos, A.C.; Eldredge, J.B.; Anand, L.N.; Zhang, M.; Qiu, M.; Nourabadi, S.; Rosenberg, D.J. External Validation of a Venous Thromboembolic Risk Score for Cancer Outpatients with Solid Tumors: The COMPASS-CAT Venous Thromboembolism Risk Assessment Model. *Oncologist* **2020**, *25*, e1083–e1090. [CrossRef] [PubMed]
66. Pestana, R.M.C.; Alves, M.T.; de Oliveira, A.N.; Oliveira, H.H.M.; Soares, C.E.; Sabino, A.P.; Silva, L.M.; Simões, R.; Gomes, K.B. Interleukin-10 levels and the risk of thromboembolism according to COMPASS-Cancer associated thrombosis score in breast cancer patients prior to undergoing doxorubicin-based chemotherapy. *Blood Coagul. Fibrinolysis* **2023**, *34*, 70–74. [CrossRef] [PubMed]
67. Cella, C.A.; Di Minno, G.; Carlomagno, C.; Arcopinto, M.; Cerbone, A.M.; Matano, E.; Tufano, A.; Lordick, F.; De Simone, B.; Muehlberg, K.S.; et al. Preventing Venous Thromboembolism in Ambulatory Cancer Patients: The ONKOTEV Study. *Oncologist* **2017**, *22*, 601–608. [CrossRef]
68. Cella, C.A.; Knoedler, M.; Hall, M.; Arcopinto, M.; Bagnardi, V.; Gervaso, L.; Pellicori, S.; Spada, F.; Zampino, M.G.; Ravenda, P.S.; et al. Validation of the ONKOTEV Risk Prediction Model for Venous Thromboembolism in Outpatients with Cancer. *JAMA Netw. Open* **2023**, *6*, e230010. [CrossRef]
69. Godinho, J.; Casa-Nova, M.; Moreira-Pinto, J.; Simões, P.; Paralta Branco, F.; Leal-Costa, L.; Faria, A.; Lopes, F.; Teixeira, J.A.; Passos-Coelho, J.L. ONKOTEV Score as a Predictive Tool for Thromboembolic Events in Pancreatic Cancer—A Retrospective Analysis. *Oncologist* **2020**, *25*, e284–e290. [CrossRef]
70. Xiong, W.; Zhao, Y.; Du, H.; Wang, Y.; Xu, M.; Guo, X. Optimal authoritative risk assessment score of Cancer-associated venous thromboembolism for hospitalized medical patients with lung Cancer. *Thromb. J.* **2021**, *19*, 95. [CrossRef]
71. Pfrepper, C.; Knödler, M.; Schorling, R.M.; Seehofer, D.; Petros, S.; Lordick, F. Predictors for thromboembolism in patients with cholangiocarcinoma. *J. Cancer Res. Clin. Oncol.* **2022**, *148*, 2415–2426. [CrossRef] [PubMed]
72. Zhang, L.; Fang, Y.; Xing, J.; Cheng, H.; Sun, X.; Yuan, Z.; Xu, Y.; Hao, J. The Efficacy of the Systemic Immune-Inflammation Index and Prognosis Nutritional Index for the Diagnosis of Venous Thromboembolism in Gastrointestinal Cancers. *J. Inflamm. Res.* **2022**, *15*, 4649–4661. [CrossRef] [PubMed]
73. Tort, M.; Sevil, F.C.; Sevil, H.; Becit, N. Evaluation of systemic immune-inflammation index in acute deep vein thrombosis: A propensity-matched. *J. Vasc. Surg. Venous Lymphat. Disord.* **2023**, *11*, 972–977.e1. [CrossRef]
74. Zhang, L.; Liu, X.; Yang, R.; Yang, Y.; Chen, X. The Diagnostic Value of the Systemic Immune-Inflammation Index for Venous Thromboembolism in Lung Cancer Patients: A Retrospective Study. *Mediat. Inflamm.* **2022**, *2022*, 9215311. [CrossRef] [PubMed]
75. Li, A.; La, J.; May, S.B.; Guffey, D.; da Costa, W.L., Jr.; Amos, C.I.; Bandyo, R.; Milner, E.M.; Kurian, K.M.; Chen, D.C.R.; et al. Derivation and Validation of a Clinical Risk Assessment Model for Cancer-Associated Thrombosis in Two Unique US Health Care Systems. *J. Clin. Oncol.* **2023**, *41*, 2926–2938. [CrossRef] [PubMed]
76. Castellón Rubio, V.E.; Segura, P.P.; Muñoz, A.; Farré, A.L.; Ruiz, L.C.; Lorente, J. High plasma levels of soluble P-Selectin and Factor VIII predict venous thromboembolism in non-small cell lung cancer patients: The Thrombo-Nsclc risk score. *Thromb. Res.* **2020**, *196*, 349–354. [CrossRef] [PubMed]
77. Li, H.; Tian, Y.; Niu, H.; He, L.; Cao, G.; Zhang, C.; Kaiweisierkezi, K.; Luo, Q. Derivation, validation and assessment of a novel nomogram-based risk assessment model for venous thromboembolism in hospitalized patients with lung cancer: A retrospective case control study. *Front. Oncol.* **2022**, *12*, 988287. [CrossRef]
78. Antic, D.; Milic, N.; Nikolovski, S.; Todorovic, M.; Bila, J.; Djurdjevic, P.; Andjelic, B.; Djurasinovic, V.; Sretenovic, A.; Vukovic, V.; et al. Development and validation of multivariable predictive model for thromboembolic events in lymphoma patients. *Am. J. Hematol.* **2016**, *91*, 1014–1019. [CrossRef]
79. Kirkizlar, O.; Alp Kirkizlar, T.; Umit, E.G.; Asker, I.; Baysal, M.; Bas, V.; Gulsaran, S.K.; Demirci, U.; Demir, A.M. The Incidence of Venous Thromboembolism and Impact on Survival in Hodgkin Lymphoma. *Clin. Lymphoma Myeloma Leuk.* **2020**, *20*, 542–547. [CrossRef]
80. Abdel-Razeq, H.; Ma'koseh, M.; Mansour, A.; Bater, R.; Amarin, R.; Abufara, A.; Halahleh, K.; Manassra, M.; Alrwashdeh, M.; Almomani, M.; et al. The Application of the ThroLy Risk Assessment Model to Predict Venous Thromboembolism in Patients with Diffuse Large B-Cell Lymphoma. *Clin. Appl. Thromb. Hemost.* **2021**, *27*, 10760296211045908. [CrossRef]
81. Rupa-Matysek, J.; Brzeźniakiewicz-Janus, K.; Gil, L.; Krasiński, Z.; Komarnicki, M. Evaluation of the ThroLy score for the prediction of venous thromboembolism in newly diagnosed patients treated for lymphoid malignancies in clinical practice. *Cancer Med.* **2018**, *7*, 2868–2875. [CrossRef] [PubMed]

82. Bastos-Oreiro, M.; Ortiz, J.; Pradillo, V.; Salas, E.; Marínez-Laperche, C.; Muñoz, A.; Buño, I.; Diéz-Martin, J.L.; Soria, J.M.; Pascual Izquierdo, C. Incorporating genetic and clinical data into the prediction of thromboembolism risk in patients with lymphoma. *Cancer Med.* **2021**, *10*, 7585–7592. [CrossRef] [PubMed]
83. López Sacerio, A.; Tejeda Ramón, M.C.; Morales Helguera, A.; Pérez Castillo, Y.; Cruz Rodríguez, J.; Guerra Rodríguez, J.F.; Falanga, A. Validation of venous thromboembolism predictive model in hematologic malignancies. *Ann. Hematol.* **2023**, *102*, 3613–3620. [CrossRef]
84. Sanfilippo, K.M.; Luo, S.; Wang, T.F.; Fiala, M.; Schoen, M.; Wildes, T.M.; Mikhael, J.; Kuderer, N.M.; Calverley, D.C.; Keller, J.; et al. Predicting venous thromboembolism in multiple myeloma: Development and validation of the IMPEDE VTE score. *Am. J. Hematol.* **2019**, *94*, 1176–1184. [CrossRef] [PubMed]
85. Sanfilippo, K.M.; Fiala, M.; Feinberg, D.; Tathireddy, H.; Girard, T.; Vij, R.; Di Paola, J.; Gage, B.F. D-dimer predicts venous thromboembolism in multiple myeloma: A nested case-control study. *Res. Pract. Thromb. Haemost.* **2023**, *7*, e102235. [CrossRef] [PubMed]
86. Wolpert, F.; Berghoff, A.S.; Grossenbacher, B.; Lareida, A.; Löb, R.; Roth, P.; Neidert, M.C.; Andratschke, N.; Le Rhun, E.; Preusser, M.; et al. Venous thromboembolic events in patients with brain metastases: The PICOS score. *Eur. J. Cancer* **2020**, *134*, 75–85. [CrossRef] [PubMed]
87. Kubo, K.; Nakamura, K.; Okamoto, K.; Matsuoka, H.; Ida, N.; Haruma, T.; Ogawa, C.; Masuyama, H. The Combination of D-dimer and Glasgow Prognostic Score Can Be Useful in Predicting VTE in Patients with Stage IIIC and IVA Ovarian Cancer. *Acta Med. Okayama* **2022**, *76*, 129–135.
88. Roy, D.C.; Wang, T.F.; Carrier, M.; Mallick, R.; Burger, D.; Hawken, S.; Wells, P.S. Thrombophilia gene mutations predict venous thromboembolism in ambulatory cancer patients receiving chemotherapy. *J. Thromb. Haemost.* **2023**, *21*, 3184–3192. [CrossRef]
89. Lindström, S.; Wang, L.; Smith, E.N.; Gordon, W.; van Hylckama Vlieg, A.; de Andrade, M.; Brody, J.A.; Pattee, J.W.; Haessler, J.; Brumpton, B.M.; et al. Genomic and transcriptomic association studies identify 16 novel susceptibility loci for venous thromboembolism. *Blood* **2019**, *134*, 1645–1657. [CrossRef]
90. de Haan, H.G.; Bezemer, I.D.; Doggen, C.J.; Le Cessie, S.; Reitsma, P.H.; Arellano, A.R.; Tong, C.H.; Devlin, J.J.; Bare, L.A.; Rosendaal, F.R.; et al. Multiple SNP testing improves risk prediction of first venous thrombosis. *Blood* **2012**, *120*, 656–663. [CrossRef]
91. Skille, H.; Paulsen, B.; Hveem, K.; Gabrielsen, M.E.; Brumpton, B.; Hindberg, K.; Gran, O.V.; Rosendaal, F.R.; Braekkan, S.K.; Hansen, J.B. Combined effects of five prothrombotic genotypes and cancer on the risk of a first venous thromboembolic event. *J. Thromb. Haemost.* **2020**, *18*, 2861–2869. [CrossRef] [PubMed]
92. Jakobsen, L.; Frischmuth, T.; Brækkan, S.K.; Hansen, J.B.; Morelli, V.M. Joint Effect of Multiple Prothrombotic Genotypes and Mean Platelet Volume on the Risk of Incident Venous Thromboembolism. *Thromb. Haemost.* **2022**, *122*, 1911–1920. [CrossRef] [PubMed]
93. Guman, N.A.M.; Mulder, F.I.; Ferwerda, B.; Zwinderman, A.H.; Kamphuisen, P.W.; Büller, H.R.; van Es, N. Polygenic risk scores for prediction of cancer-associated venous thromboembolism in the UK Biobank cohort study. *J. Thromb. Haemost.* **2023**, *21*, 3175–3183. [CrossRef] [PubMed]
94. Muñoz Martín, A.J.; Ortega, I.; Font, C.; Pachón, V.; Castellón, V.; Martínez-Marín, V.; Salgado, M.; Martínez, E.; Calzas, J.; Rupérez, A.; et al. Multivariable clinical-genetic risk model for predicting venous thromboembolic events in patients with cancer. *Br. J. Cancer* **2018**, *118*, 1056–1061. [CrossRef] [PubMed]
95. Neto, B.V.; Tavares, V.; da Silva, J.B.; Liz-Pimenta, J.; Marques, I.S.; Carvalho, L.; Salgado, L.; Pereira, D.; Medeiros, R. Thrombogenesis-associated genetic determinants as predictors of thromboembolism and prognosis in cervical cancer. *Sci. Rep.* **2023**, *13*, 9519. [CrossRef]
96. Muñoz, A.; Ay, C.; Grilz, E.; López, S.; Font, C.; Pachón, V.; Castellón, V.; Martínez-Marín, V.; Salgado, M.; Martínez, E.; et al. A Clinical-Genetic Risk Score for Predicting Cancer-Associated Venous Thromboembolism: A Development and Validation Study Involving Two Independent Prospective Cohorts. *J. Clin. Oncol.* **2023**, *41*, 2911–2925. [CrossRef]
97. Xu, Q.; Lei, H.; Li, X.; Li, F.; Shi, H.; Wang, G.; Sun, A.; Wang, Y.; Peng, B. Machine learning predicts cancer-associated venous thromboembolism using clinically available variables in gastric cancer patients. *Heliyon* **2023**, *9*, e12681. [CrossRef]
98. Nudel, J.; Bishara, A.M.; de Geus, S.W.L.; Patil, P.; Srinivasan, J.; Hess, D.T.; Woodson, J. Development and validation of machine learning models to predict gastrointestinal leak and venous thromboembolism after weight loss surgery: An analysis of the MBSAQIP database. *Surg. Endosc.* **2021**, *35*, 182–191. [CrossRef]
99. Ting Sim, J.Z.; Fong, Q.W.; Huang, W.; Tan, C.H. Machine learning in medicine: What clinicians should know. *Singap. Med. J.* **2023**, *64*, 91–97.
100. Ferroni, P.; Zanzotto, F.M.; Scarpato, N.; Riondino, S.; Nanni, U.; Roselli, M.; Guadagni, F. Risk Assessment for Venous Thromboembolism in Chemotherapy-Treated Ambulatory Cancer Patients. *Med. Decis. Mak.* **2017**, *37*, 234–242. [CrossRef]
101. Ferroni, P.; Zanzotto, F.M.; Scarpato, N.; Riondino, S.; Guadagni, F.; Roselli, M. Validation of a Machine Learning Approach for Venous Thromboembolism Risk Prediction in Oncology. *Dis. Markers* **2017**, *2017*, 8781379. [CrossRef] [PubMed]
102. Jin, S.; Qin, D.; Liang, B.S.; Zhang, L.C.; Wei, X.X.; Wang, Y.J.; Zhuang, B.; Zhang, T.; Yang, Z.P.; Cao, Y.W.; et al. Machine learning predicts cancer-associated deep vein thrombosis using clinically available variables. *Int. J. Med. Inform.* **2022**, *161*, 104733. [CrossRef] [PubMed]

103. Lei, H.; Zhang, M.; Wu, Z.; Liu, C.; Li, X.; Zhou, W.; Long, B.; Ma, J.; Zhang, H.; Wang, Y.; et al. Development and Validation of a Risk Prediction Model for Venous Thromboembolism in Lung Cancer Patients Using Machine Learning. *Front. Cardiovasc. Med.* **2022**, *9*, 845210. [CrossRef] [PubMed]
104. Mantha, S.; Chatterjee, S.; Singh, R.; Cadley, J.; Poon, C.; Chatterjee, A.; Kelly, D.; Sterpi, M.; Soff, G.; Zwicker, J.; et al. Application of Machine Learning to the Prediction of Cancer-Associated Venous Thromboembolism. *Res. Sq.* **2023**, *rs.3.rs*, 2870367.
105. Meng, L.; Wei, T.; Fan, R.; Su, H.; Liu, J.; Wang, L.; Huang, X.; Qi, Y.; Li, X. Development and validation of a machine learning model to predict venous thromboembolism among hospitalized cancer patients. *Asia Pac. J. Oncol. Nurs.* **2022**, *9*, 100128. [CrossRef]
106. Danilatou, V.; Nikolakakis, S.; Antonakaki, D.; Tzagkarakis, C.; Mavroidis, D.; Kostoulas, T.; Ioannidis, S. Outcome Prediction in Critically-Ill Patients with Venous Thromboembolism and/or Cancer Using Machine Learning Algorithms: External Validation and Comparison with Scoring Systems. *Int. J. Mol. Sci.* **2022**, *23*, 7132. [CrossRef]
107. Sanfilippo, K.M.; Wang, T.F.; Carrier, M.; Falanga, A.; Gage, B.F.; Khorana, A.A.; Maraveyas, A.; Soff, G.A.; Wells, P.S.; Zwicker, J.I. Standardization of risk prediction model reporting in cancer-associated thrombosis: Communication from the ISTH SSC subcommittee on hemostasis and malignancy. *J. Thromb. Haemost.* **2022**, *20*, 1920–1927. [CrossRef]

*cancers*

MDPI

*Article*

# Trends and Age–Period–Cohort Effect on the Incidence of Early-Onset Colorectal Cancer (20–44 Years) from 1990 to 2021 in the United States

**Wafa A. Aldhaleei [1], Michael B. Wallace [2] and Akshaya Srikanth Bhagavathula [2,3,*]**

[1] Division of Gastroenterology and Hepatology, Mayo Clinic, Rochester, MN 55905, USA; aldhaleei.wafa@mayo.edu
[2] Division of Gastroenterology and Hepatology, Mayo Clinic, Jacksonville, FL 32224, USA; wallace.michael@mayo.edu
[3] Department of Public Health, North Dakota State University, Fargo, ND 58102, USA
* Correspondence: akshaya.bhagavathula@ndsu.edu or bhagavathula.akshaya@mayo.edu

**Simple Summary:** The incidence of colorectal cancer in people under 50 years old is rapidly increasing in the United States. Our study aims to understand how often early-onset colorectal cancer occurs and what factors contribute to its rise. By analyzing data from 1990 to 2021, we found a significant increase in cancer cases, especially among women and those born after 1983. Our findings highlight the need for targeted prevention strategies and further research to uncover the reasons behind these trends. This research can help the medical community develop better screening and prevention methods to reduce the incidence of early-onset colorectal cancer.

**Abstract:** The incidence of early-onset colorectal cancer (EO-CRC) in individuals under 50 years old is rapidly increasing in the United States. This study aims to evaluate EO-CRC incidence rates using data from the Global Burden of Disease Study (GBD) 2021, providing insights into trends from 1990 to 2021. We employed an age–period–cohort (APC) model analysis to estimate the effects of age, time period, and birth cohort on EO-CRC incidence. Our findings indicate that the number of EO-CRC cases rose from 6256 (95% UI: 6059–6456) in 1990 to 9311 (95% UI: 8859–9744) in 2021, a 49% increase from 1990 to 2021. The age-standardized incidence rate per 100,000 population increased by 34% during this period. The net drift in females (0.22%, 95% CI: 0.20–0.24) was slightly higher than in males (0.21%, 95% CI: 0.19–0.23) ($p = 0.45$). The APC analysis revealed that being over 25 years old, the period from 2005–2021, and being born after 1983 negatively impacted EO-CRC incidence rates, with a sharp rise after 2000 and a reduction among females from 2017 to 2021. Our study highlights the need for targeted prevention strategies and further research to understand these trends.

**Keywords:** colorectal cancer; early-onset; incidence; age–period–cohort; global burden of diseases; epidemiology; public health; United States

## 1. Introduction

The incidence of early-onset colorectal cancer (EO-CRC), defined as colorectal cancer diagnosed before age 50, has been increasing alarmingly in the United States (US) in recent decades [1,2]. The American Cancer Society projects that around 151,000 Americans will be diagnosed with colorectal cancer in 2024, with a rapid rise in cases among young adults [3]. Specifically, the incidence of EO-CRC has risen by 50% in the last 30 years, and by 2030, colorectal cancer (CRC) is predicted to be the leading cause of cancer death for the people under 50 in the US [4]. This escalating burden has been observed across all younger age groups from 20 to 49 years [5].

Several factors have been implicated in the rise of EO-CRC, including racial disparities, obesity, sedentary lifestyle, and environmental exposures [6,7]. African Americans have historically been at higher risk for EO-CRC compared to Caucasians [8], possibly due to socioeconomic factors and healthcare access. With the increase in the prevalence of risk factors in the younger population, the incidence of EO-CRC may continue to increase.

Recent screening guidelines for the US population have lowered the recommended CRC screening age from 45 to 50 years for the average-risk population [9,10]. This change in the screening age threshold has consequently redefined the population considered unscreened for CRC. Previous studies examining the incidences and outcomes of EO-CRC did not account for this updated screening guideline [11–13]. An updated comprehensive analysis with a focus on the age group below 45 years is needed to provide a more accurate understanding of the evolving EO-CRC epidemiology.

Numerous studies have examined the epidemiological characteristics of EO-CRC at both the regional and national levels [14–17]. CRC is influenced by age-related factors; moreover, the epidemiology of CRC can be shaped by the specific time period and the birth cohort of the population. However, there is a notable gap in research examining how age, time period, and birth cohort influence the incidence of EO-CRC. Furthermore, few studies have utilized age–period–cohort (APC) models to evaluate these effects comprehensively. The Global Burden of Disease Study 2021 (GBD 2021) [18] evaluated over 370 diseases and injuries, providing comprehensive data to examine the epidemiological patterns and characteristics of EO-CRC. The age—period–cohort (APC) model is a powerful statistical method tool that can analyze trends in disease incidence and mortality by simultaneously accounting for three time-related factors: age, period, and cohort effects. This approach helps to separate these interconnected factors, offering a clear understanding of how each contributes to the observed trends in cancer incidence. By disentangling these intertwined effects, the APC model provides a clearer picture of how each factor contributes to the observed trends in cancer incidence [19].

In this study, we applied an APC model to analyze the incidence trends of EO-CRC in the US from 1990 to 2021, aiming to provide a comprehensive insight into the age, period, and cohort effects on EO-CRC, thereby informing targeted prevention strategies and future research directions.

## 2. Materials and Methods

### 2.1. Data Sources

We used aggregated national-level data provided by the Institute of Health Metrics and Evaluation (IHME) | Global Health Data Exchange (GHDx) to collect age-standardized incidence rates for EO-CRC in the US from 1990 to 2021. These data encompass age-standardized rates aggregated across the entire country, without individual or state-level breakdowns. The International Classification of Disease 10th Revision (ICD-10) codes used to define CRC (level 3) included C-180-18.9, C19, C19.0, C19.9, C2, C20, C20.0, C20.8, C20.9, C21, C21.0, C21.1, C21.2, C21.8, and C21.9. EO-CRC was defined in this study as the incidence of CRC before the age of 45 years. Age-standardized incidence rates per 100,000 population among males and females were used in our estimates.

These rates were standardized to the World Health Organization's world standard population, allowing for adjustments to account for differences in age distribution within the population over time. This standardization is important for accurately comparing incidence rates across different demographic groups and over the study period.

### 2.2. Study Population

The study population included individuals aged 20 to 44 years diagnosed with colorectal cancer from 1990 to 2021 in the United States. The population was divided into five age groups: 20–24, 25–29, 30–34, 35–39, and 40–44 years.

### 2.3. Statistical Analysis

We used the APC model to analyze the incidence trends of EO-CRC. The APC model allows for the separation of the effects of age, period, and cohort that are often intertwined.

The incidence of EO-CRC served as the dependent variable, while age, period, and birth cohort were considered as independent variables. The APC model uses statistical methods to analyze how age-specific time periods and birth years affect EO-CRC incidence rates over time. It helps to separate the influence of each factor on the incidence rates.

The model assesses the impact of age, period, and cohort factors on the incidence rates, where the age effect reflects the difference in the EO-CRC incidence across various ages, the period effect shows the impact of different external factors during the study period (1990 to 2021) on EO-CRC incidence throughout all ages, and the cohort effect illustrates EO-CRC incidence changes caused by shared experiences or exposure to several risk factors across birth years.

The incidence ratio is a measure used to compare the incidence rates between different groups. It indicates how much more or less common EO-CRC is in one group compared to another. An incidence ratio greater than 1 suggests higher incidence, while a ratio less than 1 suggests lower incidence.

Ideally, the age and period intervals in the APC model should be equal. Because the age groups in the GBD 2021 are at five-year intervals, we displayed the incidence and population data in consecutive five-year periods (1990–1994, 1995–1999, 2000–2005, etc.), with 1990–1994 as the reference period. The population was divided into five age groups: 20–24, 25–29, 30–34, 35–39 and 40–44 years, with the medians of each interval as the reference age group.

The APC model produces two main results: net drift and local drift.

1. **Net drift** shows the overall annual increase in EO-CRC incidence rates across all birth cohorts.
2. **Local drift** indicates the annual increase in specific age groups, highlighting variations by age over time.

The cohorts are the result of participants' period minus their age. The relative risk estimates and their 95% confidence intervals (CIs) were gathered using the Age–Period–Cohort web tool provided by the National Cancer Institute [19]. Other indicators include period rate ratios (RRs), birth cohort RRs, and fitted time trends.

### 2.4. Data Quality and Robustness

The estimates were generated using incidence and population data provided by the IHME and the National Center for Health Statistics. The IHME utilizes sophisticated modeling techniques to estimate disease incidence rates, incorporating data from various sources, including vital registration systems, cancer registries, and health surveys. These models adjust for potential biases and inconsistencies in the raw data, providing robust and reliable estimates of EO-CRC incidence rates.

### 2.5. Data Analysis and Visualization

Microsoft Excel 360 was used to collect the data. Figures were generated using the APC R software (version 4.2.2; R Foundation for Statistical Computing, Vienna, Austria). The statistical significance was set at a two-sided $p$-value $< 0.05$ using the APC's Wald's chi-square test.

## 3. Results

### 3.1. EO-CRC Incidence Trends

In the US, the burden of EO-CRC increased substantially from 1990 to 2021. The number of incident cases rose from 6256 (95% uncertainty interval [UI]: 6059–6456) in 1990 to 9311 (95% UI: 8859–9744) in 2021, representing a 49% increase (95% UI: 41–56%) during this period. Concurrently, the age-standardized incidence rate per 100,000 population increased significantly from 32.9 (95% UI: 31.8–33.9) in 1990 to 43.9 (95% UI: 41.8–46.0) in 2021, equating to a 34% (95% UI: 26–41%) overall increase in incidence rates from 1990 to 2021. The incidence rates of EO-CRC are generally higher in men compared to women across all age groups. More details are in Table 1.

**Table 1.** Early-onset colorectal cancer incidence and percentage change from 1990–2021.

| | Incident Cases (95% UI) | | Percentage Change (95% UI) | Incidence Rate per 100,000 (95% UI) | | Percentage Change (95% UI) |
|---|---|---|---|---|---|---|
| **Overall** | 1990 | 2021 | 1990–2021 | 1990 | 2021 | 1990–2021 |
| 20–24 | 159 (154–164) | 200 (190–209) | 0.26 (0.18–0.33) | 0.81 (0.78–0.84) | 0.92 (0.87–0.96) | 0.13 (0.06–0.19) |
| 25–29 | 457 (475–440) | 591 (557–620) | 0.29 (0.20–0.38) | 2.10 (2.02–2.19) | 2.62 (2.48–2.75) | 0.25 (0.16–0.33) |
| 30–34 | 1034 (1001–1068) | 1409 (1336–1477) | 0.36 (0.28–0.45) | 4.63 (4.48–4.78) | 6.13 (5.81–6.42) | 0.32 (0.24–0.41) |
| 35–39 | 1736 (1684–1787) | 2554 (2431–2664) | 0.47 (0.39–0.55) | 8.52 (8.27–8.77) | 11.57 (11.01–12.07) | 0.36 (0.28–0.43 |
| 40–44 | 2870 (2789–2954) | 4557 (4354–4774) | 0.59 (0.50–0.67) | 15.88 (15.43–16.35) | 21.69 (20.73–22.72) | 0.37 (0.29–0.44) |
| **Females** | | | | | | |
| 20–24 | 70 (67–73) | 92 (87–97) | 0.31 (0.21–0.41) | 0.73 (0.70–0.76) | 0.86 (0.81–0.91) | 0.17 (0.09–0.27) |
| 25–29 | 209 (200–219) | 270 (251–287) | 0.29 (0.18–0.39) | 1.93 (1.85–2.02) | 2.42 (2.25–2.57) | 0.25 (0.15–0.36) |
| 30–34 | 475 (451–497) | 625 (582–667) | 0.32 (0.20–0.45) | 4.24 (4.03–4.44) | 5.44 (5.07–5.81) | 0.28 (0.17–0.41) |
| 35–39 | 764 (735–795) | 1154 (1080–1235) | 0.51 (0.38–0.63) | 7.45 (7.16–7.75) | 10.40 (9.73–11.12) | 0.40 (0.28–0.51) |
| 40–44 | 1310 (1259–1365) | 2060 (1942–2183) | 0.57 (0.46–0.68) | 14.33 (13.77–14.93) | 19.41 (18.30–20.56) | 0.35 (0.26–0.44) |
| **Male** | | | | | | |
| 20–24 | 89 (85–92) | 108 (102–114) | 0.22 (0.13–0.31) | 0.89 (0.85–0.92) | 0.97 (1.03–0.92) | 0.09 (0.01–0.17) |
| 25–29 | 248 (237–259) | 321 (102–114) | 0.30 (0.20–0.41) | 2.27 (2.17–2.37) | 2.82 (2.63–3.00) | 0.24 (0.15–0.35) |
| 30–34 | 559 (537–583) | 784 (300–341) | 0.40 (0.30–0.51) | 5.02 (4.82–5.23) | 6.81 (6.41–7.19) | 0.36 (0.26–0.46) |
| 35–39 | 971 (932–1010) | 1400 (1317–1482) | 0.44 (0.34–0.54) | 9.61 (9.22–9.99) | 12.76 (12.00–13.51) | 0.33 (0.24–0.42) |
| 40–44 | 1560 (1506–1617) | 2497 (2351–2636) | 0.60 (0.50–0.71) | 17.47 (16.86–18.10) | 24.02 (22.62–25.35) | 0.38 (0.29–0.47) |

UI: uncertainty interval.

In females, the 40–44 years age group saw an increase in incident EO-CRC cases from 1310 (95% UI: 1259–1365) in 1990 to 2060 (95% UI: 1942–2183) in 2021 (Figure 1). EO-CRC incidence in the 35–39 years age group rose from 764 to 1154 cases, while incidence in the 30–34 and 25–29 years groups increased from 500 and 300 cases to 700 and 500 cases, respectively. The 20–24 years group showed a slight rise from 70 to 92 cases. In males, the 40–44 years age group increased from 1560 to 2500 EO-CRC cases in 2021. The 35–39 years group rose from 1000 to 1400 cases, while the 30–34 and 25–29 years groups increased from 559 and 248 cases to 784 and 341 cases, respectively. The 20–24 years group saw a rise from 89 to 321 cases.

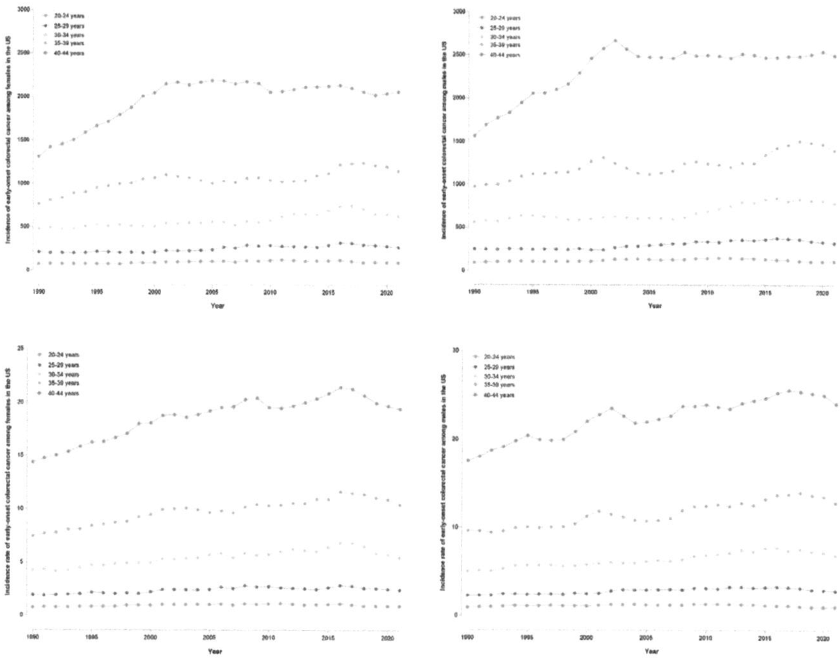


**Figure 1.** Trends in incident cases and incidence rate of early-onset colorectal cancer by age group and gender in the United States, 1990–2021 (females—left, and males—right).

The mounting burden was observed across all younger age groups from 20 to 44 years. The largest percentage increase was observed among those aged 40–44 years, with a 59% escalation in incident cases overall (60% in males, 57% in females), coupled with a 37% increase in the incidence rate. Notably, even the youngest group, 20–24 years of age, exhibited a 26% surge in EO-CRC cases and a 13% higher incidence rate. Among individuals aged 35–39 years, cases increased by 47% overall, 51% in females, and 44% in males, while incidence rates increased by approximately 36–40% in both sexes. In the 30–34 years age group, a 36% increase in EO-CRC cases and a 32% elevation in incidence rate were noted across sexes. Although percentage increases tended to be higher among males across most age groups, females exhibited slightly greater increases in the 35–39 years age group.

### 3.2. *Net and Local Drifts by Age Groups*

The net and local drifts were evaluated by age group, where net drift represents the overall annual percentage change across the study period, and the local drift represents the annual percentage change in the EO-CRC incidence rates relative to the net drift for each age group (Figure 2). The overall annual increase in EO-CRC incidence rates (net drift) was slightly higher in females (0.22% per year, 95% CI: 0.20 to 0.24) compared to males (0.21% per year, 95% CI: 0.19 to 0.23). However, this difference was not statistically significant ($p = 0.45$). The annual increase in specific age groups (local drift) was above average for both males and females, especially noticeable in individuals aged 22 years and older, indicating a worsening trend in EO-CRC incidence rates until around age 37.

### 3.3. *APC Analysis*

The figures illustrating changes in rates provide additional insights through the APC model analysis. This model isolates the effects of age, period, and cohort, offering a more nuanced understanding of EO-CRC incidence trends than simple incidence rate graphs.

Figure 3 demonstrates the effect of age, period, and cohort on the EO-CRC incidence. Overall, the incidence of EO-CRC exhibits a rapid increase after the age of 25 years, irrespective of sex. However, the highest incidence is seen in males aged 42 years, around 21 per 100,000 population. From 2005, the incidence ratio of EO-CRC was greater than 1, indicating worsening EO-CRC incidence during these periods. However, the 2019–2021 period effect positively impacted the incidence rates in females. The cohort effect shows that individuals born in 1983 onwards had an incidence ratio greater than 1, with a bell-shaped curve indicating worsening incidence rates until 1996, followed by gradual reduction.

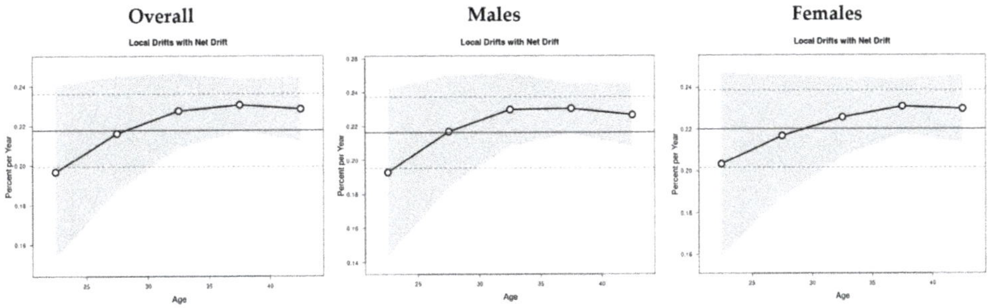


**Figure 2.** The net and local drifts of EO-CRC incidence from 1990 to 2021.

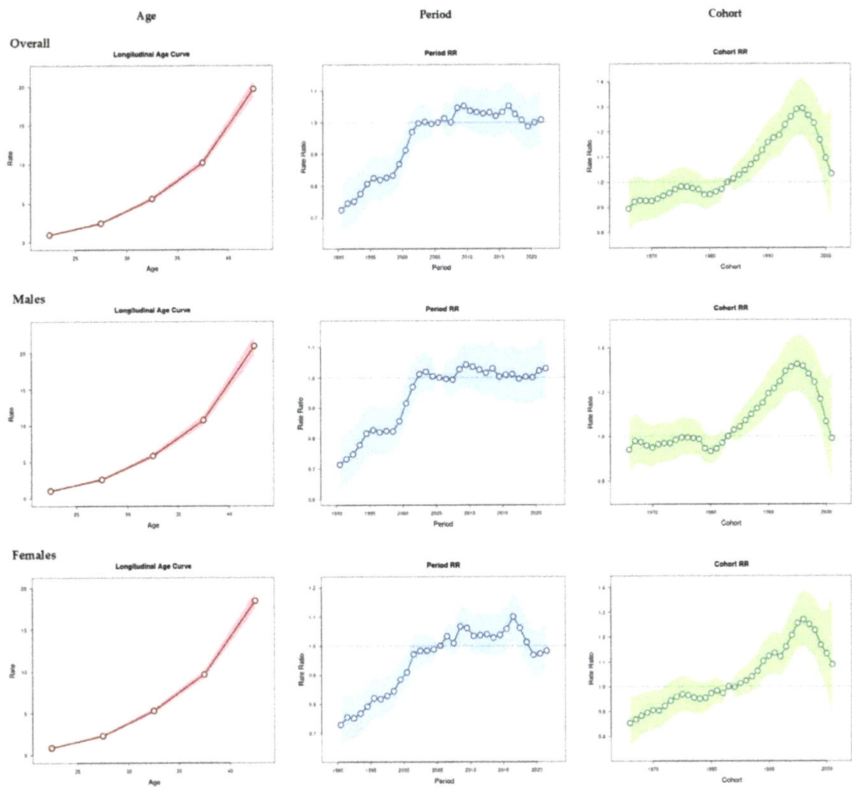


**Figure 3.** Age–period–cohort effects on EO-CRC incidence rates (males and females) from 1990 to 2021.

The APC analysis revealed that being over 25 years old, the period from 2005–2021, and being born after 1983 were important factors influencing EO-CRC incidence rates.

The fitted time trend represents the change in expected EO-CRC incidence over time for the reference age, adjusted for the cohort effects. The fitted time trend is increasing with a sharp increase after 2000, with an acute decrease in females from 2017 to 2021 (Figure 4).

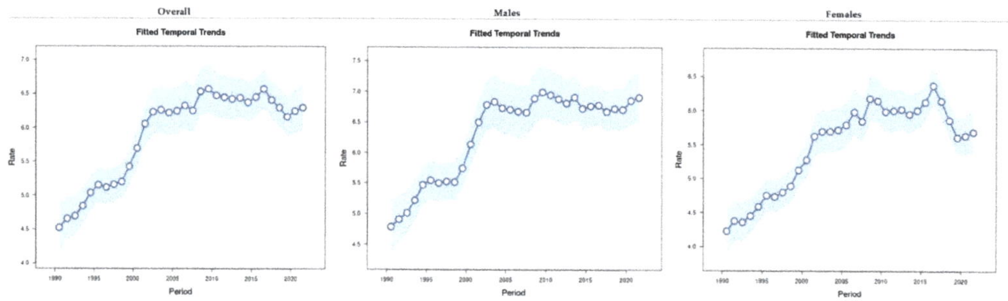


**Figure 4.** The overall age, period, and cohort effects on the EO-CRC incidence rates (per 100,000 population) by sex group from 1990 to 2021.

## 4. Discussion

To the best of our knowledge, this is the first study to examine the long-term trends and APC effects of EO-CRC in the US from 1990 to 2021, using comprehensive data from the GBD 2021 study. Our study revealed a significant increase in EO-CRC incidence over the past three decades, with a 34% rise in age-standardized incidence rates from 32.9 per 100,000 in 1990 to 43.9 per 100,000 in 2021. The greatest increase was observed in individuals aged 40–44. The APC analysis highlighted critical factors influencing EO-CRC incidence, including being over 25 years old, the period from 2005–2021, and being born after 1983. These findings align with previous research, emphasizing the impact of lifestyle changes and genetic predispositions on EO-CRC trends.

The greatest increase was observed in individuals aged 40–44, with incident cases rising by 59% and incidence rates by 37%. This substantial rise highlights a growing public health concern that necessitates urgent attention. Local drift analysis indicated an increase in EO-CRC incidence among those aged 22 and above, peaking at age 42. The cohort effect showed that individuals born after 1983 were at elevated risk, with the incidence ratio peaking around 1996 before declining. This suggests that younger cohorts may be experiencing different or additional risk factors compared to older cohorts.

Our findings are consistent with previous research showing a significant global rise in EO-CRC incidence. Patel et al. (2021) emphasized the rising burden in individuals under 50, linking EO-CRC trends to lifestyle changes and genetic predispositions [20]. Their recommendations led to updated guidelines for colorectal cancer screening, advocating for earlier screening starting at age 45 due to the high prevalence of neoplasia in the young population. Similarly, a global systematic review also documented an increase in young-onset CRC across multiple countries, particularly in North America and Europe [21–23].

Multiple studies have emphasized that the increased incidence in EO-CRC is primarily attributed to shifts in dietary patterns and increasingly sedentary lifestyle, which exacerbate CRC risk [20,24–30]. A case-control study by Low et al. identified obesity, diabetes, and smoking as prominent risk factors for EO-CRC among US veterans aged 18–49 [24]. Additionally, the study highlighted the complex interplay of diet and metabolic health, identifying regular alcohol consumption, hypertension, higher BMI, and increased fish consumption as key contributors to EO-CRC in a Chinese population [25]. While fish consumption was initially identified as a potential risk factor, this finding is unusual. Most CRC epidemiological studies indicate that fish is either neutral or protective, except in specific regions like northern Iceland where fish contamination is an issue. Furthermore, sedentary behavior, unhealthy diet, and family history, increased metabolic risk factors such as hypertension, dyslipidemia, and type 2 diabetes significantly raise the likelihood of developing colorectal adenocarcinoma [26–30].

Findings from our APC analysis highlighted the importance of distinguishing between age, period, and cohort effects in understanding EO-CRC trends. The rapid increase in incidence after age 25, irrespective of sex, suggests that interventions targeting young adults could be crucial. Moreover, the period effect from 2005 onwards, which showed a worsening trend, indicates that recent environmental or lifestyle changes are likely contributors to the rising incidence. This aligns with the observed increase in incidence rates among individuals born after 1983, peaking around 1996, which could reflect generational shifts in risk factors.

Although our study did not assess EO-CRC by cancer location due to data constraints, it is essential to note that a combination of sigmoidoscopy and fecal immunochemical test (FIT) is most appropriate for distal/rectal cancer screening, while colonoscopy and/or FIT are adequate for proximal colon screening. Future studies should aim to include cancer location to provide more specific screening recommendations.

Considering the risk factors associated with EO-CRC, they underscore the importance of adopting a multifaceted approach to prevention. Dietary guidelines should emphasize a balanced and nutrient-rich diet, as a well-rounded nutritional intake plays a critical role in reducing EO-CRC risk. Coupled with the promotion of regular physical activity, these lifestyle modifications can significantly mitigate the risk of this condition. Furthermore, targeted health screening, particularly among high-risk cohorts born between 1983 and 2016, is crucial for early detection and timely treatment, which can further aid in the prevention and management of EO-CRC.

The escalating burden of EO-CRC necessitates immediate action from healthcare policymakers and clinicians. While current screening guidelines recommend colorectal cancer screening from age 45 onwards for the average-risk populations, evidence suggests that even younger individuals may be at significant risk, particularly those with a family history or known genetic predispositions. Therefore, a comprehensive understanding of lifestyle factors impacting EO-CRC risk across different demographics and age groups is crucial. Analyzing genetic markers can help identify specific high-risk populations that would benefit from targeted screening and preventive measures. Additionally, evaluating the effectiveness of current screening guidelines and considering lowering the recommended screening age for certain high-risk groups under 45 is imperative. Furthermore, investigating socioeconomic disparities in healthcare access can shed light on the reasons behind delayed diagnoses and worse outcomes, enabling the development of targeted interventions to address these inequalities. By conducting multifaceted research, tailored strategies for prevention, early detection, and improved outcomes can be developed to combat the rising burden of EO-CRC.

*Strengths and Limitations*

A significant strength of this study is its use of the comprehensive GBD 2021 dataset, providing long-term data across 31 years for robust analysis. The APC model allowed a detailed exploration of age, period, and cohort effects on EO-CRC incidence. However, the study is limited by its reliance on aggregated national data, which may obscure regional disparities in EO-CRC trends. The GHDx dataset did not provide information on cancer location (proximal colon, distal colon, or rectal cancers). Additionally, lifestyle risk factors and genetic predispositions were not directly analyzed due to data constraints. We acknowledge the importance of analyzing ethnicity in CRC incidence studies. While our current study does not include this analysis due to data limitations, we plan to address this significant aspect in future research. Furthermore, reliance on public data might have introduced inaccuracies or inconsistencies in cancer classification.

## 5. Conclusions

Our study delivers important insights into the increasing incidence of EO-CRC in the US over the past three decades. Our findings reveal a consistent and substantial rise in incidence rates, particularly among individuals aged 40–44. The APC analysis underscores the complex interplay between age, period, and cohort effects. Our research strengthens the call for refining early detection strategies, increasing public awareness, and expanding studies into the genetic and lifestyle factors contributing to the growing EO-CRC burden. Addressing these issues through targeted research and public health interventions will be crucial in mitigating the future impact of this disease.

**Author Contributions:** Conceptualization, W.A.A. and A.S.B.; methodology, A.S.B.; software, A.S.B.; validation, W.A.A. and A.S.B.; formal analysis, A.S.B.; investigation, A.S.B.; resources, W.A.A. and A.S.B.; data curation, A.S.B.; writing—original draft preparation, W.A.A. and A.S.B.; writing—review and editing, W.A.A., M.B.W. and A.S.B.; visualization, A.S.B.; supervision, M.B.W.; project administration, A.S.B.; funding acquisition, A.S.B. All authors have read and agreed to the published version of the manuscript.

**Funding:** This research received no external funding.

**Institutional Review Board Statement:** Not applicable.

**Informed Consent Statement:** Not applicable.

**Data Availability Statement:** The data related to this research is available from https://ghdx.healthdata.org/gbd-2021.

**Acknowledgments:** We gratefully acknowledge the Institute for Health Metrics and Evaluation (IHME) for their dedication to global health research and for providing access to the Global Burden of Disease (GBD) 2021 study data. The availability of such high-quality data has been instrumental in enabling our analysis and has significantly contributed to the robustness of our findings. We extend our sincere thanks to all the researchers and contributors involved in the GBD 2021 study for their invaluable work.

**Conflicts of Interest:** W.A.A. and A.S.B.: No conflicts of interest exist. M.B.W: Michael B. Wallace has no conflicts of interest directly related to the subject of this manuscript. However, over the past 36 months, he had the following conflicts of interest: He has been a consultant for Verily, Boston Scientific, Endiatix, Fujifilm, Medtronic, Surgical Automations. He receives grant support from Fujifilm, Boston Scientific, Olympus, Medtronic, Ninepoint Medical, Cosmo/Aries Pharmaceuticals. He has stock/stock options in Virgo Inc., Surgical Automations. He has been consulting on behalf of the Mayo Clinic for Boston Scientific. Microtek. He receives general payments/minor food and beverage from Synergy Pharmaceuticals, Boston Scientific, Cook Medical.

## References

1. Rex, D.K.; Boland, C.R.; Dominitz, J.A.; Giardiello, F.M.; Johnson, D.A.; Kaltenbach, T.; Levin, T.R.; Lieberman, D.; Robertson, D.J. Colorectal cancer screening: Recommendations for physicians and patients from the US Multi-Society Task Force on Colorectal Cancer. *Gastroenterology* **2017**, *153*, 307–323. [CrossRef]
2. Patel, S.G.; Karlitz, J.J.; Yen, T.; Lieu, C.H.; Boland, C.R. The rising tide of early-onset colorectal cancer: A comprehensive review of epidemiology, clinical features, biology, risk factors, prevention, and early detection. *Lancet Gastroenterol. Hepatol.* **2022**, *7*, 262–274. [CrossRef] [PubMed]
3. Siegel, R.L.; Giaquinto, A.N.; Jemal, A. Cancer statistics, 2024. *CA Cancer J. Clin.* **2024**, *74*, 12–49. [CrossRef]
4. Bailey, C.E.; Hu, C.Y.; You, Y.N.; Bednarski, B.K.; Rodriguez-Bigas, M.A.; Skibber, J.M.; Cantor, S.B.; Chang, G.J. Increasing disparities in the age-related incidences of colon and rectal cancers in the United States, 1975–2010. *JAMA Surg.* **2015**, *150*, 17–22. [CrossRef]
5. Montminy, E.M.; Zhou, M.; Maniscalco, L.; Penrose, H.; Yen, T.; Patel, S.G.; Wu, X.C.; Karlitz, J.J. Trends in the Incidence of Early-Onset Colorectal Adenocarcinoma Among Black and White US Residents Aged 40 to 49 Years, 2000–2017. *JAMA Netw. Open* **2021**, *4*, e2130433. [CrossRef]
6. Wu, C.W.; Lui, R.N. Early-onset colorectal cancer: Current insights and future directions. *World J. Gastrointest. Oncol.* **2022**, *14*, 230–241. [CrossRef]

7. Ullah, F.; Pillai, A.S.B.; Omar, N.; Dima, D.; Harichand, S. Early-Onset Colorectal Cancer: Current Insights. *Cancers* **2023**, *15*, 3202. [CrossRef] [PubMed]
8. Carethers, J.M. Screening for colorectal cancer in African Americans: Determinants and rationale for an earlier age to commence screening. *Dig. Dis. Sci.* **2015**, *60*, 711–721. [CrossRef] [PubMed]
9. Wolf, A.M.D.; Fontham, E.T.H.; Church, T.R.; Flowers, C.R.; Guerra, C.E.; LaMonte, S.J.; Etzioni, R.; McKenna, M.T.; Oeffinger, K.C.; Shih, Y.T.; et al. Colorectal cancer screening for average-risk adults: 2018 guideline update from the American Cancer Society. *CA Cancer J. Clin.* **2018**, *68*, 250–281. [CrossRef] [PubMed]
10. US Preventive Services Task Force; Davidson, K.W.; Barry, M.J.; Mangione, C.M.; Cabana, M.; Caughey, A.S.B..; Davis, E.M.; Donahue, K.E.; Doubeni, C.A.; Krist, A.H.; et al. Screening for Colorectal Cancer: US Preventive Services Task Force Recommendation Statement. *JAMA* **2021**, *325*, 1965–1977.
11. Montminy, E.M.; Zhou, M.; Maniscalco, L.; Heda, R.; Kim, M.K.; Patel, S.G.; Wu, X.C.; Itzkowitz, S.H.; Karlitz, J.J. Shifts in the Proportion of Distant Stage Early-Onset Colorectal Adenocarcinoma in the United States. *Cancer Epidemiol. Biomark. Prev.* **2022**, *31*, 334–341. [CrossRef]
12. Gabriel, E.; Attwood, K.; Al-Sukhni, E.; Erwin, D.; Boland, P.; Nurkin, S. Age-related rates of colorectal cancer and the factors associated with overall survival. *J. Gastrointest. Oncol.* **2018**, *9*, 96–110. [CrossRef]
13. Gabriel, E.; Ostapoff, K.; Attwood, K.; Al-Sukhni, E.; Boland, P.; Nurkin, S. Disparities in the Age-Related Rates of Colorectal Cancer in the United States. *Am. Surg.* **2017**, *83*, 640–647. [CrossRef]
14. Shah, R.R.; Millien, V.O.; da Costa, W.L., Jr.; Oluyomi, A.O.; Gould Suarez, M.; Thrift, A.P. Trends in the incidence of early-onset colorectal cancer in all 50 United States from 2001 through 2017. *Cancer* **2022**, *128*, 299–310. [CrossRef]
15. Abualkhair, W.H.; Zhou, M.; Ahnen, D.; Yu, Q.; Wu, X.C.; Karlitz, J.J. Trends in incidence of early-onset colorectal cancer in the United States among those approaching screening age. *JAMA Netw. Open* **2020**, *3*, e1920407. [CrossRef]
16. Cercek, A.; Chatila, W.K.; Yaeger, R.; Walch, H.; Fernandes, G.D.S.; Krishnan, A.; Palmaira, L.; Maio, A.; Kemel, Y.; Srinivasan, P.; et al. A Comprehensive Comparison of Early-Onset and Average-Onset Colorectal Cancers. *J. Natl. Cancer Inst.* **2021**, *113*, 1683–1692. [CrossRef] [PubMed]
17. Akimoto, N.; Ugai, T.; Zhong, R.; Hamada, T.; Fujiyoshi, K.; Giannakis, M.; Wu, K.; Cao, Y.; Ng, K.; Ogino, S. Rising incidence of early-onset colorectal cancer—A call to action. *Nat. Rev. Clin. Oncol.* **2021**, *18*, 230–243. [CrossRef] [PubMed]
18. GBD 2021 Diseases and Injuries Collaborators. Global incidence, prevalence, years lived with disability (YLDs), disa-bility-adjusted life-years (DALYs), and healthy life expectancy (HALE) for 371 diseases and injuries in 204 countries and territories and 811 subnational locations, 1990–2021: A systematic analysis for the Global Burden of Disease Study 2021. *Lancet.* **2024**, *403*, 2133–2161. [CrossRef]
19. Rosenberg, P.S.; Check, D.P.; Anderson, W.F. A web tool for age-period-cohort analysis of cancer incidence and mortality rates. *Cancer Epidemiol. Biomark. Prev.* **2014**, *23*, 2296–2302. [CrossRef]
20. Patel, S.G.; May, F.P.; Anderson, J.C.; Burke, C.A.; Dominitz, J.A.; Gross, S.A.; Jacobson, B.C.; Shaukat, A.; Robertson, D.J. Updates on age to start and stop colorectal cancer screening: Recommendations from the U.S. Multi-Society Task Force on Colorectal Cancer. *Gastrointest. Endosc.* **2022**, *95*, 1–15. [CrossRef]
21. Saad El Din, K.; Loree, J.M.; Sayre, E.C.; Gill, S.; Brown, C.J.; Dau, H.; De Vera, M.A. Trends in the epidemiology of young-onset colorectal cancer: A worldwide systematic review. *BMC Cancer* **2020**, *20*, 288. [CrossRef]
22. Voigtländer, S.; Hakimhashemi, A.; Grundmann, N.; Rees, F.; Meyer, M.; Algül, H.; Müller-Nordhorn, J. Trends of colorectal cancer incidence according to age, anatomic site, and histological subgroup in Bavaria: A registry-based study. *Front. Oncol.* **2022**, *12*, 904546. [CrossRef]
23. Schell, D.; Ullah, S.; Brooke-Smith, M.E.; Hollington, P.; Yeow, M.; Karapetis, C.S.; Watson, D.I.; Pandol, S.J.; Roberts, C.T.; Barreto, S.G. Gastrointestinal Adenocarcinoma Incidence and Survival Trends in South Australia, 1990–2017. *Cancers* **2022**, *4*, 275. [CrossRef] [PubMed]
24. Low, E.E.; Demb, J.; Liu, L.; Earles, A.; Bustamante, R.; Williams, C.D.; Provenzale, D.; Kaltenbach, T.; Gawron, A.J.; Martinez, M.E.; et al. Risk Factors for Early-Onset Colorectal Cancer. *Gastroenterology* **2020**, *159*, 492–501.e7. [CrossRef] [PubMed]
25. Pan, Z.; Huang, J.; Huang, M.; Yao, Z.; Huang, J.; Chen, J.; Yu, X.; Wang, R. Risk factors for early-onset colorectal cancer: A large-scale Chinese cohort study. *J. Natl. Cancer Cent.* **2023**, *3*, 28–34. [CrossRef]
26. O'Sullivan, D.E.; Sutherland, R.L.; Town, S.; Chow, K.; Fan, J.; Forbes, N.; Heitman, S.J.; Hilsden, R.J.; Brenner, D.R. Risk Factors for Early-Onset Colorectal Cancer: A Systematic Review and Meta-analysis. *Clin. Gastroenterol. Hepatol.* **2022**, *20*, 1229–1240.e5. [CrossRef] [PubMed]
27. Hua, H.; Jiang, Q.; Sun, P.; Xu, X. Risk factors for early-onset colorectal cancer: Systematic review and meta-analysis. *Front. Oncol.* **2023**, *13*, 1132306. [CrossRef]
28. Li, Q.; Weitz, J.; Li, C.; Schardey, J.; Weiss, L.; Wirth, U.; Zimmermann, P.; Bazhin, A.V.; Werner, J.; Kühn, F. Smoking as a risk factor for colorectal neoplasms in young individuals? A systematic meta-analysis. *Int. J. Color. Dis.* **2023**, *38*, 114. [CrossRef]

29. Khoa Ta, H.D.; Nguyen, N.N.; Ho, D.K.N.; Nguyen, H.D.; Ni, Y.C.; Yee, K.X.; Pan, S.R.; Nguyen, H.S.; Thai Hoang Phuoc, T.; Chen, M.-J.; et al. Association of diabetes mellitus with early-onset colorectal cancer: A systematic review and meta-analysis of 19 studies including 10 million individuals and 30,000 events. *Diabetes Metab. Syndr.* **2023**, *17*, 102828. [CrossRef]
30. Schumacher, A.J.; Chen, Q.; Attaluri, V.; McLemore, E.C.; Chao, C.R. Metabolic Risk Factors Associated with Early-Onset Colorectal Adenocarcinoma: A Case-Control Study at Kaiser Permanente Southern California. *Cancer Epidemiol. Biomark. Prev.* **2021**, *30*, 1792–1798. [CrossRef]

cancers

MDPI

*Review*

# Influence of Rurality on Oral Cancer Trends among Organisation for Economic Co-Operation and Development (OECD) Member Countries—A Scoping Review

**Poornima Ramamurthy [1,2,*], Dileep Sharma [1,3,*], Alan Clough [4] and Peter Thomson [5]**

1 College of Medicine and Dentistry, James Cook University, Cairns 4870, Australia
2 Eleanor Duncan Aboriginal Services, Mardi 2259, Australia
3 School of Health Sciences, The University of Newcastle, Ourimbah 2258, Australia
4 College of Public Health, Medical and Veterinary Sciences, James Cook University, Cairns 4870, Australia; alan.clough@jcu.edu.au
5 School of Medicine and Dentistry, Griffith University, Southport 4215, Australia; p.thomson@griffith.edu.au
* Correspondence: poornima.ramamurthy@my.jcu.edu.au (P.R.); dileep.sharma@newcastle.edu.au (D.S.)

**Simple Summary:** Oral cancer affects the mouth and throat areas. It is a major cause of death for older people in developed countries. This review looked at how living in rural areas influences oral cancer trends in these countries. The studies from these countries showed increasing rates of oral cancer in rural areas of the US, Australia, Canada, and Europe. Older people are more affected by these cancers than younger groups. The main risk factors are tobacco use, alcohol consumption, and HPV infections. People in rural areas often do not know much about HPV-related cancers. They also tend to use more tobacco and alcohol than city dwellers. Even in developed countries, living in rural areas can lead to shorter lifespans for oral cancer patients. This is mainly because it is harder for them to access specialized cancer treatment centres and advanced medical care. In summary, where people live can significantly impact their chances of surviving oral cancer, even in wealthy nations.

**Abstract:** Oral cancer is the general term used to describe cancers of the oral cavity and oropharyngeal region. These cancers are one of the leading causes of death in elderly residents within the Organisation for Economic Co-operation and Development (OECD) member countries in the 21st century. This scoping review was carried out to assess the influence of rurality on oral cancer trends and patterns among OECD member countries. Four online databases (Medline, PubMed, Scopus, and CINAHL) were searched for studies that reported on oral cancer trends in rural and remote areas in OECD member countries. A total of 1143 articles were obtained initially; among them, 995 papers were screened to include 18 articles for this scoping review. Studies have reported increasing incidence and prevalence in the United States, Australia, Canada, and European countries wherein risk factors such as tobacco, alcohol, and human papilloma virus (HPV) infections were associated with oral and oropharyngeal cancers. Awareness among people living in rural areas about HPV-related cancers was very low, while rates of tobacco and alcohol abuse were noted to be rising more rapidly than among their urban counterparts. Furthermore, the ageing population was most affected compared to the younger age groups of people with oral and oropharyngeal cancer that are prevalent in these regions. Overall, despite living in developed countries, rurality was noted to be a significant factor in the lower life expectancy of oral cancer patients, mainly due to the limited accessibility to tertiary cancer care centres and advanced medical care.

**Keywords:** oral cancer; incidence; prevalence; risk factors; rural and remote population; OECD member countries

## 1. Introduction

Oral cancer is one of the leading causes of death among head and neck cancers worldwide [1]. Malignancies can occur in any tissue in the head and neck region, but most tumours in this region develop from the mucosa lining the upper aerodigestive tract and are more likely to be classified as squamous cell carcinoma (SCC) [2]. The recent literature suggests an increasing trend in the development of oral cancer among rural populations around the globe [3,4]. Notably, residents of rural areas experience below-average life expectancy compared to urban dwellers attributable to various sociodemographic and geographic factors, such as age, gender, rurality, low health awareness, and educational and employment levels, along with limited access to healthcare services [5–11].

The Organisation for Economic Co-operation and Development (OECD) member countries and key partners represent 80% of world trade and investment [12]. In regard to rural and remote populations in OECD member countries, the available evidence indicates that several factors contribute to an increasing trend of oral and oropharyngeal cancers [13]. In case of OECD member countries, rural populations are at a high risk of head and neck carcinoma (HNC) and lower life expectancy in comparison to their urban counterparts, either due to their remoteness from the tertiary healthcare centres or the increased burden from family life, work, financial, and educational factors which influence the overall quality of life [13].

Since the beginning of the 21st century, multiple studies have been conducted globally to assess the trends of oral and oropharyngeal cancers in rural and remote communities, including a recent systemic review focusing on rural United States [14]. In the United States, cancer is the second leading cause of death with an estimated 370,300 people diagnosed with some form of head and neck cancer [15]. Multiple studies conducted in the USA suggested that increased oral cancer incidence was associated with rurality and poverty in men of African-American ethnicity [5,16–21]. In another study, lifetime HPV risk in young adults was noted to be higher in males (91.3%) than females (84.6%) [22]. Other factors that play an important role include the following: reduced access to healthcare facilities; unemployment; sedentary lifestyle; and lower community cohesion [23]. Interestingly, oral cavity cancers were common in older males, particularly in African-American men, but oropharyngeal cancers were more commonly noted in younger Caucasian males [24]. The association between HPV and oropharyngeal cancer showed significant variation with increased knowledge about HPV in Caucasians compared to African Americans [17,18]. However, tobacco and alcohol abuse were the dominant risk factors for SCC among both the races [18]. A 225% increase in HPV-associated oropharyngeal cancer between 2010 and 2016 was also noted [25]. Studies conducted in Florida confirmed that rural residents lacked knowledge of oral and oropharyngeal cancer compared to their urban counterparts, suggesting a need to educate the population in rural areas about the risk factors and symptoms of oral cancer [26].

In Europe, oral and pharyngeal cancers are the seventh leading type of cancer. In Germany alone, there are more than 10,000 new cases diagnosed annually [12]. A total of 3127 new cases of oral and pharyngeal cancer were recorded between 2000 and 2006 within the state of Schleswig–Holstein, Germany, with more than 80% of all cases diagnosed as SCC [12]. Another German study conducted in rural communities with a high prevalence of HPV infection showed its significant influence and resulted in highly variable numbers of incidence rates of SCC [27]. Overall, studies conducted in the USA, Canada, Germany, Spain, French territories, and in Australia all reported an increased rate of incidence in rural communities compared to their urban counterparts [2,12,13,15,18,23,25–42].

Australian studies point towards an increasing number of oral cancer cases diagnosed in the advanced stages of the disease with reasons for a delay in diagnosis including regional isolation, a lack of knowledge about the risk factors and symptoms, tobacco and alcohol abuse, and HPV-related oropharyngeal squamous cell carcinoma [38,40,41]. A high prevalence of tobacco and alcohol consumption along with betel (areca) nut consumption was noted among Chinese, South Asian, and Taiwanese immigrants living in regional

Canada with low socioeconomic profiles, which contributed significantly to the increased incidence of oral cavity cancer among older age group men [23].

While there are multiple studies that have been published from OECD countries, there is no clear consensus on the influence of rurality on oral and oropharyngeal cancer trends in most OECD member countries. Hence, this scoping review focuses on the oral cancer trends in the rural and remote communities of the OECD member countries. The objective of this review is to identify the gap in research on oral cancer trends and the influence of rurality on these trends.

## 2. Methods

The framework for this scoping review, described below, was adapted from the methodology described by Arksey and O'Malley and Sucharew et al. to ensure comprehensive and reproducible, structured literature searches were completed for relevant information, with minimal bias [2,43,44]. All the steps for conducting a scoping review as outlined by Arksey and O'Malley were followed except the optional consultation, since this was not feasible in our context [43,44]. The scoping review and the search strategy were driven by the following research question.

How does rurality influence oral cancer trends in OECD member countries?

### 2.1. Inclusion Criteria

Retrospective and observational studies which assessed the oral cancer trends, such as risk factors, incidence, and prevalence of oral cancer, with no age or gender restrictions, published in the English language, and studies carried out in rural populations of OECD member countries from 2000 onwards were included in this scoping review, to assess the OSCC trends in the 21st century.

### 2.2. Exclusion Criteria

Any type of studies carried out in countries other than OECD member countries, focusing on cancer in regions other than the oral cavity and oropharynx, systematic, scoping or narrative literature reviews, animal studies, opinion papers, conference papers, case reports, case series, and articles published in non-English languages were excluded. Additionally, studies that included interventions or solely focusing on the urban population were also excluded from this review.

### 2.3. Search Strategy

After discussion with a research librarian, the formulation of the search strategy was finalised to identify suitable keywords for electronic database searches. The Medline (Ovid), PubMed, Scopus, and CINAHL databases were searched using the relevant keywords. Supplementary Table S1 consists of the search strategy and the search strings used to retrieve studies included in this review.

### 2.4. Study Selection

Two of the reviewers independently screened all the titles and abstracts and excluded the studies which did not meet the inclusion criteria. Disagreements between the two reviewers were resolved by the third reviewer. The Endnote (v20.3 Clarivate, Philadelphia, PA, USA) bibliographic software was used to import, screen, and manage the references.

## 3. Results

The initial search from all the four databases yielded a total of 1143 articles. After removing the duplicates, 995 articles were screened for inclusion by title and abstract review. The reviewers agreed to consider 22 articles for full text review and final inclusion. Based on the predetermined inclusion and exclusion criteria, 18 papers were included for this scoping review. Additionally, reference lists of these papers were searched to ensure that all the relevant studies were included in this review. The Preferred Reporting Items for

Systematic review and Meta-analysis (PRISMA) flow chart illustrates the literature search and selection process followed in this scoping review (Figure 1). The main findings and basic characteristics of the articles included in this scoping review are presented in Table 1.

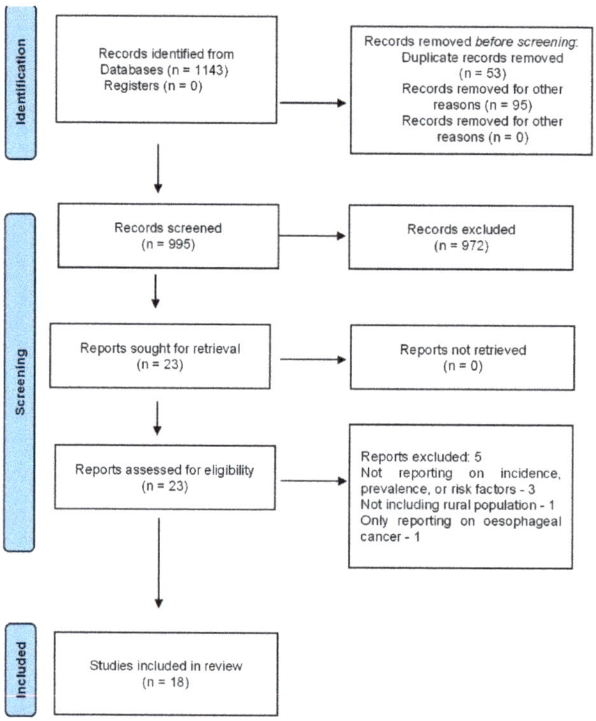


**Figure 1.** PRISMA diagram of the literature search strategy for scoping review.

Studies conducted on cancer databases from Canada, USA, France, Germany, and Australia have reported incidence of oral and oropharyngeal cancers and the factors contributing to the increase in incidence and mortality, such as, socioeconomic deprivation, suburbanisation, aged population, rurality, and tobacco and alcohol abuse, along with HPV-related oral cancer. Eleven of the studies focused on the incidence rates including data on some or all the above parameters [14,16,17,20,23,34,35,40,41,45,46]. The incidence, i.e., the reported cases of oral and oropharyngeal cancers, in the studies included in this review ranged from 34 to 154,525, with the latter utilizing multiple data sources such as the National Cancer Surveillance, epidemiology, and Surveillance, Epidemiology, and End Results (SEER) registries [14,16]. Within the studies reviewed, only nine included a comparison group, such as the urban population, while the rest collected data from the rural population alone. Most of the incidence reports consist of a significant rise in the percentage of the population affected by oral cancer in people above 40 years of age ranging from 45 to 88.6% of the people affected, compared to fewer being affected in the younger age group [14,40]. In the studies conducted in the USA, the range of percentage increase in incidence of oral cancer compared to the urban population was between 15.7% and 6.5% [20,47], while the highest increase due to rurality was reported in an Australian study affecting the Aboriginal rural population at 37.5% [42].

**Table 1.** Overview of studies included in the scoping review.

| Citation | Participants | Data Analysis Sites | Methodology/Data Sources | Outcomes and Factors Identified |
|---|---|---|---|---|
| Benard et al. (2008) [20] | 9464 | Centers for Disease Control and Prevention<br>National Program of Cancer Registries | Retrospective analysis<br>Registers and county SES data and Surveillance, Epidemiology, and End Results (SEER) data from 1998 to 2003 | Rurality—6.5% higher rates<br>High school education—higher incidence in areas with <85% high school education<br>Ethnicity—Hispanic and Asian/Pacific Islander race females showed lower ASR *<br>Caucasians—lower rates in rural areas<br>African Americans—higher rates than Caucasians in both rural and urban areas<br>Income—lower income groups had higher incidence in males<br>Poverty—higher poverty<br>Current smoking—increased OSCC risk |
| Abreu et al. (2010) [40] | 1197 | The University of Western Australia | Retrospective analysis<br>Western Australian Cancer Registry from 1982 to 2006 | Rurality—11% higher rates in men in country areas<br>Gender—men 2.4 times higher than women ASR *<br>Age—88% in <40 years<br>Indigenous status—non-indigenous 70% (men) and 55% (women) higher rates than indigenous |
| Frydrych et al. (2014) [42] | 424 | The University of Western Australia<br>Curtin University | Retrospective analysis<br>Western Australian Cancer Registry from 1990 to 1999 | Rurality—higher incidence (68.8%) in rural Aboriginals<br>Smoker—higher (44%) in Aboriginals<br>Gender—higher (68.6%) in non-Aboriginal males<br>Age at diagnosis—higher in 50–59 yrs (37.5%) Aboriginals<br>Non-Aboriginal—higher in 60–69 yrs (30.2%) |
| Krupar et al. (2014) [27] | 34 | Department of Otolaryngology of the University Hospital Regensburg | Tissue analysis<br>Cases from hospital records of OSCC patients diagnosed between 1993 and 2010 | HPV prevalence: 50%<br>Disease stage: advanced OSCC in 58.3% HPV positives |
| | 85 | Southern Germany<br>Otolaryngology private practice OSCC | Tissue analysis | HPV prevalence: 16.1%<br>Disease stage: advanced OSCC in 33.3% HPV positives |
| Walker et al. (2015) [23] | 5473 | University of British Columbia | Retrospective analysis<br>British Columbia Cancer Registry from 1981 to 2009 | Rurality: suburban cases increase 200%; rural—12%<br>Gender: higher in males (64%) |
| Derbi et al. (2016) [41] | 2801 | The University of Western Australia | Retrospective analysis<br>Western Australian Cancer Registry between 1982 and 2009 | Tongue SCC<br>Rurality: higher in rural (57%) ASR * increase—1.4 to 3.8 (1982 vs. 2009)<br>Gender: males higher (69.2%)<br>Age: highest ASR in 60–79 yrs (208.1) |
| Javadi et al. (2017) [17] | Reported on age-adjusted rates (per 100,000) | Southern Illinois University School of Medicine | Retrospective trend analysis<br>Surveillance, Epidemiology, and End Results (SEER) 9 data from 1973 to 2012 and SEER-18 data from 2000 to 2012 | Rurality: rural areas had sharpest increase in SCC trends<br>Gender: male SCC rates higher than females in all rural areas<br>Race: Whites significant decrease (1.85%) in trends |

**Table 1.** *Cont.*

| Citation | Participants | Data Analysis Sites | Methodology/Data Sources | Outcomes and Factors Identified |
|---|---|---|---|---|
| Delagranda et al. (2018) [35] | 599 | Public and private healthcare sectors | French data protection commission from 2009 to 2013 | Gender: males higher (88.6%)<br>Age: mean, 60 yrs (males), 62 yrs (females)<br>Smoking: 89.6% (OPSCC) and 76.8% (OCSCC)<br>Alcohol: 83.7% (OPSCC) and 71.6% (OCSCC)<br>HPV infection: 32.4% (OPSCC) and 12.2% (OCSCC) |
| Radespiel-Tröger et al. (2018) [34] | 18,947 (MPC) | Bavarian Health and Food Safety Authority | Retrospective analysis<br>Bavarian cancer registry from 2003 to 2012 | Rurality: higher (51.4%) cases<br>Gender: males, overall (74.5%); rural (76%) |
| Pagedar et al. (2019) [14] | 36,183 (OCC)<br>32,793 (OPC) | University of Iowa | Retrospective analysis<br>National Cancer Institute Surveillance and Epidemiology (SEER) data from 1975<br>to 2015 | Rurality: lower annual decline in incidence 0.5% vs. 2.6% (urban) for OCC; 4.6% increase vs. 2.6% (urban) for OPC<br>Age: 45% in rural at 55–69 yrs<br>Race: 99% White<br>Stage: 47.9% localised SCC |
| Ghazawi et al. (2020) [33] | 21,685 (OCC)<br>15,965 (OPC) | McGill University | Retrospective analysis<br>Canadian Cancer Registry, Le Registre Quebecois du Cancer, Canadian Vital Statistics from 1992 to 2010 | Gender: males higher 1.69 times (OCSCC) and 3.26 times (OPSCC)<br>Age: highest incidence ≥90 yrs (OCSCC) and 60–69 yrs (OPSCC) |
| Harris et al. (2020) [47] | 40,678 | Harvard School of Dental Medicine | Retrospective analysis<br>Surveillance, Epidemiology, and End Results (SEER) data from 1990 to 2015 | Rural: increase in incidence 57.8% in rural vs. 42.1% in urban (2015)<br>SCC grades: rural—higher grade 1 (well differentiated), urban—higher Grade 2 and 3 (moderately and poorly differentiated)<br>Higher SCC rates in men: 70.4%<br>Higher incidence: White (non-Hispanic) 96%<br>Low income (<$50k): 37.9% higher OSCC<br>Long term survival better in rural population<br>SCC sites: rural—lower lip (22%); urban—base of tongue (24.9%) |
| Papenberg et al. (2020) [16] | 154,525 | West Virginia University | Retrospective analysis<br>Data from NAACCR Epidemiology and SEER from 2007 to 2013 | Sex: males higher (72.4%)<br>Race: Whites higher (92%)<br>SCC stage: stage IV (43%) HPV associated 61%<br>Smoking: 20.7% |
| Clohessy et al. (2022) [37] | 286 | Calvary Mater Hospital | Retrospective analysis<br>Data from digital medical records (DMR) from 2016 to 2017 | Sex: males higher (80.4%)<br>Age: <74 years higher (73.1%)<br>Stage 4 disease 42%<br>Patients lived 68.16 km from the multi-disciplinary team<br>Cancer sites: cutaneous (35.3%) mucosa of the oral cavity including lips (29.4%) and pharynx (19.6%) |
| Cheng et al. (2022) [45] | 92,685 | West China Hospital of Stomatology | Retrospective analysis<br>Data from Surveillance, Epidemiology, and End Results (SEER) from 1975 to 2018 | Total annual percentage change (3.2)<br>Age: >60 years (12.8)<br>Sex: males higher (6.6%)<br>Oral cancer (7.1%)<br>Oropharyngeal cancer (3.9%)<br>Black (15.2%) |

**Table 1.** *Cont.*

| Citation | Participants | Data Analysis Sites | Methodology/Data Sources | Outcomes and Factors Identified |
|---|---|---|---|---|
| Sun et al. (2023) [48] | 9887 | James Cook University | Queensland Cancer Registry: International Classification of Diseases 10th Revision from 1982 to 2018 | Sites: moderately differentiated higher (49.45%), deaths higher (63%)<br>Retromolar area higher (60.34%)<br>Sex: male–female ratio 2.51–1<br>Oral SCC cases increased by 4.49-fold during study period |
| Ramadan et al. (2023) [46] | 2000 | National Cancer Institute | Surveillance, Epidemiology, and End Results (SEER) and 18 Census Track-level SES and Rurality Database from 2006 to 2018 | Sites: oral tongue accounting for 44.6%<br>Race: White people with tongue OCC 47%, Black population 36.8%, AAPI 49.2%, Hispanic 50.50%<br>OCC highest in White Americans, 2.86 per 100,000 persons, and lowest in Black Americans 1.17 per 100,000 |
| Liu et al. (2023) [49] | 39,935 | National Cancer Institute | Surveillance, Epidemiology, and End Results (SEER) and 18 Census Track-level SES and Rurality Database from 2000 to 2016 | Race: NH White 54.8%, NH Black 36.1%, Pacific Islander 56.5%<br>Sex: male—61.4% in NH Whites, NH Blacks 59.9%<br>Age: mean age in NH Whites 66.03 and NH Blacks 62.64 |

* ASR: age-adjusted incidence rates (per 100,000); OPSCC: oropharyngeal squamous cell carcinoma; MPC: mouth and pharynx cancer; NH: non-Hispanic.

## 4. Discussion

This scoping review was conducted on studies involving oral cancer trends in rural and remote areas within the OECD member countries. All data collected in these studies included the sociodemographic profiles of rural populations, incidence and prevalence, and risk factors for oral and oropharyngeal cancers. Most of the studies included used retrospective analysis of data available from various state or national cancer registries.

It is evident that a substantially higher risk of oral cancer exists in the rural population in comparison to urban counterparts, reported to be ranging between 6.5% and 68.8% incidence in the rural population [20,42]. Generally, increasing age and long-standing tobacco and alcohol abuse are the leading causes of the increased incidence of oral cavity cancers in these regions. However, in most studies, the effect was more prominent in rural men than women. Harris et al. (2020) reported on 40,678 subjects in which they noted that a large percentage of rural men were affected by oral cancer compared to the urban population, but a similar number of women were affected in both rural and urban populations [47]. A study conducted in Queensland has shown the high prevalence of SCC in males over 60 years of age [48]. Similar trends were noted in another Australian study with 68.8% of rural men affected by oral cancer due to various risk behaviours such as tobacco and alcohol abuse along with HPV infections [42]. A study conducted in the USA presented the overall temporal trend of OC-OPC and the changes in fundamental factors, emphasising on the incidence and survival rate over the past 40 years [45]. Two studies conducted in the USA reported strong evidence to attribute rurality as the risk factor in oral cancer where a lack of awareness and the absence of prevention and early detection by healthcare providers are contributing to the soaring cases in recent decades [26,47].

The trends of oral and oropharyngeal cancers in the rural and remote areas of the OECD member countries included in this scoping review are directly related to the increasing age, gender, level of education and poverty, ethnicity, smoking status, and occupation. The advancement of age and lack of awareness about the lifestyle choices that are prevalent for a longer duration of time, along with other risk factors, such as regional isolation or remoteness, play a significant role in the increased incidence. A recent retrospective cohort study that examined the effect of remoteness on oral cancers noted that there was significant delay in the commencement of treatment from both the onset of symptoms (6 months vs. 3 months) and diagnosis (47 days vs. 36 days) in regional/remote patients, when compared to metropolitan patients in New South Wales, Australia [36]. This is particularly important since most patients undergo surgery in a metropolitan tertiary hospital through multiple specialist referrals between regional and metropolitan practices [36]. Additionally, the distance of patients' residence from a multidisciplinary hospital has recently been reported to be a contributing factor, with the risk of being diagnosed with an advanced stage of cancer increasing approximately 1.5 times when the distance is over 100 km [37].

Poverty level, ethnicity, and education levels play a key role in the increasing incidence of oral cancer trends in the 21st century in the OECD countries' rural populations. Poverty is directly associated with an increased incidence of oral cancer in countries like the USA, Canada, and Australia [20,47]. Specifically, 10–20% poverty status was associated with decreased oral and oropharyngeal cancer incidence rates [20]. Two other studies reported that the poverty level plays a role in both the increased incidence of oral cancer and the advancement of the disease [18,38]. Ethnicity is also known to be one of the significant sociodemographic factors that can affect the risk of oral cancers. Among the studies included, at least nine of the included studies reported that ethnicity was a major consideration for determining rising oral cancer cases among various ethnic groups [14,16,17,20,23,40,45,46,49]. Generally, Caucasians have a higher rate of incidence ranging from 70% in Australia to 99% in USA [14,40]. This may be partly due to the demographic variations within the study population wherein the proportion of Caucasians is significantly higher than non-Caucasians. Other ethnic groups with higher incidence include African Americans, Pacific Islanders, and Aboriginal people living in both rural and urban areas [20,41,42,48,49]. Another US study has reported that different races show significant variations in the incidence and prevalence rates of OCC and other forms of head and neck cancer [49].

The education level of the population is also known to affect the oral cancer incidence [26,28]. Specifically, higher incidence was noted in areas with under 85% of people with high school education, which can indirectly relate to lower awareness levels around the risk factors [20]. Tobacco and alcohol were identified as the main risk factors of oral cavity and oropharyngeal cancers in most countries including the USA, France, and Australia [16,20,35]. Two studies identified tobacco and alcohol as the main risk factors for oral cancer in all age groups, with particularly increased incidence of SCC in the age group between 50 and 59 years [33,42].

Various occupational factors have been associated with an increased risk of head and neck cancers, including oral cancers. In a case–control study, long term unemployment was reported to increase the risk of oral cancers by 2.9 times in one study [50,51]. Notably, the unemployed patients with oral cancer had significantly higher smoking and alcohol consumption rates, which may in part explain the higher incidence [50]. Unemployment has also been correlated with cancer mortality at both the individual and community level [52]. A large INHANCE (International Head and Neck Cancer Epidemiology) Consortium-led analysis of pooled case–control studies from Western Europe, Latin America, Germany, and France analysed the role of occupational socioeconomic risks for head and neck cancer comprehensively [53]. This study reported that occupational socioeconomic prestige, position, and manual work increased the risk of head and neck cancer, especially if employed in the industry for 10 years or over, after adjusting for smoking and alcohol use [53]. A range of professions that had an increased risk (odds) of oral and oropharyngeal cancer were identified, including loggers, dairy farmers, and manual labourers in building and construction industries like bricklayers, painters, roof workers, reinforced concreters, road (asphalt) workers, drivers (lorries, vans, and earthmovers), and cargo handlers, particularly in males, mostly due to the male-dominated industries [54–56]. Exposure to harmful chemicals and known carcinogens including cement dust, asbestos, polycyclic aromatic hydrocarbons, inorganic dusts, and solvents over a long period of time were identified as the potential reasons for this increased risk [57–59]. Additionally, two US studies included in this review also reported that occupations with low income and living in rural areas were associated with an increased risk of oral cancers [20,47].

Human papillomavirus (HPV) is increasingly recognized as a known risk for some forms of head and neck cancers, particularly oral cancers, with rates of cancers with HPV on the rise while non-HPV cancers are on a decline [29]. Traditionally, two types of clinicopathological forms of oral and oropharyngeal cancers are described in the literature, based on the presence or absence of HPV [60]. HPV-positive tumours are known to clinically present with early lymph node metastasis, albeit better responsiveness to radiation and chemotherapy has been reported with up to a 58% reduction in the risk of death [61,62]. Furthermore, a significant correlation between the sexual practices and the awareness as well as vaccination status for HPV-related oropharyngeal cancer incidences has been identified [63]. An estimated 60–70% of oropharyngeal cancers are associated with HPV infection in developed countries such as the United States, compared to under 10% in developing or underdeveloped regions [2,64–66]. At least three of the studies included in our review identified an association between HPV infection and oropharyngeal squamous cell carcinoma, with increased risk ranging from 12 to 61% [16,27,35]. Additionally, higher education levels have also been associated with increased HPV-associated oral cancers.

## 5. Conclusions

This scoping review revealed the negative influence of rurality in oral cancer trends, particularly among socioeconomically deprived, aged, and geographically distant communities. This scoping review confirmed the limited knowledge and variations in the literature around the rural remote population in many OECD member countries vulnerable to cancer, where a lack of primary healthcare centres and tertiary cancer care facilities are expected. The gaps evident in the data around incidence, prevalence, and risk factors in many other OECD countries support the need for further population-based studies in the region, specifically in regional rural and remote areas, and a comparison to the urban population is essential. Furthermore, identifying the at-risk population can assist in designing awareness programs to implement effective intervention strategies targeting specific communities.

**Supplementary Materials:** The following supporting information can be downloaded at: https://www.mdpi.com/article/10.3390/cancers16172957/s1, Table S1: Search strategy used for retrieval of records.

**Author Contributions:** Conceptualization, P.R., A.C. and P.T.; methodology, P.R. and D.S.; formal analysis, P.R., A.C. and P.T.; data curation, P.R. and D.S.; writing—original draft preparation, P.R., A.C. and P.T.; writing—review and editing, P.R., A.C., D.S. and P.T.; supervision, A.C. and P.T. All authors have read and agreed to the published version of the manuscript.

**Funding:** P.R received Australian Government Research Training Scholarship and Tom and Dorothy Cook Scholarship in Public Health and Tropical Medicine.

**Conflicts of Interest:** The authors declare no conflict of interest.

## References

1. Sung, H.; Ferlay, J.; Siegel, R.L.; Laversanne, M.; Soerjomataram, I.; Jemal, A.; Bray, F. Global Cancer Statistics 2020: GLOBOCAN Estimates of Incidence and Mortality Worldwide for 36 Cancers in 185 Countries. *CA A Cancer J. Clin.* **2021**, *71*, 209–249. [CrossRef] [PubMed]
2. Ramamurthy, P.; Sharma, D.; Thomson, P. Oral cancer awareness in patients attending university dental clinics: A scoping review of Australian studies. *Aust. Dent. J.* **2022**, *67*, 5–11. [CrossRef]
3. Matos, S.; Boakye, E.A.; Crosby, D.; Sharma, A. Prevalence and Factors Associated with Oral Cavity and Pharyngeal Cancer Screening in a Rural Population. *OTO Open* **2021**, *5*, 2473974X211065018. [CrossRef] [PubMed]
4. Zahnd, W.E.; James, A.S.; Jenkins, W.D.; Izadi, S.R.; Fogleman, A.J.; Steward, D.E.; Colditz, G.A.; Brard, L. Rural–Urban Differences in Cancer Incidence and Trends in the United States. *Cancer Epidemiol. Biomark. Prev.* **2018**, *27*, 1265–1274. [CrossRef]
5. Weisgrau, S. Issues in rural health: Access, hospitals, and reform. *Health Care Financ. Rev.* **1995**, *17*, 1–14.
6. Weil, A.R. Access to Care, Hospitals, and More. *Health Aff.* **2022**, *41*, 473. [CrossRef] [PubMed]
7. O'Kane, G. Telehealth-Improving access for rural, regional and remote communities. *Aust. J. Rural Health* **2020**, *28*, 419–420. [CrossRef]
8. Lee, L.M. Equitable Health Care and Low-Density Living in the United States. *Narrat. Inq. Bioeth.* **2019**, *9*, 121–125. [CrossRef]
9. Gorin, S.H. Health care reform and older adults. *Health Soc. Work.* **2010**, *35*, 3–6. [CrossRef]
10. Goldfield, N.I.; Fuller, R.L. Access to Affordable, High-Quality Health Insurance for Rural Residents and Its Impact on Their Health and on Rural Hospitals. *J. Ambul. Care Manag.* **2019**, *42*, 78–85. [CrossRef]
11. Diamond, M. Working to make rural health matter. *Aust. J. Rural Health* **2019**, *27*, 266–267. [CrossRef] [PubMed]
12. Hertrampf, K.; Wiltfang, J.; Katalinic, A.; Timm, O.; Wenz, H.J. Trends in incidence, tumour sites and tumour stages of oral and pharyngeal cancer in Northern Germany. *J. Cancer Res. Clin. Oncol.* **2012**, *138*, 431–437. [CrossRef] [PubMed]
13. Zhang, H.; Dziegielewski, P.T.; Jean Nguyen, T.T.; Jeffery, C.C.; O'Connell, D.A.; Harris, J.R.; Seikaly, H. The effects of geography on survival in patients with oral cavity squamous cell carcinoma. *Oral Oncol.* **2015**, *51*, 578–585. [CrossRef]
14. Pagedar, N.A.; Kahl, A.R.; Tasche, K.K.; Seaman, A.T.; Christensen, A.J.; Howren, M.B.; Charlton, M.E. Incidence trends for upper aerodigestive tract cancers in rural United States counties. *Head Neck* **2019**, *41*, 2619–2624. [CrossRef] [PubMed]
15. Akinkugbe, A.A.; Garcia, D.T.; Brickhouse, T.H.; Mosavel, M. Lifestyle risk factor related disparities in oral cancer examination in the U.S: A population-based cross-sectional study. *BMC Public Health* **2020**, *20*, 153. [CrossRef]
16. Papenberg, B.W.; Allen, J.L.; Markwell, S.M.; Interval, E.T.; Montague, P.A.; Johnson, C.J.; Weed, S.A. Disparate survival of late-stage male oropharyngeal cancer in Appalachia. *Sci. Rep.* **2020**, *10*, 11612. [CrossRef]
17. Javadi, P.; Sharma, A.; Zahnd, W.E.; Jenkins, W.D. Evolving disparities in the epidemiology of oral cavity and oropharyngeal cancers. *Cancer Causes Control* **2017**, *28*, 635–645. [CrossRef]
18. Onicescu, G.; Hill, E.G.; Lawson, A.B.; Korte, J.E.; Gillespie, M.B. Joint disease mapping of cervical and male oropharyngeal cancer incidence in blacks and whites in South Carolina. *Spat. Spatio-Temporal Epidemiol.* **2010**, *1*, 133–141. [CrossRef]
19. Logan, H.L.; Yi, G.; Emanuel, A.S.; Shepperd, J.A.; Dodd, V.J.; Marks, J.G.; Muller, K.E.; Riley, J.L., III. Determinants of First-Time Cancer Examinations in a Rural Community: A Mechanism for Behavior Change. *Am. J. Public Health* **2015**, *105*, 1424–1431. [CrossRef]
20. Benard, V.B.; Johnson, C.J.; Thompson, T.D.; Roland, K.B.; Lai, S.M.; Cokkinides, V.; Tangka, F.; Hawkins, N.A.; Lawson, H.; Weir, H.K. Examining the association between socioeconomic status and potential human papillomavirus-associated cancers. *Cancer* **2008**, *113*, 2910–2918. [CrossRef]

21. Wiener, R.C. Association of smokeless tobacco use and smoking in adolescents in the United States: An analysis of data from the Youth Risk Behavior Surveillance System survey, 2011. *J. Am. Dent. Assoc.* **2013**, *144*, 930–938. [CrossRef] [PubMed]
22. Joseph, A.W.; D'Souza, G. Epidemiology of Human Papillomavirus-Related Head and Neck Cancer. *Otolaryngol. Clin. N. Am.* **2012**, *45*, 739–764. [CrossRef] [PubMed]
23. Walker, B.B.; Schuurman, N.; Auluck, A.; Lear, S.A.; Rosin, M. Suburbanisation of oral cavity cancers: Evidence from a geographically-explicit observational study of incidence trends in British Columbia, Canada, 1981–2010. *BMC Public Health* **2015**, *15*, 758. [CrossRef]
24. LeHew, C.W.; Weatherspoon, D.J.; Peterson, C.E.; Goben, A.; Reitmajer, K.; Sroussi, H.; Kaste, L.M. The health system and policy implications of changing epidemiology for oral cavity and oropharyngeal cancers in the United States from 1995 to 2016. *Epidemiol. Rev.* **2017**, *39*, 132–147. [CrossRef]
25. Osazuwa-Peters, N.; Boakye, E.A.; Hussaini, A.S.; Sujijantarat, N.; Ganesh, R.N.; Snider, M.; Thompson, D.; Varvares, M.A. Characteristics and predictors of oral cancer knowledge in a predominantly African American community. *PLoS ONE* **2017**, *12*, e0177787. [CrossRef]
26. Riley, J.L.; Pomery, E.A.; Dodd, V.J.; Muller, K.E.; Guo, Y.; Logan, H.L. Disparities in Knowledge of Mouth or Throat Cancer Among Rural Floridians. *J. Rural Health* **2013**, *29*, 294–303. [CrossRef]
27. Krupar, R.; Hartl, M.; Wirsching, K.; Dietmaier, W.; Strutz, J.; Hofstaedter, F. Comparison of HPV prevalence in HNSCC patients with regard to regional and socioeconomic factors. *Eur. Arch. Otorhinolaryngol.* **2014**, *271*, 1737–1745. [CrossRef] [PubMed]
28. Chang, J.T.; Levy, D.T.; Meza, R. Trends and factors related to smokeless Tobacco use in the United States. *Nicotine Tob. Res.* **2016**, *18*, 1740–1748. [CrossRef]
29. Cole, L.; Polfus, L.; Peters, E.S. Examining the incidence of human papillomavirus-associated head and neck cancers by race and ethnicity in the U.S., 1995–2005. *PLoS ONE* **2012**, *7*, e32657. [CrossRef]
30. Filion, E.J.; McClure, L.A.; Huang, D.; Seng, K.; Kaplan, M.J.; Colevas, A.D.; Gomez, S.L.; Chang, E.T.; Le, Q.T. Higher incidence of head and neck cancers among Vietnamese American men in California. *Head Neck* **2010**, *32*, 1336–1344. [CrossRef]
31. Liu, L.; Kumar, S.K.S.; Sedghizadeh, P.P.; Jayakar, A.N.; Shuler, C.F. Oral squamous cell carcinoma incidence by subsite among diverse racial and ethnic populations in California. *Oral Surg. Oral Med. Oral Pathol. Oral Radiol. Endod.* **2008**, *105*, 470–480. [CrossRef] [PubMed]
32. Cattelan, L.; Ghazawi, F.M.; Le, M.; Lagacé, F.; Savin, E.; Zubarev, A.; Gantchev, J.; Tomaszewski, M.; Sasseville, D.; Waschke, K.; et al. Epidemiologic trends and geographic distribution of esophageal cancer in Canada: A national population-based study. *Cancer Med.* **2020**, *9*, 401–417. [CrossRef]
33. Ghazawi, F.M.; Lu, J.; Savin, E.; Zubarev, A.; Chauvin, P.; Sasseville, D.; Zeitouni, A.; Litvinov, I.V. Epidemiology and Patient Distribution of Oral Cavity and Oropharyngeal SCC in Canada. *J. Cutan. Med. Surg.* **2020**, *24*, 340–349. [CrossRef]
34. Radespiel-Tröger, M.; Geiss, K.; Twardella, D.; Maier, W.; Meyer, M. Cancer incidence in urban, rural, and densely populated districts close to core cities in Bavaria, Germany. *Int. Arch. Occup. Environ. Health* **2018**, *91*, 155–174. [CrossRef]
35. Delagranda, A.; Leterme, G.; Chirpaz, E.; Ferdynus, C.; Fernandez, C.; Rubin, F. Epidemiological features of cancers of the oral cavity, oropharynx, hypopharynx and larynx cancer in Réunion Island. *Eur. Ann. Otorhinolaryngol. Head Neck Dis.* **2018**, *135*, 175–181. [CrossRef]
36. Chondur, R.; Li, S.Q.; Guthridge, S.; Lawton, P. Does relative remoteness affect chronic disease outcomes? Geographic variation in chronic disease mortality in Australia, 2002–2006. *Aust. N. Z. J. Public Health* **2014**, *38*, 117–121. [CrossRef]
37. Clohessy, J.; Hoffman, G.; Cope, D. Geographic remoteness from a multidisciplinary team is associated with an increased clinical staging of head and neck cancer: A Newcastle (Australia) study. *Int. J. Oral Maxillofac. Surg.* **2022**, *51*, 862–868. [CrossRef] [PubMed]
38. Jamieson, L.M.; Antonsson, A.; Garvey, G.; Ju, X.; Smith, M.; Logan, R.M.; Johnson, N.W.; Hedges, J.; Sethi, S.; Dunbar, T.; et al. Prevalence of Oral Human Papillomavirus Infection Among Australian Indigenous Adults. *JAMA Netw. Open* **2020**, *3*, e204951. [CrossRef] [PubMed]
39. Sethi, S.; Ju, X.; Antonsson, A.; Canfell, K.; Smith, M.A.; Garvey, G.; Hedges, J.; Jamieson, L. Oral HPV Infection among Indigenous Australians; Incidence, Persistence, and Clearance at 12-Month Follow-up. *Cancer Epidemiol. Biomark. Prev.* **2022**, *31*, 604–613. [CrossRef]
40. Abreu, L.P.; Kruger, E.; Tennant, M. Oral cancer in Western Australia, 1982–2006: A retrospective epidemiological study. *J. Oral Pathol. Med.* **2010**, *39*, 376–381. [CrossRef]
41. Derbi, H.A.; Kruger, E.; Tennant, M. Incidence of oral cancer in Western Australia (1982–2009): Trends and regional variations. *Asia Pac. J. Clin. Oncol.* **2016**, *12*, e305–e310. [CrossRef]
42. Frydrych, A.M.; Slack-Smith, L.M.; Parsons, R.; Threlfall, T. Oral cavity squamous cell carcinoma—Characteristics and survival in aboriginal and non-aboriginal Western Australians. *Open Dent. J.* **2014**, *8*, 168–174. [CrossRef]
43. Arksey, H.; O'Malley, L. Scoping studies: Towards a methodological framework. *Int. J. Soc. Res. Methodol.* **2005**, *8*, 19–32. [CrossRef]
44. Sucharew, H.; Macaluso, M. Methods for Research Evidence Synthesis: The Scoping Review Approach. *J. Hosp. Med.* **2019**, *14*, 416–418. [CrossRef] [PubMed]
45. Cheng, J.; Zhou, X.; Xu, H.; Dan, H.; Li, J.; Chen, Q. Incidence and Survival of Oral Cavity and Oropharyngeal Cancer in the United States From 1975 to 2018. *J. Oral Maxillofac. Surg.* **2022**, *80*, 1294–1305. [CrossRef] [PubMed]

46. Ramadan, S.; Lee, J.J.; Wang, R.; Jackson, R.S.; Pipkorn, P.; Rich, J.; Harbison, R.A.; Zolkind, P.; Kang, S.Y.; Puram, S.V.; et al. Neighborhood socioeconomic status and race are associated with incidence disparities in oral cavity cancers. *Oral Oncol.* **2023**, *147*, 106607. [CrossRef]
47. Harris, J.A.; Hunter, W.P.; Hanna, G.J.; Treister, N.S.; Menon, R.S. Rural patients with oral squamous cell carcinoma experience better prognosis and long-term survival. *Oral Oncol.* **2020**, *111*, 105037. [CrossRef] [PubMed]
48. Sun, A.; Sharma, D.; Choi, S.W.; Ramamurthy, P.; Thomson, P. Oral cancer in Australia: Rising incidence and worsening mortality. *J. Oral Pathol. Med.* **2023**, *52*, 328–334. [CrossRef]
49. Liu, Y.; Zhong, L.; Puram, S.V.; Mazul, A.L. Neighborhood Socioeconomic Status and Racial and Ethnic Survival Disparities in Oral Cavity and Laryngeal Cancer. *Cancer Epidemiol. Biomark. Prev.* **2023**, *32*, 642–652. [CrossRef]
50. Greenwood, M.; Thomson, P.J.; Lowry, R.J.; Steen, I.N. Oral cancer: Material deprivation, unemployment and risk factor behaviour--an initial study. *Int. J. Oral Maxillofac. Surg.* **2003**, *32*, 74–77. [CrossRef]
51. O'Hanlon, S.; Forster, D.P.; Lowry, R.J. Oral cancer in the North-East of England: Incidence, mortality trends and the link with material deprivation. *Community Dent. Oral Epidemiol.* **1997**, *25*, 371–376. [CrossRef]
52. Antunes, J.L. The impact of unemployment on cancer mortality, and how to avoid it. *Ann. Transl. Med.* **2016**, *4*, 404. [CrossRef] [PubMed]
53. Conway, D.I.; Hovanec, J.; Ahrens, W.; Ross, A.; Holcatova, I.; Lagiou, P.; Serraino, D.; Canova, C.; Richiardi, L.; Healy, C.; et al. Occupational socioeconomic risk associations for head and neck cancer in Europe and South America: Individual participant data analysis of pooled case–control studies within the INHANCE Consortium. *J. Epidemiol. Community Health* **2021**, *75*, 779. [CrossRef]
54. Richiardi, L.; Corbin, M.; Marron, M.; Ahrens, W.; Pohlabeln, H.; Lagiou, P.; Minaki, P.; Agudo, A.; Castellsague, X.; Slamova, A.; et al. Occupation and risk of upper aerodigestive tract cancer: The ARCAGE study. *Int. J. Cancer* **2012**, *130*, 2397–2406. [CrossRef] [PubMed]
55. Purdue, M.P.; Järvholm, B.; Bergdahl, I.A.; Hayes, R.B.; Baris, D. Occupational exposures and head and neck cancers among Swedish construction workers. *Scand. J. Work. Environ. Health* **2006**, *32*, 270–275. [CrossRef]
56. Lipworth, L.; La Vecchia, C.; Bosetti, C.; McLaughlin, J.K. Occupational exposure to rock wool and glass wool and risk of cancers of the lung and the head and neck: A systematic review and meta-analysis. *J. Occup. Environ. Med.* **2009**, *51*, 1075–1087. [CrossRef]
57. Pukkala, E.; Martinsen, J.I.; Lynge, E.; Gunnarsdottir, H.K.; Sparen, P.; Tryggvadottir, L.; Weiderpass, E.; Kjaerheim, K. Occupation and cancer—Follow-up of 15 million people in five Nordic countries. *Acta Oncol.* **2009**, *48*, 646–790. [CrossRef]
58. Huebner, W.W.; Schoenberg, J.B.; Kelsey, J.L.; Wilcox, H.B.; McLaughlin, J.K.; Greenberg, R.S.; Preston-Martin, S.; Austin, D.F.; Stemhagen, A.; Blot, W.J.; et al. Oral and pharyngeal cancer and occupation: A case-control study. *Epidemiology* **1992**, *3*, 300–309. [CrossRef] [PubMed]
59. Behrens, T.; Schill, W.; Ahrens, W. Elevated cancer mortality in a German cohort of bitumen workers: Extended follow-up through 2004. *J. Occup. Environ. Hyg.* **2009**, *6*, 555–561. [CrossRef]
60. Leemans, C.R.; Braakhuis, B.J.; Brakenhoff, R.H. The molecular biology of head and neck cancer. *Nat. Rev. Cancer* **2011**, *11*, 9–22. [CrossRef]
61. Syrjanen, S. The role of human papillomavirus infection in head and neck cancers. *Ann. Oncol.* **2010**, *21* (Suppl. S7), vii243–vii245. [CrossRef]
62. Ang, K.K.; Harris, J.; Wheeler, R.; Weber, R.; Rosenthal, D.I.; Nguyen-Tan, P.F.; Westra, W.H.; Chung, C.H.; Jordan, R.C.; Lu, C.; et al. Human papillomavirus and survival of patients with oropharyngeal cancer. *N. Engl. J. Med.* **2010**, *363*, 24–35. [CrossRef] [PubMed]
63. Shapiro, G.K.; Guichon, J.; Kelaher, M. Canadian school-based HPV vaccine programs and policy considerations. *Vaccine* **2017**, *35*, 5700–5707. [CrossRef] [PubMed]
64. Chaturvedi, A.K.; Engels, E.A.; Pfeiffer, R.M.; Hernandez, B.Y.; Xiao, W.; Kim, E.; Jiang, B.; Goodman, M.T.; Sibug-Saber, M.; Cozen, W.; et al. Human papillomavirus and rising oropharyngeal cancer incidence in the United States. *J. Clin. Oncol.* **2011**, *29*, 4294–4301. [CrossRef] [PubMed]
65. Fakhry, C.; Westra, W.H.; Li, S.; Cmelak, A.; Ridge, J.A.; Pinto, H.; Forastiere, A.; Gillison, M.L. Improved survival of patients with human papillomavirus-positive head and neck squamous cell carcinoma in a prospective clinical trial. *J. Natl. Cancer Inst.* **2008**, *100*, 261–269. [CrossRef]
66. Herrero, R.; Castellsagué, X.; Pawlita, M.; Lissowska, J.; Kee, F.; Balaram, P.; Rajkumar, T.; Sridhar, H.; Rose, B.; Pintos, J.; et al. Human Papillomavirus and Oral Cancer: The International Agency for Research on Cancer Multicenter Study. *JNCI J. Natl. Cancer Inst.* **2003**, *95*, 1772–1783. [CrossRef]

MDPI AG
Grosspeteranlage 5
4052 Basel
Switzerland
Tel.: +41 61 683 77 34

*Cancers* Editorial Office
E-mail: cancers@mdpi.com
www.mdpi.com/journal/cancers

www.ingramcontent.com/pod-product-compliance
Lightning Source LLC
Chambersburg PA
CBHW062035220926
51850CB00010B/2560
* 9 7 8 3 7 2 5 8 4 3 8 7 9 *